GW01161790

ADOLESCENT HEALTH SERVICES

Missing Opportunities

Committee on Adolescent Health Care Services and Models of
Care for Treatment, Prevention, and Healthy Development

Robert S. Lawrence, Jennifer Appleton Gootman, Leslie J. Sim, *Editors*

Board on Children, Youth, and Families

NATIONAL RESEARCH COUNCIL AND
INSTITUTE OF MEDICINE
OF THE NATIONAL ACADEMIES

THE NATIONAL ACADEMIES PRESS
Washington, D.C.
www.nap.edu

THE NATIONAL ACADEMIES PRESS   500 Fifth Street, N.W.   Washington, DC 20001

NOTICE: The project that is the subject of this report was approved by the Governing Board of the National Research Council, whose members are drawn from the councils of the National Academy of Sciences, the National Academy of Engineering, and the Institute of Medicine. The members of the committee responsible for the report were chosen for their special competences and with regard for appropriate balance.

This study was supported by Award No. 14356 between the National Academy of Sciences and The Atlantic Philanthropies (USA), Inc. Any opinions, findings, conclusions, or recommendations expressed in this publication are those of the author(s) and do not necessarily reflect the views of the organizations or agencies that provided support for the project.

Library of Congress Cataloging-in-Publication Data

Adolescent health services : missing opportunities / Committee on Adolescent Health Care Services and Models of Care for Treatment, Prevention, and Healthy Development, Board on Children, Youth, and Families ; Robert S. Lawrence, Jennifer Appleton Gootman, Leslie J. Sim, editors.
   p. ; cm.
Includes bibliographical references and index.
ISBN 978-0-309-11467-7 (hardback)
  1. Teenagers—Medical care—United States. I. Lawrence, Robert S., 1938- II. Gootman, Jennifer Appleton. III. Sim, Leslie J. IV. National Research Council (U.S.). Committee on Adolescent Health Care Services and Models of Care for Treatment, Prevention, and Healthy Development.
  [DNLM: 1. Adolescent Health Services—United States. 2. Adolescent Development—United States. 3. Delivery of Health Care, Integrated—United States. 4. Health Status—United States. 5. Needs Assessment—United States. 6. Quality of Health Care—United States. WA 330 A239 2009]
  RJ102.A375 2009
  362.19600835—dc22
                                    2008042174

Additional copies of this report are available from the National Academies Press, 500 Fifth Street, N.W., Lockbox 285, Washington, DC 20055; (800) 624-6242 or (202) 334-3313 (in the Washington metropolitan area); Internet, http://www.nap.edu.

Copyright 2009 by the National Academy of Sciences. All rights reserved.

Printed in the United States of America

Cover photo © Getty Images.

Suggested citation: National Research Council and Institute of Medicine. (2009). *Adolescent Health Services: Missing Opportunities*. Committee on Adolescent Health Care Services and Models of Care for Treatment, Prevention, and Healthy Development, R.S. Lawrence, J. Appleton Gootman, and L.J. Sim, *Editors*. Board on Children, Youth, and Families. Division of Behavioral and Social Sciences and Education. Washington, DC: The National Academies Press.

THE NATIONAL ACADEMIES
Advisers to the Nation on Science, Engineering, and Medicine

The **National Academy of Sciences** is a private, nonprofit, self-perpetuating society of distinguished scholars engaged in scientific and engineering research, dedicated to the furtherance of science and technology and to their use for the general welfare. Upon the authority of the charter granted to it by the Congress in 1863, the Academy has a mandate that requires it to advise the federal government on scientific and technical matters. Dr. Ralph J. Cicerone is president of the National Academy of Sciences.

The **National Academy of Engineering** was established in 1964, under the charter of the National Academy of Sciences, as a parallel organization of outstanding engineers. It is autonomous in its administration and in the selection of its members, sharing with the National Academy of Sciences the responsibility for advising the federal government. The National Academy of Engineering also sponsors engineering programs aimed at meeting national needs, encourages education and research, and recognizes the superior achievements of engineers. Dr. Charles M. Vest is president of the National Academy of Engineering.

The **Institute of Medicine** was established in 1970 by the National Academy of Sciences to secure the services of eminent members of appropriate professions in the examination of policy matters pertaining to the health of the public. The Institute acts under the responsibility given to the National Academy of Sciences by its congressional charter to be an adviser to the federal government and, upon its own initiative, to identify issues of medical care, research, and education. Dr. Harvey V. Fineberg is president of the Institute of Medicine.

The **National Research Council** was organized by the National Academy of Sciences in 1916 to associate the broad community of science and technology with the Academy's purposes of furthering knowledge and advising the federal government. Functioning in accordance with general policies determined by the Academy, the Council has become the principal operating agency of both the National Academy of Sciences and the National Academy of Engineering in providing services to the government, the public, and the scientific and engineering communities. The Council is administered jointly by both Academies and the Institute of Medicine. Dr. Ralph J. Cicerone and Dr. Charles M. Vest are chair and vice chair, respectively, of the National Research Council.

www.national-academies.org

COMMITTEE ON ADOLESCENT HEALTH CARE SERVICES AND MODELS OF CARE FOR TREATMENT, PREVENTION, AND HEALTHY DEVELOPMENT

ROBERT S. LAWRENCE *(Chair)*, Bloomberg School of Public Health, The Johns Hopkins University
LINDA H. BEARINGER, School of Nursing, School of Medicine, University of Minnesota
SHAY BILCHIK, Public Policy Institute, Georgetown University
SARAH S. BROWN, National Campaign to Prevent Teen and Unplanned Pregnancy, Washington, DC
LAURIE CHASSIN, Department of Psychology, Arizona State University, Tempe
GORDON DeFRIESE,[1] University of North Carolina at Chapel Hill
NANCY DUBLER, Montefiore Medical Center, Yeshiva University, New York
BURTON L. EDELSTEIN, College of Dental Medicine, Mailman School of Public Health, Columbia University
HARRIETTE FOX, Incenter Strategies, Washington, DC
CHARLES E. IRWIN, JR., School of Medicine, University of California, San Francisco
KELLY KELLEHER, College of Medicine, College of Public Health, Nationwide Children's Hospital, The Ohio State University
GENEVIEVE KENNEY, Urban Institute, Washington, DC
JULIA GRAHAM LEAR, School of Public Health and Health Services, George Washington University
EDUARDO OCHOA, JR., College of Medicine, College of Public Health, University of Arkansas for Medical Sciences
FREDERICK P. RIVARA, School of Medicine, School of Public Health, University of Washington, Seattle
VINOD K. SAHNEY, Blue Cross Blue Shield of Massachusetts, Boston
MARK A. SCHUSTER, Children's Hospital Boston, Harvard Medical School, Harvard University
LONNIE SHERROD, Society for Research in Child Development, Ann Arbor, MI
MATTHEW STAGNER, Chapin Hall Center for Children, University of Chicago
LESLIE R. WALKER, Department of Pediatrics, University of Washington, Seattle Children's Hospital

---

[1] Member until February 2007.

THOMAS G. DeWITT (liaison from the Board on Children, Youth, and Families), Cincinnati Children's Hospital Medical Center, University of Cincinnati

JENNIFER APPLETON GOOTMAN, *Study Director*
LESLIE J. SIM, *Program Officer*
REINE Y. HOMAWOO, *Senior Program Assistant* (from August 2007)
WENDY KEENAN, *Program Associate*
APRIL HIGGINS, *Senior Program Assistant* (until July 2007)

BOARD ON CHILDREN, YOUTH, AND FAMILIES

BERNARD GUYER *(Chair)*, Bloomberg School of Public Health, The Johns Hopkins University
BARBARA L. WOLFE *(Vice Chair)*, Department of Economics and Population Health Sciences, University of Wisconsin
WILLIAM R. BEARDSLEE, Department of Psychiatry, Children's Hospital, Boston
JANE D. BROWN, School of Journalism and Mass Communication, University of North Carolina at Chapel Hill
LINDA MARIE BURTON, Sociology Department, Duke University
P. LINDSAY CHASE-LANSDALE, Institute for Policy Research, Northwestern University
CHRISTINE C. FERGUSON, School of Public Health and Health Services, George Washington University
WILLIAM T. GREENOUGH, Department of Psychology, University of Illinois
RUBY HEARN, Robert Wood Johnson Foundation *(emeritus)*, Princeton, NJ
MICHELE D. KIPKE, Saban Research Institute, USC Childrens Hospital Los Angeles
BETSY LOZOFF, Center for Human Growth and Development, University of Michigan
SUSAN G. MILLSTEIN, Division of Adolescent Medicine, University of California, San Francisco
CHARLES A. NELSON, Laboratory of Cognitive Neuroscience, Children's Hospital, Boston
PATRICIA O'CAMPO, Centre for Research on Inner City Health, St. Michael's Hospital, Toronto, Canada
FREDERICK P. RIVARA, Schools of Medicine and Public Health, University of Washington, and Children's Hospital and Regional Medical Center, Seattle
LAURENCE D. STEINBERG, Department of Psychology, Temple University
JOHN R. WEISZ, Judge Baker Children's Center and Harvard Medical School
MICHAEL ZUBKOFF, Development of Community and Family Medicine, Dartmouth Medical School

ROSEMARY CHALK, *Board Director*
WENDY KEENAN, *Program Associate*

Reviewers

This report has been reviewed in draft form by individuals chosen for their diverse perspectives and technical expertise, in accordance with procedures approved by the National Research Council's Report Review Committee. The purpose of this independent review is to provide candid and critical comments that will assist the institution in making its published report as sound as possible and to ensure that the report meets institutional standards for objectivity, evidence, and responsiveness to the study charge. The review comments and draft manuscript remain confidential to protect the integrity of the deliberative process. We wish to thank the following individuals for their review of this report: Nancy Birkhimer, Teen and Young Adults Health Program, Maine Department of Human Services, Augusta, ME; Claire D. Brindis, National Adolescent Health Information Center, Institute for Health Policy Studies, University of California, San Francisco; Angela Diaz, Adolescent Health Center, Mount Sinai School of Medicine, New York, NY; Denise Dougherty, Child Health and Quality Improvement, Agency for Healthcare Research and Quality, Gaithersburg, MD; Daniel Eisenberg, Health Management and Policy, School of Public Health, University of Michigan; Elizabeth Feldman, Pediatric/Adolescent Coordinator, UIC/Illinois Masonic Family Practice Residency, University of Illinois College of Medicine; Brandon Hayes-Lattin, Adolescent and Young Adult Oncology Program, Oregon Health and Science University Cancer Institute, Portland; Jonathan Klein, Departments of Pediatrics and Community and Preventive Medicine, University of Rochester; Vaughn I. Rickert, Clinical Population and Family Health, Mailman School of Public Health, Columbia University; and Alan Shapiro, Community Pediatrics and South Bronx Children and Family Health Center, Montefiore Medical Group, New York, NY.

Although the reviewers listed above have provided many constructive comments and suggestions, they were not asked to endorse the conclusions or recommendations nor did they see the final draft of the report before its release. The review of this report was overseen by Robert Graham, Department of Family Medicine, University of Cincinnati College of Medicine, and Nancy E. Adler, Center for Health and Community, University of California, San Francisco. Appointed by the National Research Council, they were responsible for making certain that an independent examination of this report was carried out in accordance with institutional procedures and that all review comments were carefully considered. Responsibility for the final content of this report rests entirely with the authoring committee and the institution.

Preface

Under the best of circumstances, providing appropriate and comprehensive health services to adolescents poses many challenges. In the early years of adolescence, young people struggle with what Erik Erikson has described as the life stage of Identity versus Role Confusion, with many questions about who they are and where they fit in. As they move into young adulthood, the life stage of Intimacy versus Isolation raises questions of what to do with their lives and with whom, and where and how to settle down and take on adult responsibilities. Most adolescents are healthy, with a low incidence of acute illness and low prevalence of chronic conditions. Some adolescents, however, engage in unhealthful habits and risky behavior that expose them to the harmful effects of, for example, unsafe sex and experimentation with drugs, tobacco, and alcohol. Many high school students drink heavily or "binge" drink regularly. Others succumb to violent acts directed at others or themselves. Unintentional injuries are the leading cause of death among adolescents, dominated by those due to motor vehicle crashes. Between 10 and 20 percent of adolescents have mental health problems, and overweight and obesity place an increasing number of adolescents at risk for type 2 diabetes and other health problems. Rising rates of asthma interfere with normal activities and school attendance and diminish the quality of life.

Adolescence is a period when patterns of health-promoting or health-damaging behaviors are established that will have a substantial influence on health status during adulthood, affecting rates of acute and chronic disease and life expectancy. Identification and treatment of the acute effects of health-damaging behaviors provides an opportunity to counsel and educate adolescents about the lifelong benefits of establishing a healthy lifestyle.

The current system of health services in the United States is ill suited to providing the appropriate mix of clinical and preventive services to adolescents, especially those in certain circumstances, such as those who are part of the child welfare or juvenile justice system. Even adolescents with strong family and social supports and adequate financial resources are faced with a bewildering array of separate and poorly coordinated health programs and services delivered in multiple public and private settings. This arrangement may be sufficient for the majority of adolescents who are healthy, but it is woefully inadequate to meet the acute and chronic needs of vulnerable youths, especially those suffering from mental and behavioral disorders. Still less adequate is the system's ability to mount an effective screening program to support interventions focused on risk assessment, health promotion, and fostering of positive youth development. The current health services workforce includes few adolescent health generalists, specialists, educators, and scholars, and standards for accreditation of training programs for health providers for adolescents and for licensure and certification are inadequate.

To address these issues and develop recommendations for improving health care services for adolescents, The Atlantic Philanthropies provided funding to the National Research Council/Institute of Medicine (NRC/IOM) Board on Children, Youth, and Families. Through the board, the NRC and IOM formed the Committee on Adolescent Health Care Services and Models of Care for Treatment, Prevention, and Healthy Development in 2006. This report, *Adolescent Health Services: Missing Opportunities*, is the product of a multidisciplinary collaboration among committee members, NRC/IOM staff, and consultants.

The committee held five meetings and two workshops—one for research and health care service experts, and one for community and youth leaders. Committee members and staff conducted five site visits to learn firsthand about creative approaches to providing health services to adolescents, especially underserved groups. We engaged in vigorous discussion of the best approaches to improve adolescent health services, clarifying our underlying assumptions and reconciling different perspectives and priorities. It is our hope that the findings and recommendations presented in this report will help policy makers, service providers and their professional societies, and funders and government agencies shift the current patchwork quilt of health services for adolescents from a series of individual services into a coherent system of care.

The committee could not have done its work without the outstanding guidance and support provided by NRC/IOM staff Jennifer Gootman, study director, and Leslie Sim, program officer. Wendy Keenan and Reine

Homawoo provided highly skilled logistical support. Rosemary Chalk's guidance and counsel were invaluable throughout our deliberations. Finally, the young people and health professionals who participated in our workshops and those who shared their stories during our site visits deserve special thanks. Their experience in coping with the current system of care and their aspirations for something better fueled the committee's resolve to make a difference.

Robert S. Lawrence, *Chair*
Committee on Adolescent Health Care Services and Models
of Care for Treatment, Prevention, and Healthy Development

Acknowledgments

Beyond the hard work of the committee and National Research Council/Institute of Medicine (NRC/IOM) project staff, this report reflects contributions from numerous other individuals and groups.

The committee greatly benefited from the opportunity for discussion with those who made presentations at and attended the committee's workshops and meetings, including Dr. Kristin Adams, Salvador Balcorta, Dr. Anne Beal, Dr. Christina Bethell, Dr. Robert Blum, Rhonda Braxton, Dr. Claire Brindis, Dr. Richard Catalano, Coleen DeFlorimonte, Dr. Denise Dougherty, Dr. Abigail English, Dianne Ewashko, Paul Fogle, Dr. Robert Garofalo, Dr. David Grossman, Dr. Kimberly Hoagwood, Dr. Charles Homer, Linda Juszczak, Dr. Jonathan Klein, Andrea MacKay, Matthew Morton, Dr. Kathaleen Perkins, Shawn Semelsberger, Dr. Alan Shapiro, Dr. Josh Sharfstein, Dr. Warner Slack, Dr. Connie Weisner, and Dr. Charles Wibbelsman.

This study was sponsored by The Atlantic Philanthropies. We wish to thank Jackie Williams Kaye, Gara LaMarche, Charles Roussel, Mini Sanyal, Stuart Schear, and of course Debra Delgado for their support and guidance. Paula Elbirt's early advice on the development of this project is greatly appreciated.

We appreciate the extensive contributions of Dr. Robert Blum, Tumaini Coker, Abigail English, Dr. Gerry Fairbrother, Carolyn Garcia, Jose Lascal, Stephanie Limb, Andrea McKay, Daniel Moller, Joseph Schuchter, and Katherine Suellentrop, whom we commissioned to provide technical reviews of various portions of the report. Their insight and expertise added to the quality of the evidence presented. Additionally, Rona Briere and Alisa

Decatur provided superb editorial assistance in preparing the final report. The work of Eric Slade and his colleagues at Eric Slade Productions in preparing the video/DVD on adolescent health services enhanced opportunities to dissemate this report more broadly.

The committee was grateful for the opportunity to conduct five site visits during which committee members and NRC/IOM staff toured facilities and spoke with a variety of staff members and patients to learn about the successes and challenges in delivering adolescent health services to thousands of young people.

Thanks are extended to the staff at the Howard Brown Health Center and Broadway Youth Center, including Tony Alvarado-Rivera, Daniel Alvarez, Lara Brooks, Vea Cleary, Dr. Michael Cook, Michelle Emerick, Dr. Robert Garafalo, Amy Herrick, Joseph Hollendoner, Kristin Keglovitz, Jerry Lassa, Letty Martinez, Michael McFadden, Nicole Perez, Wendell Ward, Ebonii Warren, and Linda Wesp, as well as program partners Barb Bolson from The Night Ministry and David Myers from the Teen Living Program.

Thanks are due as well to the staff at Denver Health, including Lisa Abrams, Carolyn Carter, Audrey Gill, Dr. Paritosh Kaul, Abigail Mann, Dr. Paul Melinkovich, Trisha Mestas, Adrienne Pederson, and Nancy Riordan, as well as the other staff from Sandos Westside Community Clinic who took the time to meet with us.

We also thank the staff at the State of Louisiana Office of Youth Development and the Jetson Center for Youth, including Ms. Brezina, Dr. Richard Dalton, Ms. Erwin, Dr. Ronald Feinstein, Simon Gonsoulin, Dr. Stewart Gordon, Dr. Rhonda Kendrick, Dr. Seth Kunen, Ms. Lewis, Dr. Macdonald, Philippe Magloire, Dr. Menou, Gene Perkins, and Chef Ron Sonnier and his youth staff in the culinary arts program, as well as the other staff who spent time with us.

We appreciate the contributions of the staff at the Adolescent and Sports Medicine Center and the Eating Disorders Clinic at Arkansas Children's Hospital, including Dr. Bill Bandy, Marian Casey, Dr. Elton Cleveland, Kim Cossey, Brian Cox, Dr. Yancey Craft, Jennie Freyman, Dr. Brian Hardin, Skip Hoggard, Dr. Andrew Martin, Dr. J. Darrell Nesmith, Dr. Tracie Pasold, Dr. Maria Portilla, Cynthia Pumphrey, Dr. Wendy Ward-Begnoche, Dr. Jennifer Woods, and the other staff who met with us, as well as the Central High School football coaches.

Thanks are also due to the staff at the Mt. Sinai Adolescent Health Center in New York City, including Dr. Celia Blumenthal, Kelly Celony, Rachel Cymrot, Dr. Angela Diaz, Dr. Paula Elbirt, Dr. Alison Eliscu, Zayaini Lavergne-Freedman, Arlette Louden, Dr. Anne Nucci-Sack, Ken Peake, Rich Porter, and Jimmy Rao.

Others at the NRC/IOM—Athena Abdulah, Chantel Fuqua, Stephen Mautner, Matthew McDonough, Matthew Von Hendy, and Dianne Wolman—provided support in various ways to this project. As well, we are indebted to Kirsten Sampson Snyder, DBASSE reports officer, who patiently worked with us through several revisions of this report and DBASSE production editor, Yvonne Wise, who managed the production process through final publication.

Robert S. Lawrence, *Chair*
Committee on Adolescent Health Care Services and Models
of Care for Treatment, Prevention, and Healthy Development

Contents

Summary		1
1	Setting the Stage	17
2	Adolescent Health Status	52
3	Current Adolescent Health Services, Settings, and Providers	135
4	Improving Systems of Adolescent Health Services	194
5	Preparing a Workforce to Meet the Health Needs of Adolescents	240
6	Health Insurance Coverage and Access to Adolescent Health Services	265
7	Overall Conclusions and Recommendations	293

Appendixes

A	Acronyms	311
B	Harris Interactive Omnibus Survey Questions	314
C	Biographical Sketches of Committee Members and Staff	317
Index		329

Tribute to Debra Delgado

This report is dedicated to Debra Delgado, who served as program executive for The Atlantic Philanthropies on this project until she passed away on December 2, 2007, at the age of 50. Debra was a long-time advocate for children, youth, and families, adding tremendous value over her lifetime to the work of The Atlantic Philanthropies, The Annie E. Casey Foundation, The Robert Wood Johnson Foundation's Program Office for School-Based Health Care, the Title X Family Planning Program for the District of Columbia, Planned Parenthood of Metropolitan Washington, the Los Angeles Free Clinic, and the Watts Health Foundation. Debra influenced many individuals and communities through her advocacy and support for America's most vulnerable children, youth, and families.

Debra was a strong and dedicated advocate; a leader; a gentle and loving spirit; a problem solver; a patient mentor; uncommonly wise; wonderfully fun and compassionate; vibrant, kind, honest, insightful, gracious, elegant, and joyful. Her friends and colleagues miss her tremendously.

The committee's focus and its deliberations were guided by Debra's insights. This report is dedicated to her memory.

Summary

Adolescence is a time of major transitions, when young people develop many of the habits, patterns of behavior, and relationships they will carry into their adult lives. Most adolescents in the United States are healthy. But many engage in risky behavior, develop unhealthful habits, or have chronic conditions that can jeopardize their immediate health and safety and contribute to poor health in future years. During adolescence, a range of health issues can be identified and addressed in ways that affect not only the functioning and opportunities of adolescents themselves, but also the quality of their adult lives. Moreover, adolescence is a critical period for developing habits and skills that create a strong foundation for healthy lifestyles and behavior over the full life span.

The health system—health services, the settings where these services are delivered, how the services are delivered and by whom—has an important role to play in promoting healthful behavior, managing health conditions, and preventing disease during adolescence. Yet health services and settings in the United States today are not designed to help young people at this critical time in their lives, and providers often are not adequately trained in adolescent issues. As is the case in many other parts of the nation's health system, adolescents face gaps in care, fragmented services, and missed opportunities for health promotion and disease prevention.

STUDY SCOPE AND APPROACH

To address these issues, the National Research Council (NRC) and the Institute of Medicine (IOM), through the NRC/IOM Board on Children, Youth, and Families, with funding from The Atlantic Philanthropies, formed the Committee on Adolescent Health Care Services and Models of Care for Treatment, Prevention, and Healthy Development in 2006. The 19-member committee was charged with studying adolescent health services in the United States and developing policy and research recommendations that would highlight critical health needs, promising models of health services, and components of care that could strengthen and improve health services for adolescents and contribute to healthy adolescent development. In conducting this study, the committee:

- Considered settings, systems, and policies that promote high-quality health services for adolescents, as well as barriers to the provision of such services.
- Reviewed strategies for helping adolescents—especially those at significant risk for health disorders in such areas as sexual behavior and reproductive health, substance use, mental and oral health, violence, and diet—enter and navigate the health system.
- Sought to identify approaches that link disease prevention, health promotion, and behavioral health services and show significant promise for enhancing the provision of primary care for adolescents, including those who are more vulnerable because of selected population characteristics or other circumstances.
- Considered several specific aspects of providing these services, including issues related to privacy and confidentiality, financing strategies, and provider training.

Definitions

The concept of adolescence, which emerged only at the beginning of the twentieth century, is variable and evolving. Based on its review of various definitions of adolescence and of the literature on child and adolescent behavior and development, the committee focused this report—including the data, conclusions, and recommendations presented—on those aged 10–19.[1] The report includes consideration of a number of specific groups of adolescents defined by selected population characteristics and other circumstances—such as those who are poor; members of a racial or ethnic minority; in the foster care system; homeless; in families that have recently

---

[1] The committee recognized that there is disagreement among health care providers, researchers, and policy makers on the age bracket that demarcates the period of adolescence, but decided that on balance, focusing on ages 10–19 provides the best framework for the data analysis and evidence review in this report. Therefore, "adolescence" in this report denotes this age group, except when literature that uses a somewhat different age range is discussed.

immigrated to the United States; lesbian, gay, bisexual, or transgender; or in the juvenile justice system—and examined the relationship of these characteristics to health status and health services.

In defining health, the committee considered services provided by physicians, nurses, nurse practitioners, psychologists, social workers, dentists, and other health care providers. Health services were defined to include routine checkups; health maintenance or well care visits; school and sports physicals; psychiatric and substance abuse counseling; reproductive health services; dental care; and medical care for injury or illness, including chronic conditions. The committee also considered risky behavior and its implications for adolescent health and health services.

Study Frameworks

The committee was guided by two basic frameworks in its data collection, review of the evidence, and deliberations on various dimensions of adolescent health status and health services. The first focuses on behavioral and contextual characteristics that influence how adolescents interact with the health system, and the second on the objectives of adolescent health services. Neither framework alone is sufficient to explain significant variations in adolescent health outcomes; rather, they complement each other and, in tandem, provide a more complete picture of the features of the health system that should be improved in order to provide adolescents high-quality care and thus help to improve their health status.

Framework 1: Behavioral and Contextual Characteristics

Certain sets of behavioral and contextual characteristics, listed below, matter for adolescents in the ways they approach and interact with health care services, providers, and settings. When these characteristics are addressed in the design of health services for adolescents, these services can offer high-quality care that is particularly attuned to the needs of this age group. These characteristics helped frame the chapters of this report and, where relevant and supported by the evidence, are reflected in the committee's recommendations.

- **Development matters.** Adolescence is a period of significant and dramatic change spanning the physical, biological, social, and psychological transitions from childhood to young adulthood. This dynamic state influences both the health of young people and the health services they require (Chapter 1).
- **Timing matters.** Adolescence is a critical time for health promotion. Many health problems and much of the risky behavior that under-

lies later health problems begin during adolescence. Prevention, early intervention, and timely treatment improve health status for adolescents and prepare them for healthy adulthood; such services also decrease the incidence of many chronic diseases in adulthood (Chapter 2).
- **Context matters.** Social context and such factors as income, geography, and cultural norms and values can profoundly affect the health of adolescents and the health services they receive (Chapters 2 and 3).
- **Need matters.** Some segments of the adolescent population, defined by both biology and behavior, have health needs that require particular attention in health systems (Chapter 2).
- **Participation matters.** Effective health services for young people invite adolescents and their families to engage with clinicians (Chapter 4).
- **Family matters.** At the same time that adolescents are growing in their autonomy, families continue to affect adolescents' health and overall well-being and to influence what health services they use. Young people without adequate family support are particularly vulnerable to risky behavior and poor health and therefore often require additional support in health service settings (Chapter 4).
- **Community matters.** Good health services for adolescents include population-focused as well as individual and family services since the environment in which adolescents live, as well as the supports they receive in the community, are important (Chapter 4).
- **Skill matters.** Young people are best served by providers who understand the key developmental features, health issues, and overall social environment of adolescents (Chapter 5).
- **Money matters.** The availability, nature, and content of health services for adolescents are affected by such financial factors as public and private health insurance, the amount of funding invested in special programs for adolescents, and the support available for adequate training programs for providers of adolescent health services (Chapter 6).
- **Policy matters.** Policies, both public and private, can have a profound effect on adolescent health services. Carefully crafted policies are a foundation for strong systems of care that meet a wide variety of individual and community needs (Chapter 6).

Framework 2: Objectives of Health Services for Adolescents

Research from various sources and the experiences of adolescents and health care providers, health organizations, and research centers suggest the importance of designing health services that can attract and engage adolescents, create opportunities to discuss sensitive health and behavioral issues, and offer high-quality care as well as guidance on both disease prevention and health promotion. Consistent with these findings and views, a variety of national and international organizations have defined critical elements of health systems that would improve adolescents' access to appropriate services, highlighted design elements that would improve the quality of those services, and identified ways to foster patient–provider relationships that can lead to better health for adolescents.

The World Health Organization has identified five characteristics that constitute objectives for responsive adolescent health services:

1. **Accessible.** Policies and procedures ensure that services are broadly accessible.
2. **Acceptable.** Policies and procedures consider culture and relationships and the climate of engagement.
3. **Appropriate.** Health services fulfill the needs of all young people.
4. **Effective.** Health services reflect evidence-based standards of care and professional guidelines.
5. **Equitable.** Policies and procedures do not restrict the provision of and eligibility for services.

These five objectives provided the committee with a valuable framework for assessing the use, adequacy, and quality of adolescent health services; comparing the extent to which different health services, settings, and providers meet the health needs of young people in the United States; identifying the gaps that keep services from achieving these objectives; and recommending ways to close these gaps. In general, the committee found that existing approaches to providing health services for adolescents (primary care, school-based programs, hospital-based programs, and community-based models) reflect one or more of these objectives, but none of them achieves all five.

OVERALL CONCLUSIONS

The committee's many findings presented throughout this report can be consolidated into seven overall conclusions. These conclusions serve as the basis for the committee's eleven recommendations.

Overall Conclusion 1: Most adolescents are thriving, but many engage in risky behavior, develop unhealthful habits, and experience physical and mental health conditions that can jeopardize their immediate health and contribute to poor health in adulthood.

An analysis of the 21 Critical Health Objectives for ages 10–24, a subset of the Centers for Disease Control and Prevention's Healthy People 2010, highlights how little progress has been made in the overall health status of adolescents since the year 2000. Of the 21 objectives—which encompass a broad range of concerns, from reducing deaths, reducing suicides, and increasing mental health treatment to increasing seat belt use, reducing binge drinking, and reducing weapon carrying—the only ones that have shown improvement for adolescents since 2000 are behaviors leading to unintentional injury, pregnancy, and tobacco use. Negative trends include increased mortality due to motor vehicle crashes related to alcohol, increased obesity/overweight, and decreased physical activity.

Certain groups of adolescents have particularly high rates of comorbidity, defined as the simultaneous occurrence of two or more diseases, health conditions, or risky behaviors. These adolescents are particularly vulnerable to poor health. Moreover, specific groups of adolescents—such as those who are poor; in the foster care system; homeless; in families that have recently immigrated to the United States; lesbian, gay, bisexual, or transgender; or in the juvenile justice system—may have higher rates of chronic health problems and may engage in more risky behavior when compared with the overall adolescent population. These adolescents may have especially complex health issues that often are not addressed by the health services and settings they use. Furthermore, members of racial and ethnic minorities are becoming a larger portion of the overall U.S. adolescent population. And because minority racial or ethnic status is closely linked to poverty and a lack of access to quality health services, the number of adolescents experiencing significant disparities in access to quality health services can be expected to increase as well.

Overall Conclusion 2: Many current models of health services for adolescents exist. There is insufficient evidence to indicate that any one particular approach to health services for adolescents achieves significantly better results than others.

Evidence shows that while private office-based primary care services are available to most adolescents, those services depend significantly on fee-based reimbursement and are not always accessible, acceptable, appropriate, or effective for many adolescents, particularly those who are uninsured or underinsured. Such young people often have difficulty gaining access to mainstream primary care services; require additional support in order to connect with health care providers; and may rely extensively on such "safety-net" settings as hospital-, community- and school-based health centers for their primary care. For example, adolescents are in the age group most likely to depend on emergency departments for routine health care. Indeed, evidence shows that for some adolescents, safety-net settings may be more accessible, acceptable, appropriate, effective, and equitable than mainstream services. This may be especially so for more vulnerable populations of uninsured or underinsured adolescents. Although an extensive literature on the quality of school-based health services for adolescents is available, few studies have examined the quality of services received in other safety-net settings.

Evidence also shows that existing specialty services in the areas of mental health, sexual and reproductive health, oral health, and substance abuse treatment are not accessible to most adolescents, nor do they always meet the needs of many adolescents who receive care in safety-net settings. Even when such services are accessible, many adolescents may not find them acceptable because of concerns that confidentiality is not fully ensured, especially in such sensitive domains as substance use or sexual and reproductive health.

> **Overall Conclusion 3: Health services for adolescents currently consist of separate programs and services that are often highly fragmented, poorly coordinated, and delivered in multiple public and private settings.**

The various settings, services, and providers used by adolescents often are not coordinated with each other, and the result is barriers to and gaps in care. In some areas, such as mental health services for adolescents, the system of services is in substantial disarray because of financing barriers, eligibility gaps, and both confidentiality and privacy concerns—all of which can hamper transitions across care settings. Because of this segmentation, moreover, many providers of health services are poorly equipped to foster disease prevention and health promotion for adolescents. This is especially true in the areas of mental health, oral health, and substance abuse, as well as services that address sexual behavior and reproductive health.

> **Overall Conclusion 4: Health services for adolescents are poorly equipped to meet the disease prevention, health promotion, and behavioral health needs of all adolescents. Instead, adolescent health services are focused mainly on the delivery of care for acute conditions, such as infections and injuries, or special care addressing specific issues, such as contraception or substance abuse.**

This limited, problem-oriented approach fails to meet the broader profile, needs, and behavioral challenges that characterize adolescence.

Overall Conclusion 5: Large numbers of adolescents are uninsured or have inadequate health insurance, which can lead to a lack of access to regular primary care, as well as limited behavioral, medical, and dental care. One result of such barriers and deficits is poorer health.

More than 5 million adolescents aged 10–18 are uninsured. Uninsured rates are higher among the poor and near poor, racial and ethnic minorities, and noncitizens. As is true for all Americans, uninsured adolescents are less likely to have a regular source of primary care and use medical and dental care less often than those who have insurance. Having health insurance, however, does not ensure adolescents' access to affordable, high-quality services given current shortages of health care providers and problems associated with high out-of-pocket cost-sharing requirements, limitations in benefit packages, and low provider reimbursement levels. This is especially true in areas that involve counseling or case management of multiple health conditions, and in areas that are particularly problematic for adolescents, such as obesity, intentional and unintentional injury, mental health, dental care, and substance abuse. Furthermore, uninsured adolescents aged 10–18 who are eligible for public coverage often are not enrolled either because their parents do not know they are eligible or because complexities of the enrollment processes deter participation.

Overall Conclusion 6: Health care providers working with adolescents frequently lack the necessary skills to interact appropriately and effectively with this age group.

Whether providers report on their own perceptions of their competencies or adolescents describe the care they have received, data reveal significant gaps in the achievement of a well-equipped and appropriately trained workforce ready to meet the health needs of adolescents. At all levels of professional education, health care providers in every discipline serving adolescents should receive specific and detailed education in the nature of adolescents' health problems and have in their clinical repertoire a range of effective ways to treat and prevent disease in this age group, as well as to promote healthy behavior and lifestyles within a developmental framework. Evidence suggests this currently is not the case.

Overall Conclusion 7: The characterization of adolescents and their health status by such traditional measures as injury and illness does not adequately capture the developmental and behavioral health of adolescents of different ages and in diverse circumstances.

Developing a clear definition of adolescent health status is a critical step in delivering health services and forming health systems that can respond appropriately to the specific needs of adolescents. Moreover, the ability to understand and characterize health status within this definition is dependent on available data, particularly that related to adolescent behavior. Those concerned with the health of adolescents—health practitioners, policy makers, and families—would benefit from ready access to high-quality and more precise data that would aid in better understanding the consequences of health-influencing behaviors for the health status of adolescents.

LOOKING AHEAD: RECOMMENDATIONS

Based on the overall conclusions presented above, the committee makes eleven recommendations, directed to both public and private entities, for investing in, strengthening, and improving health services for adolescents. These recommendations embody many of the behavioral and contextual characteristics that the committee explored in its evidence review and, if acted on in a coordinated and comprehensive manner, should improve the accessibility, acceptability, appropriateness, effectiveness, and equity of health services delivered to adolescents.

Primary Health Care

Recommendation 1: Federal and state agencies, private foundations, and private insurers should support and promote the development and use of a coordinated primary health care system that strives to improve health services for all adolescents.

Carrying out this recommendation would involve federal and state agencies, private foundations, and private insurers working with local primary care providers to coordinate services between primary and specialty care services. It would also entail providing opportunities for primary care services to interact with health programs for adolescents in many safety-net settings, such as schools, hospitals, and community health centers.

Recommendation 2: As part of an enhanced primary care system for adolescents, health care providers and health organizations should focus attention on the particular needs of specific groups of adolescents who may be especially vulnerable to risky behavior or poor health because of selected population characteristics or other circumstances.

Implementing this recommendation would involve focusing explicit attention on issues of access, acceptability, appropriateness, effectiveness, and equity of health services for an increasingly racially and ethnically diverse population of adolescents and for selected adolescent groups, such as those who are poor; in the foster care system; homeless; in families that have recently immigrated to the United States; lesbian, gay, bisexual, or transgender; or in the juvenile justice system.

> Recommendation 3: Providers of adolescent primary care services and the payment systems that support them should make disease prevention, health promotion, and behavioral health—including early identification, management, and monitoring of current or emerging health conditions and risky behavior—a major component of routine health services.

For this recommendation to be realized, providers of adolescent primary care services would need to give attention to the coordination and management of the specialty services young people often need. They would coordinate screening, assessment, health management, and referrals to specialty services. They would also monitor behavior that increases risk in such areas as injury, mental health, oral health, substance use, violence, eating disorders, sexual activity, and exercise. Performance measures for these services would need to be incorporated into criteria used for credentialing, pay-for-performance incentives, and quality measurement. And perhaps most important, payment systems would need to finance such services and activities.

Public Health System

> Recommendation 4: Within communities—and with the help of public agencies—health care providers, health organizations, and community agencies should develop coordinated, linked, and interdisciplinary adolescent health services.

To effect this recommendation, health care providers across communities would need to work together to encourage rapid and coordinated services through collocation or participation in regional planning and action groups organized by managed care plans, large group networks, health professional associations, or public health agencies. Beyond direct patient services, primary care providers and providers of mental health/substance abuse, reproductive, nutritional, and oral health services would have to establish public and private programs in a region for managing referrals; coordinating electronic patient information; and staffing adolescent call centers and regional services to communicate directly with adolescents, their families, and various providers. In addition, the particular health needs of adolescents, especially the most vulnerable populations, would need to be addressed in the development of electronic health records. Such records offer a significant opportunity to ensure coordinated care, as well as to provide adolescent-focused patient portals, messaging and reminder services, and electronic personalized health education services to improve interventions. An overarching principle in the implementation of this recommendation is that adolescents should be asked to give explicit consent for the sharing of information about them, a point addressed in the committee's next recommendation.

Privacy and Confidentiality

Recommendation 5: Federal and state policy makers should maintain current laws, policies, and ethical guidelines that enable adolescents who are minors to give their own consent for health services and to receive those services on a confidential basis when necessary to protect their health.

To implement this recommendation, federal and state policy makers would need to examine the variations among states in the age of consent for care for adolescents and consider the impact of such variations on adolescents' access to and use of services that are essential to protecting their health (e.g., services for contraception, sexually transmitted infections/HIV, mental health, and substance use). A balance is needed between maintaining the confidentiality of information and records regarding care for which adolescent minors are allowed to give their consent, and encouraging the involvement of parents and families in the health services received by adolescents whenever possible, both supporting and respecting their role and importance in adolescents' lives and health care.

Adolescent Health Care Providers

Recommendation 6: Regulatory bodies for health professions in which an appreciable number of providers offer care to adolescents should incorporate a minimal set of competencies in adolescent health care and development into their licensing, certification, and accreditation requirements.

To implement this recommendation, regulatory bodies would need to use national meetings of specialists and educators/scholars within relevant disciplines to define competencies in adolescent health. They would also have to require professionals who serve adolescents in health care settings to complete a minimum amount of education in basic areas of adolescent development, health issues unique to this life stage, and a life course framework that encourages providers to focus on helping their adolescent patients develop healthful habits that can be carried forward into their adult lives. Finally, agencies that fund training programs would have to adhere to the requirements of the regulatory bodies (i.e., with regard to accreditation, licensure, and certification, and to maintenance of licensure or certification where appropriate), and content on adolescent health would have to be mandatory in all relevant training programs.

> **Recommendation 7:** Public and private funders should provide targeted financial support to expand and sustain interdisciplinary training programs in adolescent health. Such programs should strive to prepare specialists, scholars, and educators in all relevant health disciplines to work with both the general adolescent population and selected groups that require special and/or more intense services.

To effect this recommendation, public and private funders would need to ensure that professionals who serve adolescents in health care settings are trained in how to relate to adolescents and gain their trust and cooperation; how to develop strong provider–patient relationships; and how to identify early signs of risky and unhealthful behavior that may require further assessment, intervention, or referral. Also essential to the training of these professionals is knowing how to work with more vulnerable adolescents, such as those who are in the foster care system; homeless; in families that have recently immigrated to the United States; lesbian, gay, bisexual, or transgender; or in the juvenile justice system. Important as well is to increase the number of Leadership Education in Adolescent Health programs that train health professionals in adolescent medicine, psychology, nursing, social work, and nutrition, and to enhance the program by adding dentistry.

Health Insurance

> **Recommendation 8:** Federal and state policy makers should develop strategies to ensure that all adolescents have comprehensive, continuous health insurance coverage.

Federal and state legislatures and governments should consider the following options for implementing this recommendation: require states to provide Medicaid or other forms of health insurance coverage for especially vulnerable or underserved groups of adolescents, particularly those who are in the juvenile justice and foster care systems, and support states in meeting this requirement; design and implement Medicaid and State Children's

Health Insurance Program policies to increase enrollment and retention of eligible but uninsured adolescents; and improve incentives for private health insurers to provide such coverage (e.g., by requiring school-based coverage and allowing nongroup policies tailored to adolescents). Note that while these options would increase insurance coverage among adolescents, broader health care reform efforts would be required to ensure universal coverage. A consequence of allowing more segmentation in nongroup health insurance policies across age groups could be increased costs for older adults if younger, healthier adults are removed from the risk pool. In addition, expanding access to and election of coverage among poor adolescents would be necessary to increase the rates of insured adolescents.

Recommendation 9: Federal and state policy makers should ensure that health insurance coverage for adolescents is sufficient in amount, duration, and scope to cover the health services they require. Such coverage should be accessible, acceptable, appropriate, effective, and equitable.

Public and private health plans, including self-insured plans, should consider several options for carrying out this recommendation. First, they could see that benefit packages cover at a minimum the following key services for adolescents: preventive screening and counseling, at least on an annual basis; case management; reproductive health care that includes screening, education, counseling, and treatment; assessment and treatment of mental health conditions, such as anxiety disorders and eating disorders, and of substance abuse disorders, including those comorbid with mental health conditions; and dental services that include prevention, restoration, and treatment. Second, they could ensure coverage for mental health and substance abuse services at primary or specialty care sites that provide integrated physical and mental health care, and require Medicaid to cover mental health rehabilitation services. Third, they could make certain that providers are reimbursed at reasonable, market-based rates for the adolescent health services they provide. Finally, they could ensure that out-of-pocket cost sharing (including mental health and other health services) is set at levels that do not discourage receipt of all needed services.

Research Agenda

Recommendation 10: Federal health agencies and private foundations should prepare a research agenda for improving adolescent health services that includes assessing existing service models, as well as developing new systems for providing services that are accessible, acceptable, appropriate, effective, and equitable.

Federal health agencies should consider a number of options for carrying out this recommendation. First, they could identify performance standards and operational criteria that could be used to compare the strengths and limitations of different models of health service delivery in meeting the needs of all young people, as well as specific groups. In developing such standards and criteria, an effort should be made to translate the features of accessibility, acceptability, appropriateness, effectiveness, and equity into clear standards and ways to measure their achievement. Second, they could determine the effectiveness (not just the efficacy) of selected mental health, behavioral, and developmental interventions for adolescents. This research should be aimed at identifying individual, environmental, and other contextual factors that significantly affect the likelihood of establishing, operating, and sustaining effective interventions in a variety of service settings. Third, they could assess and compare the health status (defined by selected population characteristics and other circumstances) and health outcomes of young people who receive care through different service models and in different health settings, as well as of those who are difficult to reach and serve. Fourth, they could identify effective ways to reach more underserved and vulnerable adolescents with appropriate and accessible health services. Such research might also consider how to integrate the features of accessibility, acceptability, appropriateness, effectiveness, and equity into the primary care environment for all adolescents, as well as into the training of providers who interact with adolescents. Finally, they could evaluate the validity and reliability of various screening tools and counseling techniques for selected groups of adolescents.

Monitoring Progress

Recommendation 11: The Federal Interagency Forum on Child and Family Statistics should work with federal agencies and, when possible, states to organize and disseminate data on the health and health services, including developmental and behavioral health, of adolescents. These data should encompass adolescents generally, with subreports by age, selected population characteristics, and other circumstances.

To implement this recommendation, federal agencies would need to adopt consistent age brackets that cluster data by ages 10–14 and 15–19 and consistent identifiers of socioeconomic status, geographic location, gender, and race and ethnicity. Also needed are consistent identifiers of specific vulnerable adolescent populations, including those in the foster care system; those who are homeless; those who are in families that have recently immigrated to the United States; those who are lesbian, gay, bisexual, or transgender; and those in the juvenile justice system. Important as well is to track emerging disparities in access to and utilization of health services, with attention to specific components of health care, such as screening, assessment, and referral, as well as an emphasis on racial and ethnic differences. Finally, longitudinal studies are needed on the effects of both health-promoting and health-compromising behaviors that often emerge in the second decade of life and continue into adulthood.

CLOSING THOUGHTS

While the gaps and problems in the health services used by young people discussed in this report are not unique to this age group, a compelling case can be made for improving health services and systems both to support the healthy development of adolescents and to enhance their transitions from childhood to adolescence and from adolescence to adulthood. Current interest in restructuring the way health care is delivered and financed in the United States—and defining the content of care itself more broadly—is based on a growing awareness that existing health services and systems for virtually all Americans have important and costly shortcomings. In the midst of these discussions, the distinct deficits faced by adolescents within the health system deserve particular attention. Their developmental complexities and risky behavior, together with the need to extend their care beyond the usual disease- and injury-focused services, are key considerations in any attempt to reform the nation's chaotic health care system—especially if adolescents are to benefit. Even if the larger systemic issues of access to the health system were resolved, more would likely need to be done to achieve better health for adolescents during both the adolescent years and the transition to adulthood.

1

Setting the Stage

SUMMARY

- Adolescents aged 10–19 made up 14 percent (42 million) of the total population of the United States in 2006.
- The racial and ethnic makeup of the U.S. adolescent population is becoming more diverse. The correlations among minority racial and ethnic status, poverty, and lack of access to quality health services for adolescents are strong. Without specific attention to disparities in access to quality health services among adolescent members of minority racial and ethnic groups and actions to reduce them, such disparities may increase.

Adolescence[1] is a critical period of transition between childhood and adulthood. It is a period when significant physical, psychological, and behavioral changes occur and when young people develop many of the habits, behavioral patterns, and relationships they will carry into their adult lives. This chapter demonstrates how the healthy development of adolescents matters. While most adolescents in the United States appear to be healthy, many engage in risky behavior and develop unhealthful habits that can jeopardize their immediate health and safety and contribute to

---

[1] As will be elucidated later in this chapter, adolescence is defined in this report as ages 10–19.

poor health in future years. Others experience physical and mental illnesses, including chronic conditions, during adolescence and into adulthood. At the same time, adolescence is a critical period for developing positive behavioral patterns, healthful habits, and independent decision-making skills that create a strong foundation for healthy lifestyles and behavior over the full life span. Therefore, receiving quality health promotion and disease prevention services, supportive counseling, and chronic care treatment and management, as well as engaging in positive activities and personal skill building, plays a crucial role in nurturing healthy adolescents, as well as in reducing their risk for many adult diseases and injuries. Indeed, according to a joint report by the World Health Organization, United Nations Population Fund, and United Nations Children's Fund (1995, p. 3), "One of the most important commitments a country can make for future economic, social, and political progress and stability is to address the health and development needs of its adolescents."

It is of concern, therefore, that adolescents have one of the lowest rates of primary care use of any age group in the United States (Hing, Cherry, and Woodwell, 2006) and one of the highest rates of being under- or uninsured (Agency for Healthcare Research and Quality, 2006; U.S. Census Bureau, 2006b). Moreover, some aspects of adolescent health—such as the escalating rate of adolescent obesity and related illnesses—have become increasingly problematic over time (Institute of Medicine, 2005). In addition, certain groups within the adolescent population characterized by selected circumstances—for instance, those who are in the foster care system; homeless; lesbian, gay, bisexual, or transgender (LGBT)[2]; or in the juvenile justice system—may be especially prone to participate in risky behavior and lack community, family, or economic support. Consequently they may face special challenges that put them at particular risk for poor health outcomes (D'Augelli, Hershberger, and Pilkington, 1998; Saewyc et al., 1999, 2006; Tonkin, 1994). Being part of a racial or ethnic minority group, being poor, or being in a family that has recently immigrated to the United States may also contribute to decreased access to quality and appropriate health services (Weinick and Krauss, 2000; Wise, 2004).

There is some disagreement as to whether health status is dependent more on health services or on other factors, such as genetics, income, or behavior (Association of Maternal and Child Health Programs and the National Network of State Adolescent Health Coordinators, 2005; Fuchs, 1974, 1991; Garfinkel, Hochschild, and McLanahan, 1996). Nonetheless,

---

[2]The group referred to as "lesbian, gay, bisexual, and transgender" sometimes also encompasses the term "questioning" and is commonly referred to by the acronym LGBT (or GLBT) or LGBTQ (or GLBTQ). For the purposes of this report, the identifier "lesbian, gay, bisexual, and transgender" or LGBT is used.

it is clear that a number of potential impediments to quality health services for adolescents exist, including a lack of financial support, insurance, physicians and other health professionals who are trained in adolescent health, and transportation; cultural and language barriers; discomfort with or lack of understanding of who provides adolescent health services; and concern about the confidentiality of health services (Hock-Long et al., 2003; Kodjo, Auinger, and Ryan, 2002; Perloff, 1992; Sanci, Kang, and Ferguson, 2005; St. Peter, Newacheck, and Halfon, 1992).

Another barrier to quality adolescent health care is the fact that adolescents do not fit easily into current models of health care. There are two prevailing models of health care: one focused on children and the other on adults. In a pediatric approach to medicine, the parent is the responsible agent, and the focus is on nurturing the patient in a family context. In an adult-centered approach, the patient is the responsible agent; the provider offers information with which the patient makes decisions; and the focus is on the individual, not the family. The treatment of adolescents does not fit well into either model, and their needs change as they progress through adolescence. While some practitioners focus on caring for adolescents, their numbers are few. A third model—family medicine, in which the family, including children, adolescents, and adults, is cared for by a family physician or nurse practitioner—may offer another alternative, but the number of family medicine practices is limited.

Over the past decade, numerous published studies have addressed particular aspects of adolescent health (Ozer et al., 2003; Park et al., 2005, 2006). Much of that research, however, is focused on specific health domains, injuries or illnesses, special interests, or problem behavior—such as mental health, teen pregnancy, sexually transmitted infections, substance abuse, tobacco use, violence, diet and exercise, or oral health. Often neglected is a more comprehensive strategy for adolescent health services that integrates behavioral, psychological, physical, and social aspects of health. Moreover, much of the research available to help understand different types of services, organizational models, service settings, and provider skills that influence the health, safety, and well-being of today's adolescents is scattered among different disciplines and literatures, including pediatrics, reproductive health, social work, mental health, and education (The Center for Development and Population Activities, 2003; Chung et al., 2006; Committee on Adolescence, 2008; Kopelman, 2004; Lear, 2002; National Association of Social Workers, 2002; Rand et al., 2007).

Experimentation with different models for providing health services to adolescents has occurred at the local, state, and national levels, and the health, safety, and well-being of adolescents are receiving attention from diverse public and private agencies. Fundamentally, however, the research being conducted is not always comprehensive, the health service approaches are not always the same, and the services or systems are not always integrated. Gaps in the service delivery system for today's adolescents are common, particularly for those who are most vulnerable to risky behavior and poor health or who face major barriers in gaining access to primary and preventive services.

STUDY CHARGE, APPROACH, AND SCOPE

Study Charge

Concerned about these issues, the National Academies' Board on Children, Youth, and Families formed the Committee on Adolescent Health Care Services and Models of Care for Treatment, Prevention, and Healthy Development, with funding from The Atlantic Philanthropies. The National Research Council (NRC) and the Institute of Medicine (IOM) appointed the 19-member committee in May 2006 to study adolescent health services in the United States and develop policy and research recommendations that would highlight critical health needs, promising service models, and components of care that could strengthen and improve health services for adolescents and contribute to healthy adolescent development. Committee members brought to this task expertise in the areas of adolescent health; general pediatrics; health care services; adolescent development; school-based health services; health care finance; mental health; alcohol, tobacco, and drug abuse treatment; sexual health; oral health; nursing; public policy; statistics/epidemiology; preventive medicine; program evaluation; injury research; law; and immigrant/minority adolescents (see Appendix C for biographies of the committee members). The committee was asked to explore the following issues:

- **Features of quality adolescent health services.** What does the evidence base suggest constitutes high-quality health care and health promotion services for adolescent populations? What do parents, community leaders, and adolescents themselves perceive to be essential features of such services?
- **Approaches to the provision of adolescent health services.** What are the strengths and limitations of different service models in addressing adolescent health care needs? What lessons have been learned in efforts to promote linkages and integration among adolescent health care, health promotion, and adolescent development services? What service approaches show significant promise in offering primary care as well as prevention, treatment, and health promotion services for adolescents with special health care needs and for selected adolescent populations?

- **Organizational settings and strategies.** What organizational settings, finance strategies, and communication technologies promote engagement with, access to, and use of health services by adolescents? Are there important differences in the use and outcomes of different service models among selected adolescent populations on the basis of such characteristics as social class, urbanicity, ethnicity, gender, sexual orientation, age, special health care needs, and risk status?
- **Adolescent health system supports.** What policies, mechanisms, and contexts promote high-quality health services for adolescents? What innovative strategies have been developed to address such concerns as decision making, privacy, confidentiality, consent, and parental notification in adolescent health care settings? What strategies help adolescents engage with and navigate the health care system, especially those at significant risk for health disorders in such areas as sexual and reproductive health, substance use, mental health, violence, and diet? What barriers impede the optimal provision of adolescent health services?
- **Adolescent health care providers.** What kinds of training programs for health care providers are necessary to improve the quality of health care for adolescent populations?

Study Approach

A variety of sources informed the committee's work. Five formal committee meetings and two public workshops were held during the course of the study. A community forum on adolescent health care revealed the views of both those who consume and those who provide adolescent health services so the committee could learn about adolescent and provider perspectives, as well as organizational and contextual factors that diminish or enhance the delivery and quality of adolescent health services. A research workshop on adolescent health care services and systems highlighted the views of those who are familiar with current research on the organization and delivery of adolescent health services, as well as identified research needs and gaps in the literature base. The National Academies published a summary report of these two meetings in 2007.

The committee also reviewed literature from a range of disciplines and sources. Data and research on adolescents, their families, and health practitioners who treat adolescents were analyzed. The committee considered research on various health services, the features of settings that serve adolescents, and the utilization of health services by adolescents. Public policies related to adolescent health, health services, health care provider training, and financing were studied. Private-sector health funding mechanisms were reviewed.

Additionally, the committee visited several institutions and organizations focused on providing adolescent health services. The sites visited were chosen because they represent different institutional structures and service delivery locations, types, and models. The limited evaluation of these services and the lack of a standard against which to study them make it impossible to designate any of them as exemplary models of adolescent health care. However, these visits provided examples of health services being delivered specifically to adolescents, and they helped the committee gain insight into various services, settings, financing arrangements, partnerships, approaches to coordination of care, and care models used in the United States to meet the health service needs of adolescents. A description of each site and what was learned from these visits is presented in Chapter 4.

The sites visited were Denver Health, Denver, Colorado; Broadway Youth Center, Chicago, Illinois; Jetson Center for Youth, Baton Rouge, Louisiana; Arkansas Children's Hospital, Little Rock; and Mt. Sinai Adolescent Health Center, New York City, New York. Each visit encompassed a tour of the program site or sites; meetings with leaders of the sponsoring institution to discuss institutional objectives and program operations, as well as reflections on successes, challenges, lessons learned, and research related to their efforts; and meetings with the institution's various health practitioners to discuss the nature of the adolescents who receive services in their setting, the primary health issues being addressed, obstacles to service delivery, and clinical and program management issues. Meetings involved clinical leadership; key program staff (managers, relevant senior staff, and others identified by the site); clinical/agency partners; and health care providers working with adolescents in the setting, such as physicians, nurses, counselors, and office assistants.

The committee also made various efforts to understand the perspectives of adolescents on their health and their experiences with health services. During the site visits, the committee met with groups of adolescents to discuss their perceptions of adolescent health issues and health service needs in their community and to gather first-hand accounts of experiences illustrating how health programs have successfully reached out to this population. The adolescents were also encouraged to suggest ways in which adolescent health services in general could better serve their needs and those of their peers. As well, questions were posed in an online Harris Interactive poll of a nationally representative sample (in terms of geographic location, age, race/ethnicity, and socioeconomic status) of adolescents aged 10–18. (The results of this poll are described later in this chapter, and the list of questions included in the poll is provided in Appendix B.)

Challenges and Limitations

The committee was challenged by the limited data and existing scientific literature in a number of key areas. There are no comprehensive national indicators of the health status of adolescents that place particular emphasis on behavioral and developmental health. Specifically, information is lacking by selected population characteristics (e.g., income, racial and ethnic status, geographic location) and other circumstances (e.g., LGBT, in the foster care system) that would provide longitudinal trends and enable comparison of the health behaviors of selected adolescent populations as they grow. Health services for adolescents are delivered in myriad settings and through varied institutional structures, and data on and evaluation of services are limited, thus making comprehensive assessment of the quality of service delivery, as well as comparison of different settings and services, a further challenge. Information on issues related to the adolescent health workforce, such as competency requirements for health professionals who work with adolescents, is also difficult to obtain. Finally, while there may be costs associated with the recommendations presented in this report, the committee did not address these economic implications. Such an analysis was beyond the scope of the study charge and the committee's expertise. A future topic for research, therefore, is whether implementing the committee's recommendations would require additional resources or could be financed through reallocation of current investments.

Study Scope

The committee was charged broadly with an examination of adolescent health and health services. However, the charge did not specify what ages fall within the period of adolescence and what "health" should encompass. Therefore, one of the committee's early tasks was to reach consensus on how to define these terms in reviewing the literature.

Defining Adolescence

The period of adolescence is influenced by social, cultural, economic, and physical elements, and the boundaries of this life phase are not precise. As a period in the life span, adolescence is a fairly new concept, recognized first at the beginning of the twentieth century. Psychologist G. Stanley Hall wrote a two-volume book in 1904 in which he described the nature of teens and argued that their specific developmental period required particular types of supports. The concept of adolescence became increasingly popular throughout the twentieth century as society changed its perspective on children. The view of children shifted from their being simply members of a family during agrarian times (Hernandez, 1993) to their being economic assets working in factories during the period of industrialization (Zelizer, 1985). As the rate of industrialization decreased, the need for workers also decreased, and society began to become aware of the awful conditions to which child factory workers were subjected. As a result, numerous laws were passed at the end of the nineteenth century to protect children. Public education through mass schooling originated early in the twentieth century. These profound changes led to society's view of adolescents as valued members of society with future intellectual and economic contributions to make, a view that has continued into the twenty-first century (Brown, 2001; Larson, Wilson, and Mortimer, 2003). Research on behavior and development during the adolescent period also emerged in the twentieth century, further highlighting the unique aspects of adolescence and the importance of health services and systems that would support the healthy development of adolescents into adulthood.

Adolescence is characterized by profound changes at many levels—physical, social, emotional, and behavioral; it is also a time of transition between childhood and adulthood. Dramatic biological changes are associated with pubertal development: the body grows physically; adult facial appearance develops; and production of the hormones estrogen, progesterone, and testosterone begins. These biological changes generally result in burgeoning sexual interest and may lead to health issues, such as the development of acne and weight loss or gain. For a variety of reasons, the period that delineates adolescence has expanded over time, starting earlier because of early pubertal development and lasting longer because of such factors as changes in employment and education and later ages at both marriage and childbearing (Arnett, 2006).

Adolescence is also characterized by identity formation, with individuals starting to make independent choices and experiment with new behavior and experiences. During this time, adolescents often select their peer group and decide for themselves how to spend time out of school. Peer group acceptance becomes increasingly important, and adolescents may focus on conforming to their peers and be susceptible to peer influence. For some adolescents, these decisions can result in rebellious, independent, thrill-seeking, and sometimes risky attitudes and behaviors (National Research Council and Institute of Medicine, 1999). For many adolescents, risk taking and experimentation are simply an important stage in their development, and when not taken to an extreme, do not result in problems. And of course some young people experience adolescence as a tranquil transition into adulthood. For others, however, these attitudes and behaviors can have negative impacts on health and development.

Adolescents also often begin to make independent purchases that may affect their health. Among these purchases, food and beverages—particularly high-calorie and low-nutrient candy, carbonated soft drinks, and salty snacks—consistently dominate (Institute of Medicine, 2006). Once they reach age 18, adolescents also may be purchasing health care independently, with additional potential impacts on health.

Research conducted in the last decade suggests that the brain is not completely developed until late in adolescence, and until that time, the connections between neurons affecting emotional, physical, and mental abilities are incomplete. Some adolescent behavior, such as inconsistency in controlling emotions, impulses, and judgments, may be attributable to this incomplete brain development, and much of that behavior is associated with unhealthful and risky adolescent activities (Dahl, 2003; Giedd et al., 1999; National Institute of Mental Health, 2001).

The committee recognized that among health care providers, researchers, and policy makers, different age brackets often demarcate the period of adolescence, ranging from as young as 10 to as old as 25. In most cases, those at the upper end of this age range are identified separately as "young adults" or "emerging adults." Even within the U.S. government, several definitions are in use. Examples include the following:

- U.S. Department of Health and Human Services (2007) (Healthy People 2010)
  - Adolescents (ages 10–19)
  - Young adults (ages 20–24)
- Substance Abuse and Mental Health Services Administration (2007) (National Survey on Drug Use and Health)
  - Youths (ages 12–17)
  - Young adults (ages 18–25)
- Centers for Disease Control and Prevention (2006) (STD Surveillance)
  - Adolescents (ages 10–19)
    Young adults (ages 20–24)
- U.S. Department of Justice (2006) (Criminal Victimization)
  - Age clustering: ages 12–15, 16–19, 20–24
- Youth Risk Behavior Survey (Centers for Disease Control and Prevention, 2007)
  - Young people (grades 9–12)
- Society for Adolescent Medicine (1995) (position statement)
  - Adolescent medicine (ages 10–25)
- National Longitudinal Study of Adolescent Health (Carolina Population Center, 2007)
  - Adolescents (grades 7–12)
- Office of Technology Assessment (OTA) (U.S. Congress and Office of Technology Assessment, 1991)
  - Adolescents (ages 10–18)
  - Young adults (ages 18–26)

- National Initiative to Improve Adolescent Health (NIIAH 2010, or the National Initiative) (National Adolescent Health Information Center, 2004)
  – Youth (ages 10–14)

The committee reviewed these and other delineations of the period of adolescence, as well as literature on child and adolescent behavior and development, and examined health service needs, health service options, health financing issues, and issues regarding legal autonomy for those aged 10–24. This broad age range encompasses the most critical years of adolescent development, as well as the sometimes complex transitions from childhood to adolescence and from adolescence to adulthood. Ultimately, given the marked differences in health issues, developmental needs, health service needs, health financing issues, and legal status between adolescents and young adults, the committee found it difficult to address adequately the health service needs of such a broad age group. The committee also found that most evidence was limited regarding the health status, health services, and health service needs of those at the upper end of this age range.

The committee therefore focused this report on adolescents aged 10–19. This age range allows the discussion to include the lower bound of puberty, as well as the age at which most adolescents embark on adult paths, such as college, employment, military service, or marriage. This target population is referred to throughout the report primarily by the term "adolescents," but that term is sometimes used interchangeably with others, including "youths," "young people," and "teens" or "teenagers." Where appropriate and possible, the committee broke the available data down into two subsets: early adolescence (ages 10–14) and adolescence (ages 15–19). In addition, some issues salient for those aged 18–19 do not apply to those aged 10–17 since the former are legally defined as adults; where relevant, this distinction is made.

Having decided to focus this study on those aged 10–19, however, the committee faced a significant challenge arising from the variation in age ranges used to define adolescence among the various professional organizations, authorities (federal, state, and local), researchers, and advocacy groups that take an interest in, enact public policy for, and collect data and conduct research on adolescents. This variation made it impossible for the committee to rely exclusively on data and research on those aged 10–19. Throughout this report, therefore, the committee uses the best available evidence for adolescents aged 10–19, but notes that there are inconsistencies in the data and cases in which parallel data were not available. At times, moreover, the report refers to late adolescence or early adulthood (ages 20–24). For example, the health service needs of this older age group are included in the discussion of insurance coverage in Chapter 5 since the available evidence tends to distinguish between issues related to those aged 10–18 and those aged 19–24. Since the committee's definition includes those aged 19, data on insurance eligibility and coverage for the full older age range are included to demonstrate the major transitions and striking shortcomings in access to health services that occur as adolescents grow older.

The committee's decision to focus on ages 10–19 was difficult and problematic. The lack of attention to the health and health service needs of older adolescents or emerging adults is a major concern that lies beyond the scope of this report, but one that the committee believes deserves careful attention in its own right in future studies.

Selected Adolescent Subpopulations

The range of subpopulations of adolescents in the United States results in broad variation among adolescents and their health status. The health and development and health service needs of adolescents vary by gender, race and ethnicity, social and economic environment, information and skills, and access to health services, as well as other factors. When possible, the committee considered a variety of population variables and their relationship to adolescent health status and health services. In addition, the committee considered the specific issues and needs of adolescents in various circumstances, such as those who are in the foster care system, are homeless, are in families that have recently immigrated to the United States, identify themselves as LGBT, or are in the juvenile justice system. Data on the number of adolescents who fall into these subpopulations are sparse, and in many cases there is overlap among groups. Where possible, however, the committee attempted to quantify the numbers of adolescents in these specific groups.

Finally, it is important to note that, while there is recognition in the literature and among experts that certain groups of adolescents have differing needs, risks, and resources related to health, there is no agreement on the specific subpopulations within the adolescent population (Knopf et al., 2007). As will be discussed further in subsequent chapters, this lack of agreement creates challenges in addressing the unique health and health service needs of selected subpopulations and tailoring service delivery accordingly. As well, much of the evidence on health status and health objectives for specific adolescent subpopulations is based on limited data and likely represents an underestimation of the challenges involved (Knopf et al., 2007).

Defining Health

Beyond defining the adolescent population, the committee recognized the importance of defining adolescent health. A report of the NRC and the IOM defines children's health as "the extent to which individual children or groups of children are able or enabled to (a) develop and realize their potential, (b) satisfy their needs, and (c) develop the capacities that allow them to interact successfully with their biological, physical, and social environments" (National Research Council and Institute of Medicine, 2004a, p. 4). The committee further delineated three distinct but related domains of health: health conditions, which captures disorders or illnesses of body systems; functioning, which focuses on the manifestation of health in an individual's daily life; and health potential, which denotes the development of assets and positive aspects of health, such as competence, capacity, and developmental potential. The World Health Organization's definition of health as "a state of complete physical, mental, and social well-being and not merely the absence of disease or infirmity" (World Health Organization, 1948, p. 100) is consistent with the committee's strong interest in looking broadly at health. The committee defined oral health as a part of physical health, and identified behavior as an element of health and well-being.

The committee focused on the influence of health services and settings on adolescent health while also recognizing that a broad range of individual factors—biological (demographic, genetic, special needs), behavioral (sexual activity, diet, physical activity, use of weapons, substance use), attitudinal (values and personal preferences), social environmental (peers, schools, families), and immediate context or environment (neighborhood, media, geographic location, built environment)—all affect the health of adolescents. Health services, in turn, are affected by providers (training, types, and diversity), the overall system (funding, coverage and insurance, accessibility, acceptability, content and structure of care, service models, comprehensiveness of care, confidentiality, Medicaid, the State Children's Health Insurance Program [SCHIP], school policies), and the overall sociocultural environment (culture and values, income and inequality, the role of government, content and confidentiality, and political values).

Within this web of influences, the committee's specific focus was on health services and settings. The committee considered health services broadly, encompassing those services provided by doctors, nurses, mental health professional, dentists, or other health care providers. These services include health maintenance visits,[3] school physicals, sports physicals, dental

---

[3]Defined as clinical preventive services that incorporate screening, immunizations, and counseling about potential health problems and address prevention of future illness and injury; may also be called a well-care visit, a physical examination, a well-child examination, or ambulatory care.

care, psychiatric care, and medical care when an adolescent is sick, injured, or managing a chronic condition. Health care can also occur in many different settings—a traditional medical or dental office, community-based health center, hospital or medical outpatient department, school, or pharmacy.

NOTABLE PAST WORK

Research and public policies aimed at better understanding and promoting adolescent health and health services served as an important starting point for this study.

The most notable and comprehensive policy work to date on adolescent health is probably that conducted more than 15 years ago by the OTA. The OTA identified three major policy options for Congress that would demonstrate the nation's commitment to a new approach to adolescent health issues and provide tangible, appreciable assistance to adolescents with health needs (U.S. Congress and Office of Technology Assessment, 1991):

- Take steps to improve adolescents' access to appropriate health and related services.
- Take steps to restructure and invigorate the federal government's efforts to improve adolescents' health.
- Support efforts to improve adolescents' environments.

The OTA report observed that there were numerous potential strategies for implementing each of these policy options. The overarching goal, however, would be to craft a health system that could move beyond the problem-specific services and health centers that characterized much of the delivery system for adolescent health services. The report concluded that federal and other policy makers should follow the basic guiding principle of providing a prolonged protective and appropriately supportive environment for adolescents. This effort should include a strategic vision of the ultimate purposes and features of a health system, as well as specific, concrete improvements to a broad range of health and related services, policies, and care settings. Although leadership to implement these recommendations never emerged, they still serve as an important framework for thinking about adolescent health.

More recently, the Health Resources and Services Administration's Maternal and Child Health Bureau and the Centers for Disease Control and Prevention (CDC) within the U.S. Department of Health and Human Services launched the National Initiative to Improve Adolescent Health. The purpose of this initiative is to stimulate a wide array of public and private partnerships aimed at focusing on and improving the health, safety, and well-being of adolescents, young adults, and their families by increasing access to quality health care and eliminating health disparities. A variety of health organizations are participating, including the Partners in Program Planning for Adolescent Health, the Association of Maternal and Child Health Programs, the National Assembly on School-Based Health Care, the National 4-H Council, the Children's Safety Network, and the National Network of State Adolescent Health Coordinators, as well as academic centers at the University of Minnesota, Baylor College of Medicine, the University of California, San Francisco, the University of Maryland, Indiana University, The Johns Hopkins University, the University of Alabama, Boston Children's Hospital, and the University of California, Los Angeles. The initiative takes a broad view of adolescent health, recognizing that healthful outcomes for adolescents involve more than access to health services. A number of other components—including behavioral strategies; counseling, support, and referral services; and safe, nurturing environments—are important to healthy adolescent development and also help adolescents make healthful decisions.

The National Academies has prepared several reports presenting conclusions about the health and well-being of adolescents and recommendations as to the types and features of settings that are successful in promoting adolescent health. *Community Programs to Promote Youth Development* (National Research Council and Institute of Medicine, 2002) provides a framework for thinking about adolescent development in the context of the various settings where adolescents live, learn, and work. Discussed in more detail in Chapter 4, this report identifies a set of personal and social assets that foster the healthy development and well-being of adolescents and facilitate a successful transition from childhood through adolescence and into adulthood. A comprehensive and interdisciplinary synthesis of the literature conducted to inform this report revealed a specific set of characteristics—regardless of setting—that support the development of these assets in adolescents. These include such features as supportive relationships, appropriate program structure, safety, and opportunities for skill building.

Various other reports of the National Academies provide insight into specific aspects of adolescent development and health. *Reducing Underage Drinking* (National Research Council and Institute of Medicine, 2004b) reviews the dangerous behavior of underage alcohol use and its association with traffic fatalities, violence, unsafe sexual activities, suicide, educational failure, and health risks. It offers recommendations for how this behavior can be prevented and for what individuals and groups can do to have an impact in promoting positive change to this end.

Preventing Childhood Obesity: Health in the Balance (Institute of Medicine, 2005) looks specifically at the epidemic of obesity in children and adolescents. It explores the underlying causes of this serious health problem and the actions needed to initiate, support, and sustain the societal and lifestyle changes that can reverse the trend toward obesity among the nation's children and adolescents. A follow-up to this report, *Food Marketing to Children and Youth: Threat or Opportunity* (Institute of Medicine, 2006), considers the specific impact of food and beverage marketing on the dietary patterns and health status of American children and adolescents and offers recommendations for how government agencies, educators and schools, health professionals, industry companies, industry trade groups, the media, and those involved in community and consumer advocacy can promote healthful food and beverage messages to children and adolescents.

Preventing Teen Motor Crashes: Contributions from the Behavioral and Social Sciences (National Research Council, Institute of Medicine, and Transportation Research Board, 2007) explores the role of behavioral and social factors in teenage driving and considers prevention strategies to reduce the burden of injury and death from teen motor vehicle crashes. The report identifies several key opportunities for applying research knowledge to teen driving practices, especially in such areas as coaching and novice driving practices, parental supervision, error detection, peer interactions, adolescent decision making, and the development of incentives to foster safe-driving skills. The social context of teen driving that influences cognitive development and the acquisition of driving expertise is identified as an important sphere that has received little attention in prevention strategies.

Children's Health, The Nation's Wealth (National Research Council and Institute of Medicine, 2004a) reviews the information about children's health that is needed by policy makers and program providers at the federal, state, and local levels. This information can be used to assess both current conditions and possible future threats to children's health, as well as to identify what is needed to expand the knowledge base on adolescent health.

As a part of the IOM's Quality of Health Care in America project, *Crossing the Quality Chasm: A New Health System for the 21st Century* (Institute of Medicine, 2001) examines the sizable gap between the quality of health services that exist in the United States and that which Americans should expect. The report documents the causes of this gap, identifies current practices that impede quality care, and explores how systemic approaches can be used to implement change. It recommends a redesign of the American health system and identifies performance expectations for the system. The report is focused broadly on the U.S. population. The health service needs of adolescents, however, are relevant within several of the report's priority areas, such as immunization, asthma, pregnancy and childbirth, mental illness, and obesity—specifically through the report's focus on children with special needs and as an element of its system-level recommendations, such as those for coordination of care.

STUDY CONTEXT

Adolescents in the United States

In 2006 there were nearly 42 million adolescents aged 10–19 in the United States—14 percent of the total U.S. population. According to the U.S. Census Bureau (n.d., 2004, 2006b, 2007), the number of adolescents in the United States is expected to increase by 28 percent through 2050 (see Figure 1-1). Although this is a much smaller increase than that projected for the overall population, it represents an additional 11.5 million adolescents.

Finding: Adolescents aged 10–19 made up 14 percent (42 million) of the total population of the United States in 2006.

Of the total adolescent population, 51.2 percent are male and 48.8 percent female. The majority of adolescents aged 10–19 are white (76 per-

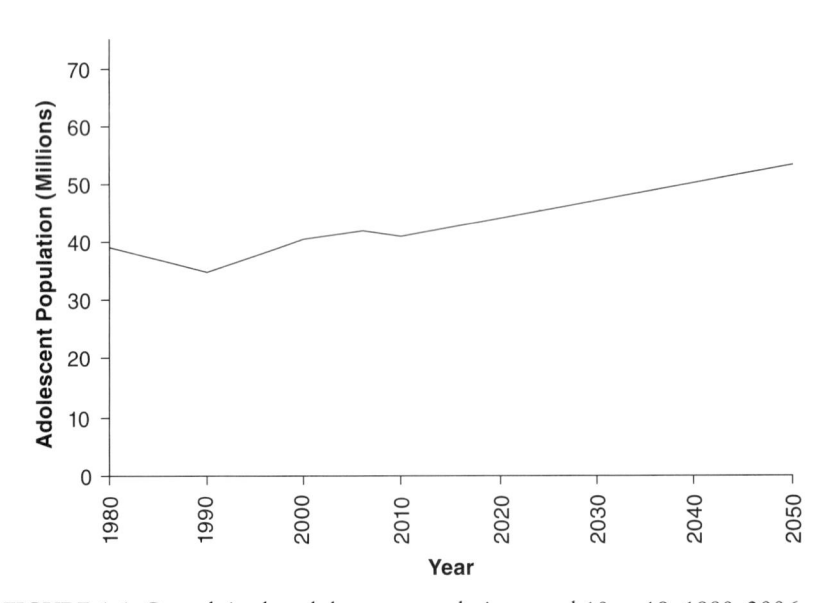

FIGURE 1-1 Growth in the adolescent population, aged 10 to 19, 1980–2006 and 2006–2050 (projected).
SOURCE: U.S. Census Bureau (n.d., 2004, 2006b, 2007).

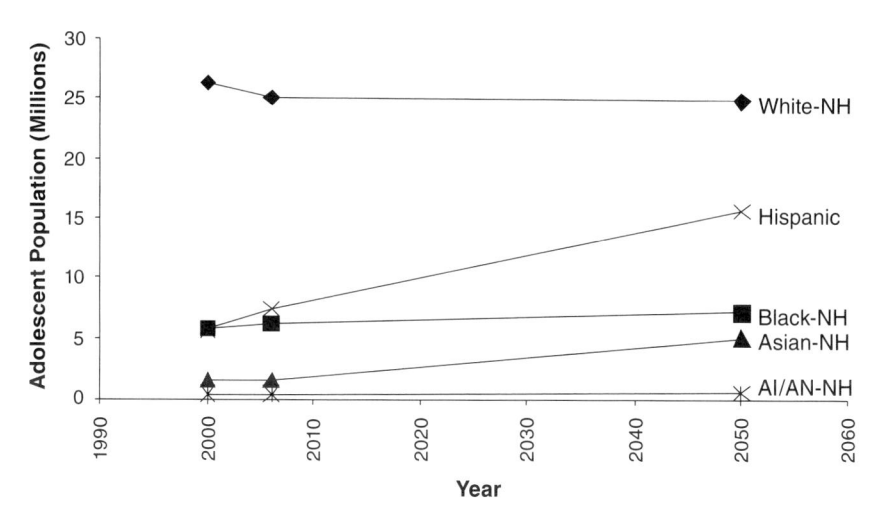

FIGURE 1-2 Changing racial/ethnic composition of the U.S. adolescent population, aged 10 to 19, 2000–2006 and 2006–2050 (projected).
NOTE: AI/AN = American Indian/Alaskan Native; NH = non-Hispanic.
SOURCE: U.S. Census Bureau (2006b, 2007).

cent), including non-black Hispanics, followed by black/African American (16 percent), Asian (3.8 percent), two or more races (2.5 percent), American Indian/Alaskan Native (1.2 percent), and Native Hawaiian and other Pacific Islander (less than 1 percent). Adolescents of Hispanic origin are also increasing in number. They currently make up approximately 18 percent of the U.S. adolescent population, but that figure is expected to increase to 30 percent by 2050 (compared with the white non-Hispanic population, expected to decrease from 60 to 47 percent) (see Figure 1-2) (U.S. Census Bureau, 2006b, 2007). In 2004, nearly 7 percent of adolescents aged 10–19 were foreign born; 85 percent of those foreign born are not U.S. citizens (U.S. Census Bureau, 2005).

> *Finding: The racial and ethnic makeup of the U.S. adolescent population is becoming more diverse. The correlations among minority racial and ethnic status, poverty, and lack of access to quality health services for adolescents are strong. Without specific attention and actions to reduce them, disparities in access to quality health services among minority racial and ethnic groups may increase.*

There is a correlation between poverty and the lack of access to quality health services for adolescents (Agency for Healthcare Research and Quality and Health Resources and Services Administration, 2000; Reading, 1997; Stevens et al., 2006; Zeni et al., 2007). This fact is particularly distressing when viewed in light of the most recent data related to adolescents living in poverty. In 2005, the U.S. Census Bureau reported that 17.6 percent of adolescents under age 18 were living in poverty. Black and Hispanic adolescents under age 18 experience poverty at a higher rate than their Asian and white non-Hispanic counterparts. This is a consistent trend seen since 1980 (see Figure 1-3) (DeNavas-Walt, Proctor, and Hill Lee, 2006).

Where adolescents live and with whom may also directly affect health status, health-related behavior, health needs, and health services because of the potential impact of these variables on financial stability and stress level. In 2006, 35 percent of those aged 9–17 lived either in one-parent households or in households where no parent was present (U.S. Census Bureau, 2006a).

Access to quality health services may be a particular challenge in rural areas (Gamm, Hutchison, and Bellamy, 2002), which have fewer health services within a reasonable distance of where people live. Of U.S. adolescents aged 12–17, 19 percent, or 4.6 million, live in rural areas (nonmetropolitan counties including no city with a population of greater than 10,000) (Fields,

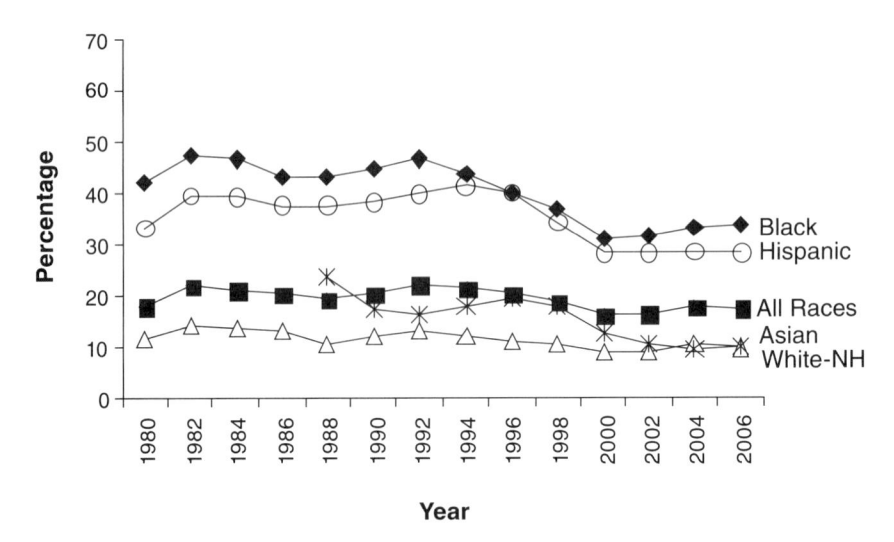

FIGURE 1-3 Percentage of adolescents under age 18 in poverty by race/ethnicity, 1980–2006.
NOTES: Poverty is defined by the U.S. Census Bureau using the Office of Management and Budget's Statistical Policy Directive 14. NH = non-Hispanic.
SOURCE: DeNavas-Walt, Proctor, and Hill Lee (2006).

2003). The population of rural adolescents increased from 1990 to 2002 (U.S. Census Bureau, 1992, 2003).

A portion of the adolescent population is disconnected from basic opportunities and supports that provide for their health, well-being, and economic self-sufficiency. These adolescents include those who are homeless, are transitioning from foster care, are recent immigrants to the United States, and are involved in the juvenile justice system.

Of the U.S. population under age 18, 0.5 percent live in group quarters— either institutionalized (e.g., correctional institutions, nursing homes, hospital wards and hospices for the chronically ill, mental [psychiatric] hospitals or wards, juvenile institutions, other institutions) or noninstitutionalized (e.g., college dormitories; military quarters; other noninstitutionalized group quarters, such as group homes and shelter facilities). Correctional and juvenile facilities are the two leading group quarters for both male and female adolescents under age 18 living in institutions. There are twice as many adolescent males as females living in institutions (U.S. Census Bureau, 2000). While this factor is important, it is notable that, according to the National Survey of Child Health, family income and mother's own health status are more likely to be correlated with adolescent health status than is place of residence (Maternal and Child Health Bureau, 2005a,b).

Data on runaway and homeless adolescents are difficult to capture given this population's inclination to be invisible or difficult to find. The National Runaway Switchboard collects data on calls to its crisis line. In 2006, it handled 113,916 calls from adolescents aged 12–21, 76 percent of whom were female (National Runaway Switchboard, 2006). These adolescents are frequently in a precarious living situation as a result of their being involved in systems of care such as the foster care or juvenile justice system, or their being recent immigrants to the United States or being disenfranchised socially, as may be the case for LGBT adolescents. They generally lack primary health care and may have increased health problems because of either factors that influenced their being homeless or the increased risk and exposure that result from living on the street (Shapiro, 2006).

How adolescents use their time may also affect their health, both positively and negatively. Adolescents who have a substantial amount of unsupervised time during nonschool hours may be at risk of participating in health-damaging behavior (National Research Council and Institute of Medicine, 2002); there is evidence that these adolescents are more likely to engage in sexual activity, smoke, use alcohol and drugs, and participate in violent and gang-related activities (Zill, Nord, and Loomis, 1995). Moreover, involvement with electronic media leads to increased sedentary time and less active playing (Institute of Medicine, 2005), which may contribute to obesity. Besides work time (4 to 6 hours a day), which includes schoolwork, household labor, and paid labor, adolescents in the United States have 6.5 to 8 hours of free time a day, much of which is unstructured discretionary time (Larson, 2001; Larson and Verma, 1999). A great deal of this discretionary time is spent watching television, playing video games, using computers, and engaging with other electronic media (Rideout, Vandewater, and Wartella, 2003; Roberts et al., 1999). Multiple televisions, radios, tape players, video cassette and DVD players, video game players, and computers are common in American homes (Rideout, Vandewater, and Wartella, 2003). Fully 70 percent of adolescents aged 10–17 have access to the Internet at home (Cheeseman Day, Janus, and Davis, 2005), and yet there is no evidence to help understand the extent to which adolescents have access to electronic communication with their health care providers.

Adolescent Health and Health Services

The past century of medical advances in research and treatment has improved the understanding of physical and hormonal changes, psychological development, and risk-taking behavior that define puberty and the major psychological, cognitive, and behavioral developments that characterize the transition from childhood to adulthood. Historically, the medical care of adolescents was subsumed under the disciplines of pediatrics, psychiatry, internal medicine, and gynecology, but none of these focused exclusively on adolescents. During this century—likely as a response to the rapidly expanding adolescent population; increases in adolescent morbidity and mortality; advances in understanding of adolescent physical, emotional, and cognitive development; and societal influences that have made the adolescent environment less restrictive—the subspecialty of adolescent medicine has emerged (Alderman, Rieder, and Cohen, 2003).

In 1941 the American Academy of Pediatrics held a symposium on adolescence, a first effort to incorporate adolescent medicine into the domain of pediatric practice. This was followed by the development of a few medical school academic divisions focused on adolescents. Ten years later, J. Roswell Gallagher, often credited as the founder of adolescent medicine, began the first inpatient adolescent health unit at Boston Children's Hospital. Early in his career he worked as a school physician, studying adolescent growth and development, and ultimately helping to highlight the need for health services that included comprehensive preventive services, as well as diagnosis and treatment of physical health and "mental hygiene" or emotional health issues (Prescott, 1998).

Since the 1960s, several important developments have further improved the knowledge base on and drawn attention to adolescent health and health services. Adolescent medicine training programs funded by the federal government, the Society of Adolescent Medicine, the American Academy of Pediatrics' Committee on Adolescence, and various other organizations with a primary focus on adolescents have made important contributions to research, training, and the formulation of policies focused on adolescent health and health services.

In addition to the development of a better understanding of how to treat and cure medical illnesses, adolescent health care has examined the effects of high-risk adolescent behavior and investigated strategies for reducing such risks and limiting their impact. There has also been a movement toward promoting healthy adolescent development rather than simply preventing adolescent problems.

In addition to adolescent medical specialists, a broad range of medical practitioners continue to provide health services to adolescents. They include pediatricians, family physicians, and dentists, with the involvement of such subspecialty fields as gynecology, infectious diseases, sports medicine, psychology, and endocrinology. As well, the settings where adolescent health services are delivered have evolved from doctors' offices to community and specialized clinics, school based health centers, and mobile vans. These multiple entry points into the system of care offer both opportunities and challenges.

Perceptions and Attitudes About Adolescent Health

Many people and groups—adolescents, their parents, other adults, and the various practitioners who deliver health services—have perceptions about adolescent health status and behavior and perspectives on appropriate and needed adolescent health services. Understanding the perceptions and attitudes of these many stakeholders is important to the successful development of adolescent health policies and services that are well supported by the public and respond appropriately to the needs and interests of those who are served. As well, those engaged in adolescent health (adolescent themselves, parents, health practitioners, schools) face complex and sometimes controversial issues with regard to the right to and importance of confidentiality of care. Chapter 4 includes a full discussion of these issues.

Adolescents sometimes appear to be a difficult group for the public to embrace. They may also be blamed for the health conditions that result from such behavior as drug and alcohol use, risky sexual conduct, and risky driving. Moreover, negative attitudes may be more intense toward certain subpopulations of adolescents, such as those who are homeless, LGBT, or in the juvenile justice system. And, the public often perceives these adolescents as someone else's problem—a problem for which the government should not have to take responsibility or on which their tax dollars should not be spent.

There is a limited literature of varying quality and significance on perceptions and attitudes regarding adolescent health and health services, and much of that work is based on surveys. Nonetheless, the committee selected some examples that highlight adolescent, parent, and practitioner perspectives.

Adolescents

It is important for the design and delivery of adolescent health services to appeal to adolescents and be responsive to their needs and concerns. In that spirit, the committee included questions in an online Harris Interactive poll aimed at understanding the health perspectives and interests of adolescents themselves. Nearly 1,200 adolescents responded to questions about their access to medical services, barriers to receiving care, communication about health services, the extent to which their parents or other adults or peers are involved in helping them obtain health services, their interest in using technology for health information and health reminders, and their perspective on how health services could be more helpful to them. Respondents reported that their parents are quite often involved in their health care and that they view this involvement positively. The majority of respondents indicated that they experience no access barriers to health services. When barriers were reported, cost and scheduling were cited most frequently, along with a lack of insurance. Respondents frequently mentioned having access to affordable, convenient, and high-quality dental care as what they would most like to change about health services to make them more helpful. Although confidentiality appeared to be of low concern, 10 percent of respondents worry that their parents will learn information they do not want their parents to have. (Privacy and confidentiality issues are discussed further below.) About 20 percent of respondents are extremely or very interested in using technology (e.g., mobile phones, the Internet) to obtain health information.

Differences in adolescent perspectives may be attributable to certain demographic variables. Family values and structures, for instance, may play a role in the health behavior and attitudes of adolescents. A study of urban adolescent males found that family circumstances influenced attitudes toward sexual behavior. Young male adolescents who were raised by a single parent with no father present or had a mother who was a teenage parent reported little concern about sexual responsibility. By contrast, urban adolescent males with two parents in the home or father-figure relationships expressed concern about their sexual health and the possibility of becoming a teenage father (Gohel, Diamond, and Chambers, 1997).

Gender may also have an impact on adolescent perspectives. In a study conducted by Pleck and O'Donnell (2001), male adolescents reported more risky health behavior than did female adolescents. Another study found that while 87 percent of healthy adolescents were satisfied with the general health services they received, 13 percent were dissatisfied because of the gender of the provider, embarrassment, or an uncomfortable atmosphere in the provider's office (Jacobson et al., 2000).

Some limited work has been done to collect data on the perspectives of adolescents regarding mental health services (Garland and Besinger, 1996; Shapiro, Welker, and Jacobson, 1997). More commonly, however, parents are surveyed about their satisfaction with their children's services (Magura and Moses, 1984). In a study of adolescents in foster care conducted by Lee and colleagues (2006), adolescents were asked to share their experiences with mental health services and specific providers, with the goal of identifying and describing the characteristics they valued in relationships with mental health professionals and the services they received. The relationship with their provider, the professionalism of the provider, and the effects of the treatment were the areas the adolescents identified as critical to receiving quality care.

Adolescents using drugs do not typically perceive a need for or seek treatment for substance abuse. In the National Survey on Drug Use and Health (Substance Abuse and Mental Health Services Administration 2003–2004), among those who were classified as needing such treatment but had received none in the past year, only 2.2 percent perceived a need for treatment for alcohol use problems and only 3.5 percent for drug use problems (note that the criminal justice system is a major source of referral for such treatment). According to data from the Treatment Episode Data Set (Substance Abuse and Mental Health Services Administration, 2006), in 2004 the criminal justice system accounted for 52 percent of referrals for those aged 12–17, 52 percent for those aged 18–21, and 45 percent for those aged 22–25. In the Cannabis Youth Treatment Study, 80 percent of adolescents saw no need for treatment. Those who viewed treatment as most relevant, who liked their therapist, who felt comfortable discussing their problems with their therapist, and who perceived fewer practical obstacles to treatment attended more drug abuse treatment sessions (Mensinger et al., 2006). Another study found that adolescents who experienced more negative consequences from their substance use showed more motivation to change (Battjes et al., 2003; Breda and Heflinger, 2004).

Parents

Parents' perspectives on adolescent health status and behavior frequently differ from those of adolescents. For instance, in a 2006 Phillip Morris Teenage Attitudes and Behavior Survey, fewer than half of adolescent smokers aged 11–14 reported that their parents were aware that they smoked (Phillip Morris USA, 2006). Similarly, according to the National Survey of Child Health, 83 percent of parents believed their adolescent children (aged 12–17) were in excellent or very good health. Yet the definition of good health may vary tremendously among parents, in some cases being based on traditional medical measures and in others simply on the absence of a noticeable illness.

Sexual behavior and reproductive health is an area that elicits particularly strong opinions, and one in which parents' perceptions of behavior and reports of behavior by adolescents are often inconsistent. Many parents underestimate the number of adolescents who are sexually active (Hutchinson et al., 2003; Miller and Whitaker, 2000). A national survey conducted by the Society for Adolescent Medicine in 2004 found that while 60 percent of parents were concerned about the consequences of adolescent sexual activity, 84 percent of these parents did not believe their own child was sexually active (Society for Adolescent Medicine, 2004). According to CDC, however, nearly half of adolescents in grades 9–12 have had sex (Grunbaum et al., 2004). Similarly, a study by the National Campaign to Prevent Teen Pregnancy revealed that two-thirds of parents of sexually active 14-year-olds had no idea their children were having sex (Albert, Brown, and Flanigan, 2003). Moreover, while parents value the information they receive from health practitioners about their children's health, practitioners believe parents often misunderstand the benefits of sex education versus the costs of irresponsible sexual behavior (Deptula et al., 2006). For example, parents may not want their children to receive information about the human papillomavirus vaccine or methods of birth control because they believe this will promote early sexual activity or are opposed on religious grounds (Zimet, 2005). In fact, it is now clear that comprehensive sex education does not hasten the onset of sexual activity at all (Kirby, 2007).

There may also be differences in adolescent perspectives among racial and ethnic groups. A study of adults in rural North Carolina found that black parents were more than 50 percent more likely than white parents to believe that public schools should provide adolescents with general health services, including pregnancy testing and treatment of sexually transmitted diseases. However, they were only half as likely to approve of sexual experimentation by adolescents (Horner et al., 1994).

Practitioners

Health practitioners believe more work is needed to ensure that adolescents and their parents are aware of the health services available to them in the community and that health care providers have a positive approach to adolescent health services (Burack, 2000). At the same time, some providers believe adolescents are best served at medical clinics focused on specific health needs, such as mental health, substance abuse treatment, healthy eating/obesity, injuries/orthopedics, sexual behavior and reproductive health, and safety/domestic issues (McDonagh et al., 2006).

Some health care providers (physicians, nurses, nurse practitioners) lack confidence that they have the training needed to provide the best health services to adolescents. Fewer than half of providers who care for adolescents on a regular basis have received formal training in doing so (Burack, 2000).

Communication between health care providers and adolescents is also important. In one study, 43 percent of physicians reported that they did not believe adolescents would tell the truth about their sexual activity. This was the case even though the physicians indicated that they had discussed sexual health needs, sex education, and/or birth control and condoms with nearly 75 percent of their patients (Igra and Millstein, 1994).

Many health care providers fail to realize that the health concerns of adolescents can vary greatly by gender and are much more diverse than might be expected, with social and psychological concerns being just as important as traditional medical concerns. Without rigorous and diligent inquiry on the part of providers regarding social and emotional as well as physical issues, adolescents may not reveal important information that relates to their total well-being (Kowpak, 1991).

Pharmacists have an important role in assessing, initiating, monitoring, and modifying medications, one that often leads to interactions with patients and creates opportunities to assist in providing adolescent health services. In a survey of close to 1,000 pharmacists, however, a substantial portion reported inadequate training in issues related to adolescent health (Conard et al., 2003). Many of the pharmacists expressed interest in gaining a better understanding of these issues, which could improve their interactions with adolescent patients. Given the important role of pharmacists as an integral part of a health care team, Conard and colleagues (2003) suggest that the role of pharmacists in adolescent health receive increased attention during pharmacy training and in postgraduate forums.

Policy Environment

Whether adolescents receive quality health services, preventive health services, and supportive counseling is affected by the policy environment in which the need for and cost of these services are debated. There is disagreement among policy makers on whether there should be universal access to health services in the United States. There is also no agreement on the appropriate role of government-supported health services versus those that should be financed by private health insurance. The result has been a haphazard system for providing these services for adolescents, as well as other children and adults. With much of the ultimate determination of the quality and extent of care being left to the states, and with federal and state funding for health services frequently being limited, many adolescents fall through the cracks of the health system. This situation is exacerbated by the fact that there is no national policy consensus in the United States on how to deal with adolescents except with regard to education.

The operation of Medicaid and SCHIP provides an example of this problem. These programs provide health coverage that, in theory, should be adequate for children and adolescents. In reality, however, both programs have flaws that result in many adolescents being covered not at all or inadequately as states adjust eligibility, the extent of service provision, and the requirements for copayments that adolescents and their families may not be able to afford. The federal government has focused on private health care and insurance that covers care for more vulnerable populations not currently served by Medicaid or SCHIP, and has therefore encouraged changes to the tax code to make private insurance affordable and state action to monitor the adequacy of coverage. As a result, a variety of proposals for the reform of state health insurance have surfaced that are currently being considered to increase health insurance coverage for children and adolescents.

Privacy and Confidentiality

Beyond attitudes and perceptions about adolescent health and health services, legal considerations of confidentiality and informed consent are central to any discussion of the interests and rights of adolescents with respect to their health. These matters are ethically and legally complex, and a great deal is at stake in these discussions. Although the ethical and legal complexities involved have the potential to divide health care providers, parents, policy makers, and advocates for children[4] and for families,[5] there is also significant potential for defining common ground.

Some parents may believe that their authority and their ability to shape their children's lives and values (*Wisconsin v. Yoder* [1972], 406 U.S. 205, 234)—moral, religious, and spiritual—are threatened by the notion that adolescents themselves have independent interests and rights. Most parents, however, are concerned primarily with promoting their adolescent children's health, safety, and well-being. In that context, it can be challenging for parents to understand when and why it is appropriate for adolescents to be able to consent to their own health services and receive those services on a confidential basis, and how those interests may differ from their own.

Many adolescents perceive that they are engaged in a process of self-

---

[4]See http://www.plannedparenthood.org/.
[5]See http:///www.afa.net/prolife/articles.asp.

definition and individuation that requires—to a greater or lesser degree—the creation of a private persona with desires and behavior that, even if not forbidden by parents, are separate from parental scrutiny and supervision. For a few young people, adolescence can lead to a significant disjunction of interests that may even threaten the integrity of the family. In some families, the impetus for this disjunction comes from the adolescent, while in others the parents are motivated by their own problems or their children's behavior to initiate a break. Even so, the majority of adolescents obtain health services with the knowledge and support of their parents and benefit from that involvement.

Health professionals, both by inclination and by training, focus on the needs of their patients. For this reason, providers of health services to adolescents often view themselves as allies of the adolescent who is seeking to define a separate existence and decision-making structure. At the same time, adolescent health experts in clinical settings, research institutions, and professional organizations have repeatedly recognized the important role of parents in fostering the health of adolescents.

It is critical that these challenging issues be addressed within a current social and policy context in which there is little overt support for the adolescent experimentation and risk taking that may give rise to the need for confidentiality protection in adolescent health services. Even so, a large body of evidence, drawn from research conducted over the past several decades, serves not only to document the range and extent of behavior that affects adolescents' health, but also to provide a rationale and strong justification for protecting confidentiality in their health services.

BEHAVIORAL AND CONTEXTUAL CHARACTERISTICS

Creating successful interactions between adolescents and health service settings and systems requires a multifaceted approach. The committee was guided by two frameworks in its data collection, review of the evidence, and attention to various dimensions of adolescent health status and health services. The first focuses on behavioral and contextual characteristics that influence how adolescents interact with the health system. The second, which is described in Chapter 3, focuses on the objectives of adolescent health services. Neither framework alone is sufficient to explain significant variations in adolescent health outcomes; rather, they complement each other and, in tandem, provide a more complete picture of the features of the health system that should be improved in order to provide adolescents high-quality care and thus help to improve their health status.

The committee recognized that certain sets of behavioral and contextual characteristics shape the ways in which adolescents approach and interact with health care services, providers, and settings. When these characteristics are addressed in the design of health services for adolescents, these services can offer high-quality care that is particularly attuned to the needs of this age group. These characteristics helped frame the chapters of this report and, where relevant and supported by the evidence, are reflected in the committee recommendations.

- **Development matters.** Adolescence is a period of significant and dramatic change spanning the physical, biological, social, and psychological transitions from childhood to young adulthood. This dynamic state influences both the health of young people and the health services they require (Chapter 1).
- **Timing matters.** Adolescence is a critical time for health promotion. Many health problems and much of the risky behavior that underlies later health problems begin during adolescence. Prevention, early intervention, and timely treatment improve health status for adolescents and prepare them for healthy adulthood; such services also decrease the incidence of many chronic diseases in adulthood (Chapter 2).
- **Context matters.** Social context and such factors as income, geography, and cultural norms and values can profoundly affect the health of adolescents and the health services they receive (Chapters 2 and 3).
- **Need matters.** Some segments of the adolescent population, defined by both biology and behavior, have health needs that require particular attention in health systems (Chapter 2).
- **Participation matters.** Effective health services for young people invite adolescents and their families to engage with clinicians (Chapter 4).
- **Family matters.** At the same time that adolescents are growing in their autonomy, families continue to affect adolescents' health and overall well-being and to influence what health services they use. Young people without adequate family support are particularly vulnerable to risky behavior and poor health and therefore often require additional support in health service settings (Chapter 4).
- **Community matters.** Good health services for adolescents include population-focused as well as individual and family services since the environment in which adolescents live, as well as the supports they receive in the community, are important (Chapter 4).
- **Skill matters.** Young people are best served by providers who understand the key developmental features, health issues, and overall social environment of adolescents (Chapter 5).
- **Money matters.** The availability, nature, and content of health services for adolescents are affected by such financial factors as public

and private health care insurance, the amount of funding invested in special programs for adolescents, and the support available for adequate training programs for providers of adolescent health services (Chapter 6).
- **Policy matters.** Policies, both public and private, can have a profound effect on adolescent health services. Carefully crafted policies are a foundation for strong systems of care that meet a wide variety of individual and community needs (Chapter 6).

ORGANIZATION OF THE REPORT

This report reviews the literature on adolescent health and health service delivery; presents the committee's findings; and offers recommendations directed to both public and private entities, for investing in, strengthening, and improving the system of health services for adolescents. Chapter 2 reviews the health status of adolescents, while Chapter 3 describes the health services, settings, and providers currently available for adolescents. Chapter 4 identifies strategies for improving current health services to achieve a system that would reflect the needs and concerns of the adolescent population more accurately. Chapter 5 describes the training requirements and needs of health care providers who serve adolescents. Chapter 6 describes adolescent health insurance coverage and associated challenges in accessing health services. Finally, Chapter 7 highlights the committee's task, summarizes the committee's overall conclusions related to this task, and presents the committee's recommendations. In addition, for reference throughout the report, a list of acronyms is provided in Appendix A. The questions on the online Harris Interactive Omnibus Survey used for this study are listed in Appendix B, and Appendix C contains biographical sketches of the committee members.

REFERENCES

Agency for Healthcare Research and Quality. (2006). *Medical Expenditure Panel Survey: Table 1. Health insurance coverage of the civilian noninstitutionalized population: Percent by type of coverage and selected population characteristics, United States, first half of 2006*. Available: http://www.meps.ahrq.gov/mepsweb/data_stats/quick_tables_results.jsp?component=1&subcomponent=0&year=2006&tableSeries=4&searchText=&searchMethod=1&Action=Search [December 6, 2007].

Agency for Healthcare Research and Quality and Health Resources and Services Administration (2000). Access to Quality Health Services. *Healthy People 2010*, Volume I (second edition). Objectives for Improving Health (Part A: Focus Areas 1-14), 1–47. Available: http://www.healthypeople.gov/Document/pdf/Volume1/01Access.pdf [January 22, 2008].

Albert, B., Brown, S., and Flanigan, C. (Eds.). (2003). *14 and Younger: The Sexual Behavior of Young Adolescents (Summary)*. Washington, DC: National Campaign to Prevent Teen Pregnancy.

Alderman, E. M., Rieder, J., and Cohen, M. I. (2003). A history of pediatric specialties: The history of adolescent medicine. *Pediatric Research, 54*, 137–147.

Arnett, J. J. (2006). Emerging adulthood: Understanding the new way of coming of age. In J. J. Arnett and J. L. Tanner (Eds.), *Emerging Adults in America: Coming of Age in the 21st Century* (pp. 3–18). Washington, DC: American Psychological Association.

Association of Maternal and Child Health Programs and the National Network of State Adolescent Health Coordinators. (2005). *A Conceptual Framework for Adolescent Health*. Washington, DC: Association of Maternal and Child Health Programs.

Battjes, R., Gordon, M., O'Grady, K., Kinlock, T., and Carswell, M. (2003). Factors that predict adolescent motivation for substance abuse treatment. *Journal of Substance Abuse Treatment, 24*, 221–232.

Breda, C., and Heflinger, C. (2004). Predicting incentives to change among adolescents with substance abuse disorder. *American Journal of Drug and Alcohol Abuse, 20*, 251–267.

Brown, N. A. (2001). *Promoting Adolescent Livelihoods*. A discussion paper prepared for the Commonwealth Youth Programme and UNICEF. Available: www.unicef.org/adolescence/files/promoting_ado_livelihoods.pdf [July 29, 2008].

Burack, R. (2000). Young teenagers' attitude towards general practitioners and their provision of sexual health care. *British Journal of General Practice, 50*, 550–554.

Carolina Population Center. (2007). *Add Health: The National Longitudinal Study of Adolescent Health 2007*. Available: http://www.cpc.unc.edu/addhealth [November 27, 2007].

The Center for Development and Population Activities. (2003). *Adolescent Sexual and Reproductive Health: A Training Manual for Program Managers*. Washington, DC: The Center for Development and Population Activities.

Centers for Disease Control and Prevention. (2006). *Sexually Transmitted Disease Surveillance, 2005*. Atlanta, GA: Division of Sexually Transmitted Disease Prevention.

Centers for Disease Control and Prevention. (2007). *Youth Online: Comprehensive Results Youth Risk Behavior Survey*. Available: http://www.cdc.gov/healthyyouth/physicalactivity/ [August 8, 2007].

Cheeseman Day, J., Janus, A., and Davis, J. (2005). Computer and Internet use in the United States: 2003. *Current Population Reports, P23-208*, October.

Chung, P. J., Lee, T. C., Morrison, J. L., and Schuster, M. A. (2006). Preventive care for children in the United States: Quality and barriers. *Annual Review of Public Health, 27*, 10.1–10.25.

Committee on Adolescence. (2008). Achieving quality health services for adolescents. *Pediatrics, 121*, 1263–1270.

Conard, L. A., Fortenberry, J. D., Blythe, M. J., and Orr, D. P. (2003). Pharmacists' attitudes toward and practices with adolescents. *Archives of Pediatric and Adolescent Medicine, 157*, 361–365.

Dahl, R. E. (2003). *Adolescent Brain Development*. Key note address. Available: http://www.nyas.org/ebriefreps/main.asp?intSubsectionID=318 [April 1, 2008].

D'Augelli, A. R., Hershberger, S. L., and Pilkington, N. W. (1998). Lesbian, gay, and bisexual youth and their families: Disclosure of sexual orientation and its consequences. *American Journal of Orthopsychiatry, 68*, 361–371.

DeNavas-Walt, C., Proctor, B. D., and Hill Lee, C. (2006). *Income, Poverty, and Health Insurance Coverage in the United States, 2005*. Washington, DC: U.S. Department of Commerce, U.S. Census Bureau.

Deptula, D., Henry, D. B., Shoeny, M. E., and Slavick, M. S. (2006). Adolescent sexual behavior and attitudes: A costs and benefits approach. *Journal of Adolescent Health, 38,* 35–43.

Fields, J. (2003). Children's living arrangements and characteristics: March 2002. *Current Population Reports, P20-547,* June.

Fuchs, V. (1974). *Who Shall Live? Health, Economics, and Social Choice-Expanded Edition.* Singapore: World Scientific.

Fuchs, V. (1991). National health insurance revisited. *Health Affairs, 10,* 10–17.

Gamm, L., Hutchison, L., and Bellamy, G. (2002). Rural healthy people 2010: Identifying rural health priorities and models for practice. *Journal of Rural Health, 18,* 9–14.

Garfinkel, I., Hochschild, J., and McLanahan, S. (Eds.). (1996). *Social Policies for Children.* Washington, DC: The Brookings Institution.

Garland, A. F., and Besinger, B. A. (1996). Adolescents' perceptions of outpatient mental health services. *Journal of Child and Family Studies, 5,* 355–375.

Giedd, J., Blumenthal, J., Jeffries, N., Castellanos, F., Liu, H., Zijdenbos, A., Paus, T., Evans, A., and Rapoport, J. (1999). Brain development during childhood and adolescence: A longitudinal MRI study. *Nature Neuroscience, 2,* 861–863.

Gohel, M., Diamond, J., and Chambers, C. (1997). Attitudes toward sexual responsibility and parenting: An exploratory study of young urban males. *Family Planning Perspectives, 29,* 280–283.

Grunbaum, J. A., Kann, L., Kinchen, S., Ross, J., Hawkins, J., Lowry, R., Harris, W. A., McManus, T., Chyen, D., and Collins, J. (2004). Youth risk behavior surveillance—United States, 2003. *Morbidity and Mortality Weekly Report, 53,* 1–96.

Hernandez, D. (1993). *America's Children: Resources from Family, Government, and the Economy.* New York: Russell Sage Foundation.

Hing, E., Cherry, D. K., and Woodwell, D. A. (2006). National Ambulatory Medical Care Survey: 2004 summary. *Advance Data from Vital and Health Statistics, 374,* 1–36.

Hock-Long, L., Herceg-Baron, R., Cassidy, A. M., and Whittaker, P. G. (2003). Access to adolescent reproductive health services: Financial and structural barriers to care. *Perspectives on Sexual and Reproductive Health, 35,* 144–147.

Horner, R. D., Kolasa, K. M., Irons, T. G., and Wilson, K. (1994). Racial differences in rural adults' attitudes toward issues of adolescent sexuality. *American Journal of Public Health, 84,* 456–459.

Hutchinson, M., Jemmott III, J., Sweet Jemmott, L., Braverman, P., and Fong, G. (2003). The role of mother–daughter sexual risk communication in reducing sexual risk behavior among urban adolescent females: A prospective study. *Journal of Adolescent Health, 33,* 98–107.

Igra, V., and Millstein, S. G. (1994). *Physician Attitudes towards STD/HIV-Related Preventive Services to Teens.* The Woodlands, TX: American Pediatric Society.

Institute of Medicine. (2001). *Crossing the Quality Chasm. A New Health System for the 21st Century.* Washington, DC: National Academy Press.

Institute of Medicine. (2005). *Preventing Childhood Obesity: Health in the Balance.* Washington, DC: The National Academies Press.

Institute of Medicine. (2006). *Food Marketing to Children and Youth: Threat or Opportunity?* Washington, DC: The National Academies Press.

Jacobson, L. D., Mellanby, A. R., Donovan, C., Taylor, B., and Tripp, J. H. (2000). Teenagers' views on general practice consultations and other medical advice. *Family Practice, 17,* 156–158.

Kirby, D. (2007). *Emerging Answers 2007. Research Findings on Programs to Reduce Teen Pregnancy and Sexually Transmitted Diseases.* Washington, DC: National Campaign to Prevent Teen and Unplanned Pregnancy.

Knopf, K. D., Jane Park, M., Brindis, C. D., Mulye, T. P., and Irwin, C. E., Jr. (2007). What gets measured gets done: Assessing data availability for adolescent populations. *Maternal and Child Health Journal, 11,* 335–345.

Kodjo, C., Auinger, P., and Ryan, S. (2002). Barriers to adolescents accessing mental health services. *Journal of Adolescent Health, 30,* 101–102.

Kopelman, J. (2004). The provider system for children's mental health: Workforce capacity and effective treatment. *National Health Policy Forum Issue Brief, 801.*

Kowpak, M. (1991). Adolescent health concerns: A comparison of adolescent and health care provider perceptions. *Journal of the American Academy of Nurse Practitioners, 3,* 122–128.

Larson, R. W. (2001). How U.S. children and adolescents spend time: What it does (and doesn't) tell us about their development. *Current Directions in Psychological Science, 10,* 160–164.

Larson, R. W., and Verma, S. (1999). How children and adolescents spend time across cultural settings of the world: Work, play, and developmental opportunities. *Psychological Bulletin, 125,* 701–736.

Larson, R. W., Wilson, S., and Mortimer, J. T. (2003). Conclusions: Adolescents' preparation for the future. *Journal of Research on Adolescence, 12,* 159–166.

Lear, J. G. (2002). Schools and adolescent health: Strengthening services and improving outcomes. *Journal of Adolescent Health, 31,* 310–320.

Lee, B. R., Munson, M. R., Ware, N. C., Ollie, M. T., Scott, L. D., and McMillen, J. C. (2006). Experiences of and attitudes toward mental health services among older youths in foster care. *Psychiatric Services, 57,* 487–492.

Magura, S., and Moses, B. S. (1984). Clients as evaluators in child protective services. *Child Welfare, 63,* 99–112.

Maternal and Child Health Bureau. (2005a). *The Health and Well-Being of Children: A Portrait of States and the Nation, 2005.* Rockville, MD: U.S. Department of Health and Human Services, Health Resources and Services Administration.

Maternal and Child Health Bureau. (2005b). *The Health and Well-Being of Children in Rural Areas: A Portrait of the Nation, 2005.* Rockville, MD: U.S. Department of Health and Human Services, Health Resources and Services Administration.

McDonagh, J., Minnaar, G., Kelly, K., O'Connor, D., and Shaw, K. (2006). Unmet education and training needs in adolescent health of health professionals in a UK children's hospital. *Acta Paediatrica, 95,* 715–719.

Mensinger, J. L., Diamond, G. S., Kaminer, Y., and Wintersteen, M. B. (2006). Adolescent and therapist perception of barriers to outpatient substance abuse treatment. *American Journal of Addiction, 15,* 16–25.

Miller, M., and Whitaker, D. (2000). Parent–adolescent discussions about sex and condoms. *Journal of Adolescent Research, 15,* 251–273.

National Adolescent Health Information Center. (2004). *Improving the Health of Adolescents & Young Adults: A Guide for States and Communities.* Atlanta, GA: Centers for Disease Control and Prevention.

National Association of Social Workers. (2002). Dismantling stereotypes about adolescents: The power of positive images. *Adolescent Health NASW Practice Update, 2*(5).

National Institute of Mental Health (2001). *Teenage Brain: A Work in Progress.* Available: www.nimh.nih.gov/publicat/teenbrain.cfm [April 1, 2008].

National Research Council and Institute of Medicine. (1999). *Risks and Opportunities: Synthesis of Studies on Adolescence.* M. D. Kipke (Ed.). Washington, DC: National Academy Press.

National Research Council and Institute of Medicine. (2002). *Community Programs to Promote Youth Development*. J. Eccles and J. Appleton Gootman (Eds.). Washington, DC: The National Academies Press.

National Research Council and Institute of Medicine. (2004a). *Children's Health, the Nation's Wealth: Assessing and Improving Child Health*. Washington, DC: The National Academies Press.

National Research Council and Institute of Medicine. (2004b). *Reducing Underage Drinking: A Collective Responsibility*. R. J. Bonnie and M. E. O'Connell (Eds.). Washington, DC: The National Academies Press.

National Research Council, Institute of Medicine, and Transportation Research Board. (2007). *Preventing Teen Motor Crashes: Contributions from the Behavioral and Social Sciences, A Workshop Report*. Washington, DC: The National Academies Press.

National Runaway Switchboard. (2006). *NRS Call Statistics*. Available: http://www.1800runaway.org/news_events/call_stats.html [July 30, 2007].

Ozer, E. M., Park, M. J., Paul, T., Brindis, C. D., and Irwin, C. E., Jr. (2003). *America's Adolescents: Are They Healthy?* San Francisco: University of California and National Adolescent Health Information Center.

Park, M. J., Paul, T., Irwin, C. E., Jr., and Brindis, C. D. (2005). *A Health Profile of Adolescent and Young Adult Males*. San Francisco: University of California.

Park, M. J., Mulye, T. P., Adams, S. H., Brindis, C. D., and Irwin, C. E., Jr. (2006). The health status of young adults in the United States. *Journal of Adolescent Health, 39*, 305–317.

Perloff, J. (1992). Health care resources for children and pregnant women. *The Future of Children, 2*, 78–94.

Phillip Morris USA. (2006). *Teenage Attitudes and Behavior Survey*. Available: http://www.philipmorrisusa.com/en/ysp/tabs/results/charts/topic_5/chart_5_6.asp?navId=c1&sub=s5 [July 31, 2007].

Pleck, J., and O'Donnell, L. (2001). Gender attitudes and health risk behaviors in urban African American and Latino early adolescents. *Maternal and Child Health Journal, 5*, 265–272.

Prescott, H. M. (1998). *A Doctor of Their Own. A History of Adolescent Medicine*. Cambridge, MA: Harvard University Press.

Rand, C. M., Shone, L. P., Albertin, C., Auinger, P., Klein, J. D., and Szilagyi, P. G. (2007). National health care visit patterns of adolescents. Implications for delivery of new adolescent vaccines. *Archives of Pediatrics and Adolescent Medicine, 161*, 252–259.

Reading, R. (1997). Poverty and the health of children and adolescents. *Archives of Disease in Childhood, 76*, 463–467.

Rideout, V. J., Vandewater, E. A., and Wartella, E. A. (2003). *Zero to Six: Electronic Media in the Lives of Infants, Toddlers, and Preschoolers*. Menlo Park, CA: Henry J. Kaiser Family Foundation.

Roberts, D., Foher, U., Rideout, V., and Brodie, M. (1999). *Kids and the Media @ the New Millennium*. Menlo Park, CA: Henry J. Kaiser Family Foundation.

Saewyc, E., Bearinger, L., Blum, R., and Resnick, M. (1999). Sexual intercourse, abuse, and pregnancy among adolescent women: Does sexual orientation make a difference? *Family Planning Perspectives, 31*, 127–131.

Saewyc, E., Bearinger, L., McMahon, G., and Evans, T. (2006). A national needs assessment of nurses providing health care to adolescents. *Journal of Professional Nursing, 22*, 304–313.

Sanci, L. A., Kang, M. S. L., and Ferguson, B. J. (2005). Improving adolescents' access to primary health care. *The Medical Journal of Australia, 183*, 416–417.

Shapiro, A. (2006). *Quality Health Care for Homeless Youth: Examining Barriers to Care.* Presentation at a National Community Forum on Adolescent Health Care, November, Washington, DC.

Shapiro, J. P., Welker, C. J., and Jacobson, B. J. (1997). The Youth Client Satisfaction Questionnaire: Development, construct validation, and factor structure. *Journal of Clinical Child Psychology,* 26, 87–98.

Society for Adolescent Medicine. (1995). A position statement of the Society for Adolescent Medicine. *Journal of Adolescent Health,* 16, 413. Available: https://www.adolescenthealth.org.PositionStatement_Adolescent_Medicine.pdf [November 27, 2007].

Society for Adolescent Medicine. (2004). *New Survey Reveals Surprising Insights into Parental Attitudes Toward Teenage Sexual Behavior: Parents Share Top Concerns about Their High Schoolers.* Available: http://www.eurekalert.org/pub_releases/2004-08/cw-nsr081004.php [September 22, 2008].

St. Peter, R. F., Newacheck, P. W., and Halfon, N. (1992). Access to care for poor children. *Journal of the American Medical Association,* 267, 2760–2764.

Stevens, D., Seid, M., Mistry, R., and Halfon, N. (2006). Disparities in primary care for vulnerable children: The influence of multiple risk factors. *Health Services Research,* 41, 507–531.

Substance Abuse and Mental Health Services Administration. (2006). *Treatment Episode Data Set (TEDS). Highlights—2004. National Admissions to Substance Abuse Treatment Services,* DASIS Series: S-31, DHHS Publication No. (SMA) 06-4140. Rockville, MD: Office of Applied Studies.

Substance Abuse and Mental Health Services Administration. (2007). *Results from the 2006 National Survey on Drug Use and Health: National Findings.* FMA 07-4923. Rockville, MD: Office of Applied Studies, U.S. Department of Health and Human Services.

Tonkin, R. (1994). *Adolescent Health Survey: Street Youth in Vancouver.* Vancouver, Canada: McCreary Centre Society.

U.S. Census Bureau. (n.d.). *Intercensal Estimates of the United States Resident Population by Age and Sex: 1990.* Available: http://www.census.gov/popest/archives/EST90INTERCENSAL/US-EST90INT-07/US-EST90INT-07-1990.csv [November 6, 2007].

U.S. Census Bureau. (1992). *1990 Census of Population: General Population Characteristics, United States* (CP-1-1). Available: http://www.census.gov/prod/cen1990/cp1/cp-1-1.pdf [August 13, 2007].

U.S. Census Bureau. (2000). *American FactFinder.* Available: http://factfinder.census.gov/servlet/DatasetTableListServlet?_ds_name=DEC_2000_SF1_U&_type=table&_program=DEC&_lang=en&_ts=191842413501 [May 25, 2007].

U.S. Census Bureau. (2003). *American FactFinder, Census 1990 Summary Tape File 1* [tabulated data]. Washington, DC: Author.

U.S. Census Bureau. (2004). *National Estimates. Quarterly Population Estimates, 1980 to 1990.* Available: http://www.census.gov/popest/archives/1980s/80s_nat_detail.html [November 6, 2007].

U.S. Census Bureau. (2005). *Foreign-Born Population of the United States Current Population Survey—March 2004, Table 1.1a.* Available: http://www.census.gov/population/www/socdemo/foreign/ppl-176.html [May 22, 2008].

U.S. Census Bureau. (2006a). *America's Families and Living Arrangements: 2006.* Available: http://www.census.gov/population/www/socdemo/hh-fam/cps2006.html [May 25, 2007].

U.S. Census Bureau. (2006b). *National Population Estimates for the 2000s. Estimates by Age, Sex, Race, and Hispanic Origin: January 1, 2006.* Available: http://www.census.gov/popest/national/asrh/2005_nat_res.html [November 6, 2007].

U.S. Census Bureau. (2007). *U.S. Interim Projections by Age, Sex, Race, and Hispanic Origin.* Available: http://www.census.gov/ipc/www/usinterimproj/ [November 6, 2007].

U.S. Congress and Office of Technology Assessment. (1991). *Adolescent Health.* OTA-H-466, 467, and 468. Washington, DC: U.S. Government Printing Office.

U.S. Department of Health and Human Services. (2007). *21 Critical Health Objectives for Adolescents and Young Adults.* Available: http://www.cdc.gov/HealthyYouth/adolescenthealth/NationalInitiative/pdf/21objectives.pdf [October 17, 2007].

U.S. Department of Justice. (2006). *Criminal Victimization in the United States, 2005: Statistical Tables.* Bureau of Justice Statistics. Available: http://www.ojp.usdoj.gov/bjs/pub/pdf/cvus05.pdf [October 2, 2007].

Weinick, R., and Krauss, N. (2000). Racial/ethnic differences in children's access to care. *American Journal of Public Health, 90,* 1771–1774.

Wise, P. (2004). The transformation of child health in the United States. *Health Affairs, 23*(5), 9–25.

World Health Organization. (1948). *Constitution of the World Health Organization.* Geneva: World Health Organization.

World Health Organization, United Nations Population Fund, and United Nations Children's Fund. (1995). *Action for Adolescent Health: Towards a Common Agenda: Recommendations from a Joint Study Group.* Available: http://www.who.int/child_adolescent_health/documents/frh_adh_97_9/en/index.html [May 28, 2008].

Zelizer, V. (1985). *Pricing the Priceless Child: The Changing Social Value of Children.* New York: Basic Books.

Zeni, M. B., Sappenfield, W., Thompson, D., and Hailin Chen, H. (2007). Factors associated with not having a personal health care provider for children in Florida. *Pediatrics, 119,* (Supplement 1), S61–S67.

Zill, N., Nord, C. W., and Loomis, L. S. (1995). *Adolescent Time Use, Risky Behavior, and Outcomes: An Analysis of National Data.* Rockville, MD: Westat.

Zimet, G. (2005). Improving adolescent health: Focus on HPV vaccine acceptance. *Journal of Adolescent Health, 37,* S17–S23.

2

Adolescent Health Status

SUMMARY

- Most adolescents are considered healthy as defined by traditional medical measures of current health status, such as mortality rates, incidence of disease, prevalence of chronic conditions, and use of health services.
- Adolescence is a period of both risk and opportunity. Adolescents may take risks that can jeopardize their health during these early years, as well as contribute to the leading causes of death and disease in adulthood. During adolescence, a range of health conditions can be identified and addressed in ways that affect not only adolescents' functioning and opportunities, but also the quality of their adult lives. Adolescence also provides many opportunities to develop habits that create a strong foundation for healthy lifestyles and behavior over the full life span.
- Some specific subpopulations of adolescents defined by selected population characteristics and other circumstances—such as those who are poor or members of a racial or ethnic minority; in the foster care system; homeless; in a family that has recently immigrated to the United States; lesbian, gay, bisexual, or transgender; or in the juvenile justice system—have higher rates of chronic health problems and may engage in more risky behavior relative to the overall adolescent population.

Mortality and Morbidity

- Motor vehicle crashes, homicide, and suicide, rather than infectious or chronic diseases, are the leading causes of mortality among adolescents.
- Injuries continue to be the leading cause of mortality among adolescents; the majority of these injuries are due to motor vehicle crashes.
- The prevalence of asthma and diabetes, two common causes of chronic illness in adolescents, has increased in recent years.
- Between 10 and 20 percent of adolescents are affected annually by mental disorders, and half of all cases of adult lifetime mental disorders start by age 14. The most common mental health disorder in adolescence is anxiety.
- Sexually transmitted infections are the most commonly reported infectious diseases in adolescents and continue to increase in this population. Non-Hispanic black adolescents have higher rates of chlamydia and gonorrhea than any other racial or ethnic group.
- The most common oral health problem in adolescence is dental caries. Non-Hispanic black adolescents have a higher prevalence of untreated dental caries than non-Hispanic white adolescents.

Behavior and Health

- Behavior that is unhealthful and/or risky, rather than infectious or chronic diseases, is the leading cause of morbidity among adolescents.
- Use of alcohol, tobacco, and illicit drugs and carrying a weapon are adolescent behaviors that pose serious risk.
- Pregnancy rates among adolescents aged 13–19 have decreased since 1990; declines have been seen among all racial and ethnic groups, although the rate of pregnancy among Hispanic adolescents has been decreasing less dramatically. Pregnancy rates among Hispanic and non-Hispanic black adolescents continue to be twice as high as those among non-Hispanic white adolescents.
- The percentage of overweight adolescents has more than tripled since 1980, with more than 17 percent of adolescents aged 12–19 being considered overweight.
- Certain subpopulations of adolescents, especially those who are in the juvenile justice or foster care system, are at significantly increased risk of health and mental disorders.

- Adolescents who enter the juvenile justice system generally have preexisting health problems, particularly substance abuse, sexually transmitted infections, unplanned pregnancies, dental problems, and psychiatric disorders.
- Adolescents in foster care face more health challenges and chronic health issues—such as asthma, anemia, neurological abnormalities, emotional and behavioral problems, chronic physical disabilities, birth defects, and developmental delays—than those not in foster care. These adolescents are also at increased risk of unprotected sex and pregnancy, and have higher rates of severe mental health problems and substance use.

Most adolescents are considered healthy as defined by the traditional medical measures of health status, such as mortality rates, incidence of disease, prevalence of chronic conditions, and use of health services. According to the National Survey of Child Health, approximately 83 percent of adolescents aged 12–17 are in either excellent or very good health as reported by their parents, regardless of whether they live in urban or rural areas (Maternal and Child Health Bureau, 2005a,b). According to data from the Behavioral Risk Factor Surveillance System, 91 percent of those aged 18–24 consider themselves to be in good, very good, or excellent health (McCracken, Jiles, and Michels Blanck, 2007).

This chapter explores how *timing matters*—how adolescence is a critical time for health promotion. Many adolescents behave in risky ways or live in environments that not only affect their immediate health, but also have a significant impact on their health as adults. For example, McGinnis and Foege (1993) and more recently Mokdad and colleagues (2004) have shown that half of deaths among adults are due to health-related behaviors that for many people have their onset during adolescence. For example, tobacco use is the leading actual cause of preventable death in the United States. Other health-related behaviors that are associated with the leading causes of death include poor diet and physical inactivity, drug and alcohol abuse, risky driving, risky sexual behavior, and use of drugs. The effects of such health-compromising behaviors—and the extent to which the health system attempts to prevent and respond to them—are also influenced by socioeconomic status, living circumstances, school environment and quality, and after-school care. This chapter also considers how *context matters* for adolescents and their health and looks at how the social context and such factors as income, race/ethnicity, geography, and community efficacy may affect the health of adolescents. (The importance of context in adolescents' access to and utilization of health services is explored more fully in Chapter 3.) Moreover, this chapter addressed differences in how *need matters*, as some segments of the adolescent population, defined by biology as well as behavior, have health needs that require particular attention in health systems.

A recent analysis of the 21 Critical Health Objectives for Adolescents and Young Adults, a subset of the objectives of the Centers for Disease Control and Prevention's (CDC's) Healthy People 2010, highlights how little progress has been made in the overall health status of adolescents (Park et al., 2008; U.S. Department of Health and Human Services, 2006a). Of these 21 objectives, the only ones that have shown improvement since 2000 are unintentional injury-related behavior, pregnancy and sexually related behavior, and tobacco use (see Table 2-1). Moreover, several areas have worsened, including deaths caused by motor vehicle crashes related to alcohol use, which have risen, and obesity/overweight, which has increased along with a decrease in reported physical activity (Park et al., 2006).

With these and many other findings in mind, this chapter explores available evidence on the health status of adolescents as defined by traditional measures (mortality rates, incidence of disease, prevalence of chronic conditions, and use of health services). The chapter also offers a more complex and complete picture of health status by reviewing behaviors that may adversely affect health status not only during adolescence, but also in adulthood. Finally, the chapter highlights the current health status of various subpopulations of adolescents who are especially likely to be affected by several co-occurring health challenges, including those who behave in more than one risky way at the same time. Data on adolescents' use of health services are discussed in Chapter 3.

As discussed in Chapter 1, the committee focused this study on health services and policies for adolescents between the ages of 10 and 19, and where appropriate and possible, broke this population down into the two subsets of early adolescence (ages 10–14) and adolescence (ages 15–19). Throughout this chapter, health status is described for the adolescent population, and where data are available, is distinguished for these two subsets, adhering as closely as possible to these specific age ranges. Moreover, at some points in the chapter, the health status of those transitioning from adolescence to adulthood (those aged approximately 20–24) is included in the discussion because (1) the data do not always break off at exactly age 19, and (2) health problems in adolescence can have implications for adult health, and the progression of these problems is important to note.

Finding: Most adolescents are considered healthy as defined by traditional medical measures of current health status, such as mortality

TABLE 2-1 21 Critical Health Objectives for Adolescents and Young Adults and Progress from Healthy People 2010, Ages 10–24

Objective	Baseline[a]
MORTALITY	
Reduce deaths of adolescents and young adults	1998
10- to 14-year-olds (per 100,000)	21.5
15- to 19-year-olds (per 100,000)	69.5
20- to 24-year-olds (per 100,000)	92.7
Reduce suicide rate	1999
10- to 14-year-olds (per 100,000)	1.2
15- to 19-year-olds (per 100,000)	8.0
Reduce deaths caused by motor vehicle crashes	1999
15- to 24-year-olds (per 100,000)	25.6
Reduce deaths caused by alcohol- and drug-related motor vehicle crashes	1998
Alcohol-related deaths	
15- to 24-year-olds (per 100,000)	11.8
Reduce homicides	1999
10- to 14-year-olds (per 100,000)	1.2
15- to 19-year-olds (per 100,000)	10.4
MORBIDITY	
Sexually Transmitted Infections (STIs)	
(Developmental) Reduce the number of new cases of HIV/AIDS diagnosed among adolescents and young adults	1998
13- to 24-year-olds	16,479[d]
Reduce the proportion of adolescents and young adults with *Chlamydia trachomatis* infections	1999
15- to 24-year-olds (percent)	
Females attending family planning clinics	5.0
Females attending STI clinics	12.2
Males attending STI clinics	15.7

Midcourse Review[b]							Target[a]	Progress to
1999	2000	2001	2002	2003	2004	2005	2010	Target[c]
20.4	20.3	19.1	—	—	18.7	—	16.8	Toward
68.6	67.4	67.1	—	—	66.4	—	39.8	Toward
90.8	93.6	94.9	—	—	96.4	—	49.0	Away
—	1.5	1.3	—	—	1.3	—	TNP	TNP
—	8.0	7.9	—	—	8.2	—	TNP	TNP
—	26.3	26.3	—	—	25.8	—	TNP	TNP
11.7	12.2	12.2	12.4	—	—	—	TNP	TNP
—	1.1	—	—	—	1.0	—	TNP	TNP
—	NA	—	—	—	9.3	—	TNP	TNP
—	—	—	—	—	—	—	TNP	TNP
—	5.9	5.9	6.0	—	6.9	—	3.0	Away
—	13.5	13.3	13.5	—	15.3	—	3.0	Away
—	17.0	17.0	17.0	—	20.2	—	3.0	Away

Continued

TABLE 2-1 Continued

Objective	Baseline[a]
MENTAL HEALTH	
Increase the proportion of children and adolescents with mental health problems who receive treatment	2001
4- to 17-year-olds (percent)	59.0
Reduce the proportion of children and adolescents with disabilities who are reported to be sad, unhappy, or depressed	1997
4- to 17-year-olds (percent)	31.0
Reduce the rate of suicide attempts by adolescents that require medical attention	1999
9th- to 12th-grade students (percent)	2.6
BEHAVIOR AND HEALTH	
Injuries	
Reduce the proportion of adolescents who report that they rode during the past 30 days with a driver who had been drinking alcohol	1999
9th- to 12th-grade students (percent)	33.0
Increase use of safety belts	1999
9th- to 12th-grade students (percent)	84.0
Reduce injuries caused by alcohol- and drug-related motor vehicle crashes	1998
Alcohol-related injuries	
15- to 24-year-olds (per 100,000)	374.0
Violence	
Reduce physical fighting among adolescents	1999
9th- to 12th-grade students (percent)	36.0
Reduce weapon carrying by adolescents on school property	1999
9th- to 12th-grade students (percent)	6.9
Binge Drinking	
Reduce the proportion of adolescents engaging in binge drinking of alcoholic beverages	1998
12- to 17-year-olds (percent)	8.3

| Midcourse Review[b] | | | | | | | Target[a] | Progress to |
1999	2000	2001	2002	2003	2004	2005	2010	Target[c]
—	—	—	—	—	—	64.0	66.0	Toward
—	—	—	—	—	—	27.0	17.0	Toward
—	—	2.6	—	—	—	2.3	1.0	Toward
—	—	31.0	—	30.0	—	28.5	30.0	Met target
—	—	86.0	—	—	—	89.8	92.0	Toward
403.0	391.0	359.0	301.0	—	—	—	TNP	TNP
—	—	33.0	—	—	—	35.9	32.0	Toward
—	—	6.4	—	—	—	6.5	4.9	Toward
10.1	10.4	10.6	10.7	10.6	—	9.9	2.0	Away

Continued

TABLE 2-1 Continued

Objective	Baseline[a]
Substance Use	
Reduce past-month use of illicit substances (marijuana)	1998
12- to 17-year-olds (percent)	8.3
Reduce tobacco use by adolescents	1999
9th- to 12th-grade students (percent)	40.0
Pregnancy	
Reduce pregnancies among adolescent females	1996
15- to 17-year-olds (per 1,000 families)	67.0
Increase the proportion of adolescents who participate in responsible sexual behavior	1999
9th- to 12th-grade students (percent)	85.0
Disordered Eating	
Reduce the proportion of adolescents who are overweight or obese	1988–1994
12- to 19-year-olds (percent)	11.0
Physical Activity	
Increase the proportion of adolescents who engage in vigorous physical activity that promotes cardiovascular fitness 3 or more days per week for 20 or more minutes per occasion	1999
9th- to 12th-grade students (percent)	65.0

NOTES: — = data not available; TNP = target not provided.
[a]U.S. Department of Health and Human Services (2000).
[b]U.S. Department of Health and Human Services (2006a, 2007a).

rates, incidence of disease, prevalence of chronic conditions, and use of health services.

Finding: *Adolescence is a period of both risk and opportunity. Adolescents may take risks that can jeopardize their health during these early years, as well as contribute to the leading causes of death and disease in adulthood. During adolescence, a range of health conditions can*

Midcourse Review[b]							Target[a]	Progress to
1999	2000	2001	2002	2003	2004	2005	2010	Target[c]
8.2	8.0	8.2	7.9	—	—	6.8	0.7	Toward
—	—	34.0	—	—	—	28.4	21.0	Toward
56.0	54.0	—	44.4	—	—	—	43.0	Toward
—	—	86.0	—	88.0	—	—	95.0	Toward
—	—	1999–2000 16.0	—	—	2003–2004 17.0	—	5.0	Away
—	—	65.0	—	—	—	64.1	85.0	Away

[c]Progress to target = toward, away from, or met target compared with baseline data. Objectives without a projected target were not assessed.
[d]Includes ages 13 years and older.

be identified and addressed in ways that affect not only adolescents' functioning and opportunities, but also the quality of their adult lives. Adolescence also provides many opportunities to develop habits that create a strong foundation for healthy lifestyles and behavior over the full life span.

MORTALITY AND MORBIDITY

Mortality

More than 17,500 adolescents aged 10–19 die annually according to the National Vital Statistics System Mortality File collected by CDC's National Center for Health Statistics in 2004. In general, mortality rates increase with age even within this narrow age range. For example, those aged 15–19 have a mortality rate more than three times higher than that of those aged 10–14 (see Figure 2-1). This higher rate is attributable largely to mortality among males—more than twice that among females in this age group. American Indian/Alaskan Native non-Hispanic and black non-Hispanic adolescents generally have the highest mortality rates, while Asian/Pacific Islander non-Hispanics have the lowest (see Table 2-2).

Deaths among adolescents are caused by injuries (unintentional, such as those due to motor vehicle crashes, and intentional, such as those due to suicide or homicide) and by natural causes (such as disease or a chronic health condition). Unintentional injury (the leading cause of mortality among adolescents), homicide, and suicide accounted for almost three-quarters of all deaths among adolescents aged 10–19 in 2004 (National Center for Injury Prevention and Control, 2007; see Figure 2-2). Unintentional injury was also one of the three leading causes of death among adults aged 35–54 in 2004; in contrast with adolescents, however, malignant neo-

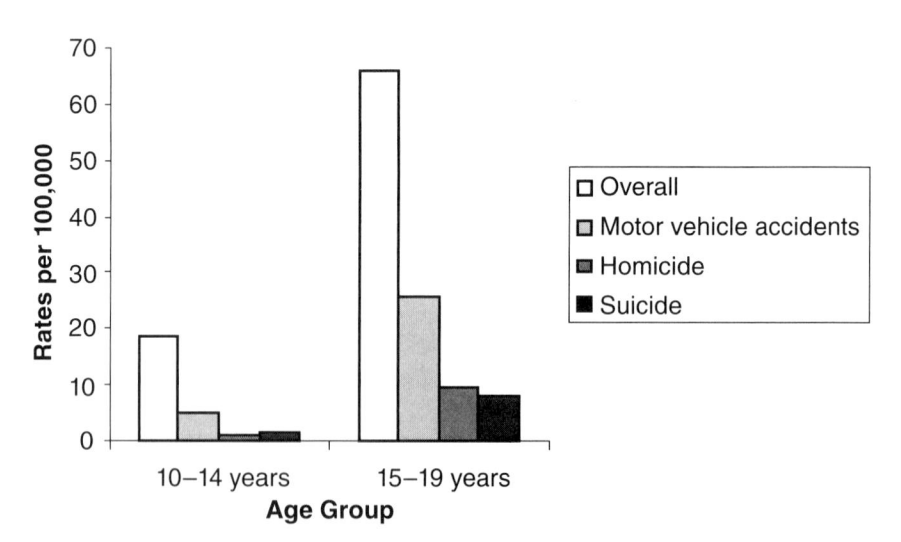

FIGURE 2-1 Adolescent mortality rates (per 100,000) in 2004 by age group.
SOURCE: National Center for Injury Prevention and Control (2007).

TABLE 2-2 Mortality Rates (per 100,000) of Adolescents by Age, Gender, and Race/Ethnicity, 2004

	Overall	Male	Female	White-NH	Black-NH	AI/AN-NH	Asian- or A/PI-NH	Hispanic
Overall								
Ages 10–14	18.7	21.8	15.4	17.4	26.5	29.7	12.6	16.3
Ages 15–19	66.1	91.0	40.0	63.4	83.7	106.2	34.7	64.3
Motor vehicle accidents								
Ages 10–14	4.8	5.6	4.0	5.0	4.7	8.4	2.8	4.2
Ages 15–19	25.3	32.6	17.6	28.6	16.2	37.8	11.3	23.3
Homicide								
Ages 10–14	1.0	1.3	0.7	0.6	2.6	1.8	0.5	1.1
Ages 15–19	9.5	15.6	3.0	2.7	32.8	11.4	4.5	15.0
Suicide								
Ages 10–14	1.3	1.7	1.0	1.4	1.4	3.6	0.9	1.0
Ages 15–19	8.2	12.7	3.5	9.2	4.8	29.4	5.7	6.4

NOTES: A/PI = Asian/Pacific Islander; AI/AN = American Indian/Alaskan Native; NH = non-Hispanic.
SOURCE: National Center for Injury Prevention and Control (2007).

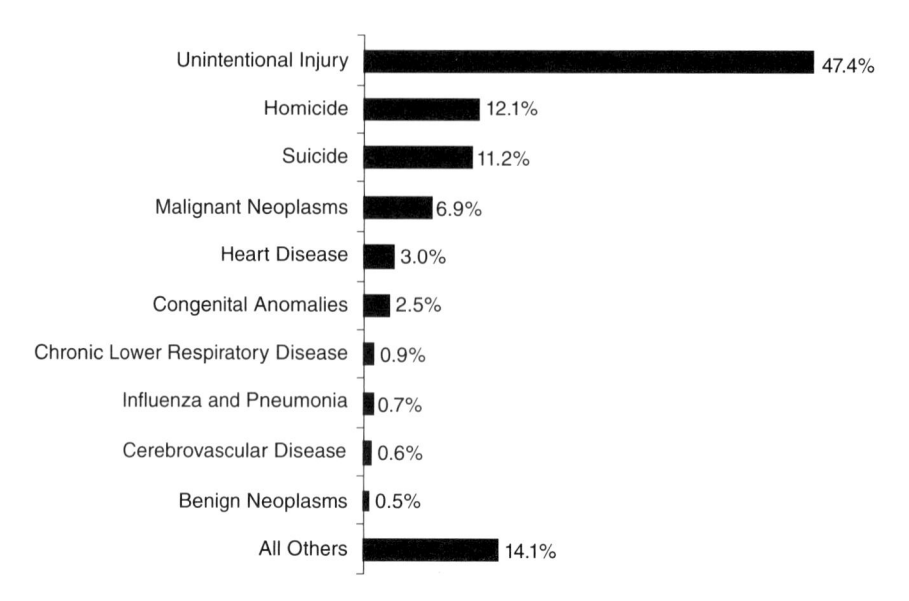

Cause	Percentage
Unintentional Injury	47.4%
Homicide	12.1%
Suicide	11.2%
Malignant Neoplasms	6.9%
Heart Disease	3.0%
Congenital Anomalies	2.5%
Chronic Lower Respiratory Disease	0.9%
Influenza and Pneumonia	0.7%
Cerebrovascular Disease	0.6%
Benign Neoplasms	0.5%
All Others	14.1%

FIGURE 2-2 Ten leading causes of death in adolescents aged 10–19, United States, 2004.
SOURCE: National Center for Injury Prevention and Control (2007).

plasms and heart disease—both physical chronic health conditions—were the cause of almost half of all deaths in adults (National Center for Injury Prevention and Control, 2007). Malignant neoplasms, heart disease, and congenital anomalies are the three leading natural causes of mortality among adolescents aged 15–19 and account for about 10 percent of deaths in this age group; they account for a higher proportion—20 percent—of deaths among younger adolescents, aged 10–14 (National Center for Injury Prevention and Control, 2007).

Homicide accounts for the high mortality rates among black non-Hispanic adolescents, whereas suicide and motor vehicle crashes are responsible for the high mortality rates among American Indian/Alaskan Native non-Hispanic adolescents; suicide rates are generally higher among non-Hispanic white than among non-Hispanic black adolescents. Much of the variation in mortality among racial and ethnic groups of adolescents has been shown to be related to differences in socioeconomic status. When analyses adjust adequately for the latter differences among individuals, families, and neighborhoods, the variations in mortality among racial and ethnic groups are much smaller, if not eliminated (Anderson et al., 1994; Gjelsvik, Zierler, and Blume, 2004).

Findings:

- *Motor vehicle crashes, homicide, and suicide, rather than infectious or chronic diseases, are the leading causes of mortality among adolescents.*
- *Injuries continue to be the leading cause of mortality among adolescents; the majority of these injuries are due to motor vehicle crashes.*

Morbidity

Chronic Health Conditions

Chronic conditions, or what are sometimes referred to as adolescents with special health care needs,[1] generally encompass learning disabilities; attention-deficit hyperactivity disorder (ADHD); other emotional or behavioral problems; developmental delay or physical impairment; asthma or breathing problems; speech problems; diabetes; depression or anxiety; bone, joint, or muscle problems; autism; severe respiratory, food, or skin allergies; frequent or severe headaches; and hearing or vision problems not correctable with glasses. In 2005, according to parental reports, nearly 10 percent of adolescents aged 12–17 in the United States had special health care needs. Among those adolescents, approximately one-fifth had a functional limitation that lasted 1 year or more, and almost half managed their special health condition with prescription medication (Child and Adolescent Health Measurement Initiative, 2008). Data for the 1980s and 1990s indicate that 10–30 percent of children and adolescents under age 20 had a chronic condition, depending on the definition of such conditions used (Gortmaker and Sappenfield, 1984, Newacheck and Taylor, 1992).

Many adolescents have more than one special health care need. According to parental reports, in 2005 more than 17 percent of adolescents with special health care needs had more than three conditions (Bethell et al., 2008). Approximately one-fifth of adolescents with a *severe* chronic condition (defined as causing limitations in major daily age-appropriate activities) had more than one condition. Although the prevalence of adolescents with special health care needs does not vary substantially among

---

[1] Adolescents with special health care needs are defined by McPherson and colleagues (1998, p. 138) as "those who have or are at increased risk for a chronic physical, developmental, behavioral, or emotional condition and who also require health and related services of a type or amount beyond that required by children generally."

income groups, adolescents in poor and near-poor families (those at less than 200 percent above the poverty threshold as defined by the U.S. Census Bureau) had substantially higher rates of severe chronic health conditions than adolescents in nonpoor families (those at more than 200 percent above the poverty threshold).

These mental and physical chronic health conditions have significant implications for adult health and health outcomes. Not only has the prevalence of chronic health conditions in children dramatically increased since the 1960s, but it is also important to understand that more children with severe chronic conditions (e.g., leukemia, cystic fibrosis, congenital heart disease) are living longer because of medical technological advances, and that some chronic conditions (e.g., obesity, asthma, ADHD) persist into adolescence and adulthood (Perrin, Bloom, and Gortmaker, 2007; Wise, 2004). This increase in the incidence and prevalence of chronic health conditions and their persistence from childhood into adolescence and into adulthood may have a major impact on health care expenditures and participation in society, including the workforce. The following sections highlight the prevalence of and trends in chronic health conditions—both physical and mental health—in adolescence and note the progression of increasing health problems into adulthood.

Asthma

Asthma is a major chronic illness among adolescents in the United States. In 2005, at least 4 million adolescents (15–17 percent) aged 10–17 were reported to have lifetime asthma, and more than 2.5 million (10–15 percent) were reported to have asthma currently; by comparison, only 7 percent of adults aged 18–44 were reported to have lifetime asthma and 10 percent to have asthma currently (Akinbami, 2006; Eaton et al., 2006; U.S. Department of Health and Human Services and Centers for Disease Control and Prevention, 2007). More recent data indicate that 20 percent of adolescents in high school have lifetime asthma (Eaton et al., 2008). In addition, the reported prevalence of chronic asthma or breathing problems causing limitations in normal daily activities is almost 6 per 100,000 adolescents aged 10–17 (MacKay and Duran, 2007).

The prevalence of lifetime asthma is generally higher among black than white adolescents, and among Puerto Rican and American Indian/Alaskan Native than white adolescents (see Table 2-3). It is generally higher among older male than older female adolescents and among younger female than older female adolescents (Eaton et al., 2006; U.S. Department of Health and Human Services and Centers for Disease Control and Prevention, 2007). Socioeconomic status has also been found to be correlated with the prevalence of asthma in adolescents. Adolescents in poor families have substantially higher rates of chronic asthma that limits normal daily activities relative to adolescents in nonpoor families (MacKay and Duran, 2007). The prevalence (total number of cases) and incidence (rate of new cases) of childhood asthma (ages 10–17) increased dramatically from 1980 to the late 1990s (Akinbami, 2006; Rudd and Moorman, 2007). The current prevalence of childhood asthma has remained at these high levels (Akinbami, 2006).

Diabetes

In 2001, more than 120,000 adolescents aged 10–19 were reported to have diabetes (Duncan, 2006; SEARCH for Diabetes in Youth Study Group, 2006). Data suggest that the prevalence of diabetes increases with advancing age: there were 2.29 cases per 1,000 adolescents aged 10–14 compared with 3.35 cases per 1,000 aged 15–19 (SEARCH for Diabetes in Youth Study Group, 2006). The reported prevalence of diabetes is higher among female than male adolescents, and is lowest overall among Asian adolescents (see Table 2-3). Of those reported to have diabetes, 71 percent are categorized as having type 1 and 29 percent as having type 2 (Duncan, 2006). Non-Hispanic white adolescents (aged 10–19) have the highest prevalence of type 1 diabetes. American Indian and black adolescents aged 10–19 have a higher prevalence of type 2 diabetes than their Hispanic and non-Hispanic white counterparts (SEARCH for Diabetes in Youth Study Group, 2006).

Research has shown that impaired fasting glucose levels have a high rate of conversion to type 2 diabetes in adults. Impaired fasting glucose levels have been reported in 11 percent of adolescents aged 12–19—with important implications for health in adulthood (Duncan, 2006).

The prevalence of diabetes in adolescents has increased in the past decade (Duncan, 2006). However, the contribution of this increase to the prevalence of type 2 diabetes, impaired fasting glucose levels, or the increasing prevalence of overweight and obesity is unclear (Duncan, 2006; Fagot-Campagna et al., 2001). Diabetes has been linked to a number of poor health outcomes in adulthood, including eye and foot problems; dental, kidney, nerve, respiratory, and cardiovascular complications; reproductive health issues; and stroke (Centers for Disease Control and Prevention, 2007a).

Cancer

As noted earlier, cancer is the leading natural cause of death in adolescence. In 2004, nearly 62,000 adolescents aged 10–19 were living with cancer (having received a diagnosis of the disease within the past 14 years),

TABLE 2-3 Prevalence of Morbidity in Adolescents by Age, Gender, and Race/Ethnicity

	Overall	Male	Female
Asthma (%)[a]			
Ages 10–17	14.9	17.1	12.5
Diabetes (per 1,000)[b]			
Ages 10–19	3.0	2.8	3.1
Mental Health Conditions (%)[c]			
(predictive symptoms)			
Anxiety Disorder			
Ages 12–17	15.0	11.4	18.9
Major Depression			
Ages 12–17	12.1	7.9	16.5
ADHD			
Ages 12–17	14.7	13.8	15.6
Conduct Disorder			
Ages 12–17	11.5	12.8	10.1
Eating Disorder			
Ages 12–17	6.1	3.7	8.7
Substance Disorders (%)[d]			
Alcohol Disorders			
Ages 12–17	5.4	5.1	5.7
Illicit Drug Disorders			
Ages 12–17	4.6	4.7	4.6
Sexually Transmitted Infections			
Chlamydia (per 100,000)[e]			
Ages 10–14	66.8	11.1	125.3
Ages 15–19	1,621.0	505.2	2,796.6
Gonorrhea (per 100,000)[e]			
Ages 10–14	20.2	6.0	35.2
Ages 15–19	438.2	261.2	624.7
HIV/AIDS[f] (cases diagnosed)			
Ages 13–19	1,255.0	64% of cases	34% of cases

White-NH	Black-NH	AI/AN-NH	Asian- or A/PI-NH	Hispanic
14.3	18.2	20.8[b]	7.7[b]	14.3[i]
3.2	3.2[b]	2.3[b]	1.4[b]	2.2
15.6	15.6	NA	NA	13.2
12.2	10.6	NA	NA	12.0
13.8	18.3	NA	NA	15.1
10.9	12.4	NA	NA	12.2
5.9	6.5	NA	NA	6.4
6.3	2.3	7.2	2.8[i]	5.1
4.7	4.3	6.9	3.3[i]	4.8
25.1	246.0	150.6	15.0	58.4
769.6	5,502.6	2675.3	499.9	1,674.9
5.4	93.5	20.0	3.0	9.4
120.0	2,106.3	369.0	74.3	219.6
15% of cases	69% of cases	<1% of cases	<1% of cases	15% of cases

Continued

TABLE 2-3 Continued

	Overall	Male	Female
Oral Health			
Untreated Cavities (%)[g]			
Ages 10–15	18.8	19.3	18.4
Ages 16–19	21.2	22.4	19.9

NOTES: ADHD = attention-deficit hyperactivity disorder; A/PI = Asian/Pacific Islander; AI/AN = American Indian/Alaskan Native; NA = not available; NH = non-Hispanic.

[a]Adolescents who had ever been told by a doctor or nurse that they had asthma. All asthma data are presented as a percentage of the population (National Center for Health Statistics, 2007).

[b]Data from Duncan (2006); SEARCH for Diabetes Youth Study Group (2006).

[c]Data indicate prevalence of specific mental health conditions among U.S. adolescents aged 12–17 within the past year. Data from 2000 National Household Survey of Drug Abuse were used to estimate prevalence rates using DISC (Diagnostic Interview Schedule for Children) predictive scales. Multiple logistic regressions were used to derive significant correlates of each domain of DPS (DISC Predictive Scale)-derived symptom cluster indicators of psychiatric problems (Chen, Killeya-Jones, and Vega, 2005).

[d]Data indicate prevalence of alcohol and illicit drug abuse or dependence disorders among U.S. adolescents aged 12–17 in the previous year based on the definition found in the *Diag-*

a prevalence twice that among infants and children from birth to age 9 (National Cancer Institute, 2008). Data on the incidence of and trends over time in new diagnoses of cancer in adolescents are not readily available. Among older adolescents aged 15–19, lymphomas, germ cell tumors, and leukemias account for the largest incidence of cancer (Bleyer et al., 2006). For these older adolescents, only a modest improvement was seen in 5-year survival rates from 1975 to 1997 compared with children and younger adolescents (birth through age 14) and adults (over age 45). This modest improvement in survival rates (and even no improvement for some ages) was seen from older adolescence into young adulthood (up to age 39). Data on differences by racial or ethnic and socioeconomic status in the incidence of cancer in adolescents are not readily available. One report on older adolescents and younger adults (ages 15–39) indicates that non-Hispanic whites have the highest incidence of cancer, but also have the highest overall 5-year survival rates; American Indians/Alaskan Natives have the lowest incidence but poorer survival rates; and non-Hispanic blacks have incidence rates between non-Hispanic white and American Indians/Alaskan Natives, but have the lowest 5-year survival rates across the age range (Bleyer et al., 2006).

White-NH	Black-NH	AI/AN-NH	Asian- or A/PI-NH	Hispanic
15.9	21.3	NA	NA	24.2[k]
17.0	30.4	NA	NA	27.9[k]

nostic and Statistical Manual of Mental Disorders, 4th edition (DSM-IV) (Substance Abuse and Mental Health Services Administration, 2007).

[e]Chlamydia and gonorrhea infections are expressed as rates per 100,000 of specific populations (Centers for Disease Control and Prevention, 2006b).

[f]HIV/AIDS cases are expressed as estimated number of cases diagnosed in 2005 for ages 10–19 from 33 states that have confidential name-based surveillance of HIV/AIDS (Centers for Disease Control and Prevention, 2007b).

[g]Indicates percentage of adolescents with one or more untreated cavities for the specific age population (MacKay and Duran, 2007).

[h]Indicates that particular race only; includes Hispanic adolescents.

[i]Puerto Rican adolescents aged 10–17 have lifetime asthma prevalence rates of 29.4 percent.

[j]Indicates Asians only; does not include Native Hawaiians or other Pacific Islanders.

[k]Indicates Mexican Americans; does not include all Hispanic adolescents.

Finding: *The prevalence of asthma and diabetes, two common chronic illnesses in adolescents, has increased in recent years.*

Chronic Mental Health Conditions

In a review of mental health policy in the United States, Frank and Glied (2006) note that there is continual debate on how to define mental disorder. They describe three ways that epidemiologists generally define people who have a mental disorder: (1) those who have symptoms and signs of a particular disorder, (2) those who have mental health–related impairment in daily life, and (3) those who have sought treatment for a mental health condition. A combination of these three criteria is generally preferred over any one alone because each selects a distinct subgroup of the population, usually with small overlap. Additionally, experts continue to argue about not only the specific mental disorders to include in diagnostic manuals, but also the combination of signs and symptoms to be used to diagnose individuals. (For a more detailed discussion, see Frank and Glied, 2006.) Although in general there is a paucity of data on the prevalence of mental disorders in the adolescent population, the data that are available are based on inconsistent measures. Many of the national surveys on the prevalence of mental disorders among the adolescent population include various predictive symptoms of a disorder, while a few measure the current clinical diagnosis of a disorder; hardly any measure impairment and the seeking of treatment. In this report, therefore, the committee describes the prevalence of mental disorders among adolescents on the basis of both predictive symptoms and clinical diagnosis where the data are available.

Most studies estimate that between 10 and 20 percent of adolescents are affected annually by mental disorders, while estimates for adults aged 25 and older are around 10 percent (depending on the ascertainment methods employed, sampling characteristics, and environmental conditions at the time of the study) (Costello et al., 1996; Kataoka, Zhang, and Wells, 2002; Roberts, Attkisson, and Rosenblatt, 1998; Shaffer et al., 1996; Substance Abuse and Mental Health Services Administration, 2007). The lifetime prevalence of mental health problems may be as high as 37 percent by age 16 (Costello et al., 2003). More important, between 5 and 10 percent of adolescents in any given year are afflicted with severe mental disorders that cause significant impairment in one or more aspects of normal functioning (Costello, 1999). Additionally, about half of those aged 18–29 have reported being diagnosed with a mental disorder at some point their life, and half of all adult lifetime cases start by age 14 (Kessler et al., 2005).

Anxiety disorders are the most common mental health problem among adolescents, 13 percent of whom meet criteria for these disorders (Costello et al., 1996). Depression affects more than 7 percent of the adolescent population, while ADHD and conduct disorder each represent a large portion of the remainder of mental disorders found in adolescents (Roberts, Roberts, and Chen, 1997; U.S. Department of Health and Human Services, 1999). Comorbid mental disorders are common among adolescents. In 2003, 21 percent of those aged 12–17 who were admitted for treatment of mental health and substance abuse disorders had a comorbid mental health problem in addition to an alcohol and/or drug problem, a finding similar to that of other research (Costello et al., 1996; Loeber et al., 2000; Substance Abuse and Mental Health Services Administration, 2005a). Rates of particular disorders vary among subpopulations.

The diversity of the symptoms, onset, and course of mental disorders across and within conditions suggests the multifactorial nature of these disorders and the corresponding variation in risk factors. Nevertheless, some risk factors appear to increase the rate of mental disorders across populations. These include poverty and low socioeconomic status, physical and emotional trauma, neurological disorders, genetic load, and substance abuse (Costello, 1999; Loeber et al., 2000; U.S. Department of Health and Human Services, 1999).

Gender is an important risk factor for mental disorders, although its influence varies by age. In childhood, boys are much more likely to be diagnosed with conduct disorder, disruptive disorders such as ADHD, and other mental health problems (Nock et al., 2006; Roberts, Roberts, and Xing, 2007; U.S. Department of Health and Human Services, 1999). Beginning in early adolescence, however, females are much more likely than males to be diagnosed with depression and anxiety (Roberts, Roberts, and Xing, 2007; Substance Abuse and Mental Health Services Administration, 2007).

An extensive body of research has examined variations in the prevalence of mental disorders among different racial and ethnic groups of adolescents. In general, rates of mental disorders are remarkably similar across different groups after controlling for income, resident status, education, and neighborhood supports (Kubik et al., 2003; Roberts, Roberts, and Chen, 1997; Roberts, Roberts, and Xing, 2007). However, service providers note large variations among adolescents referred for mental health services because of significant referral biases: minority adolescents (Hispanic and black) with mental disorders are often managed in the foster care and juvenile justice systems, while nonminority adolescents with similar presentations are much more likely to be referred to mental health services (U.S. Department of Health and Human Services, 1999).

Anxiety Disorders

As noted above, anxiety disorders are the most common mental disorders in adolescents. They include phobias, general anxiety, panic disorder, obsessive-compulsive disorder, and post-traumatic stress disorder. In 1999, 13 percent of those aged 9–17 had experienced an anxiety disorder in the past year, and in 2003, 30 percent of those aged 19–29 had been diagnosed with an anxiety disorder in their lifetime (Costello et al., 1996; Kessler et al., 2005; U.S. Department of Health and Human Services, 1999). More recently, Chen and colleagues (2005) reported that 40 percent of adolescents aged 12–17 had symptoms of an anxiety disorder according to a predictive scale of diagnosis, although not being clinically diagnosed as having such a disorder (see Table 2-3).

Depression

Major depression can appear during childhood and adolescence, and can lead to school failure and to use of alcohol, tobacco, or other drugs. Most adolescents who commit suicide have a prior history of depression. A majority of adolescents experiencing major depression also report symptoms associated with other mental disorders (Kessler and Walters, 1998). In 2006, almost 3.2 million adolescents (12.8 percent) aged 12–17 had experienced at least one major depressive episode in their lifetime, including 1.9 million who had done so in the past year (Substance Abuse and Mental

Health Services Administration, 2007). Additionally, a large number of adolescents report depressive symptoms but do not meet the diagnostic criteria for major depressive disorder. Prevalence rates vary depending on the adolescent population surveyed and the methodology employed, but depressive symptoms have been reported in from 13 to 40 percent of adolescents (Chen, Killeya-Jones, and Vega, 2005; Kubik et al., 2003; see Table 2-3).

Rates of major depressive disorder and symptoms of depression are higher for female than male adolescents. Adolescents having experienced major depressive disorder in the past year are more likely to report use of cigarettes and use of, dependence on, or abuse of illicit drugs or alcohol compared with adolescents without major depressive disorder in the past year. It is unclear whether the rates of major depression among adolescents have changed over time, or the variations are due to differences in survey methodology and sample characteristics. In the 1990s, however, 8–13 percent of adolescents (aged 11–19) reported having experienced major depression (Kessler and Walters, 1998; Roberts, Roberts, and Chen, 1997), and in 2000, 12 percent of those aged 12–17 reported having experienced predictive symptoms of major depression (not a clinical diagnosis) (Chen, Killeya-Jones, and Vega, 2005).

Attention-Deficit Hyperactivity Disorder

ADHD is a mental health problem seen mainly in children and adolescents who consistently display such behavior as inattention, hyperactivity, and impulsivity. In 2005, approximately 2.2 million adolescents (8.9 percent) aged 12–17 had ever been told that they had ADHD (Bloom, Dey, and Freeman, 2006). Additionally, almost 15 percent of adolescents aged 12–17 were reported to have had symptoms of ADHD, but did not meet clinical diagnostic criteria (Chen, Killeya-Jones, and Vega, 2005; see Table 2-3). ADHD is one of the most frequently cited chronic conditions causing activity limitations among adolescents aged 10–17, a fact that indicates its severity (MacKay and Duran, 2007). Activity limitations vary by gender, affecting males more than females. For example, male adolescents are three times more likely than females to have limitations due to ADHD.

Conduct Disorder

Conduct disorder is characterized by a persistent pattern of aggressive, deceptive, and destructive behavior that usually begins in early adolescence, around age 11 (Nock et al., 2006). Adolescents suffering from conduct disorder also are at increased risk of developing other mental disorders, such as oppositional defiant disorder, depression, and anxiety (Lahey et al.,

1999). In a recent study, 11 percent of those aged 18–29 reported meeting the criteria for conduct disorder in their lifetime (Kessler et al., 2005). The prevalence of symptoms of conduct disorder peaks in late adolescence (ages 15–17) (Chen, Killeya-Jones, and Vega, 2005). Adolescent males are more likely than females to be diagnosed with conduct disorder; there are no significant racial or ethnic differences (Chen, Killeya-Jones, and Vega, 2005; Nock et al., 2006; see Table 2-3). In the 1980s and 1990s, community studies found that the prevalence of conduct disorder in adolescents ranged from 4 to 16 percent (Cohen et al., 1993; Kashani et al., 1987). It is unclear whether the prevalence of conduct disorder in adolescents has changed over the past few decades, or the variation is due to differences in survey methodology and sample characteristics.

Eating Disorders

Eating disorders frequently co-occur with other mental disorders, such as depression, substance abuse, and anxiety disorders. The three most common eating disorders are anorexia nervosa, bulimia nervosa, and binge-eating disorder (U.S. Department of Health and Human Services, 1999). It is estimated that during 2000–2002, almost 1.5 million (6 percent) of adolescents aged 12 to 17 had predictive symptoms of an eating disorder (not a clinical diagnosis) (Chen, Killeya-Jones, and Vega, 2005; see Table 2-3). Adolescent females are more likely than males to have symptoms of an eating disorder; no significant racial or ethnic differences have been found. As reviewed later in this chapter, subclinical risky eating behaviors (e.g., vomiting or taking laxatives) and overweight are even more prevalent (see the later discussion of unhealthful and risky eating behavior). Hoek and van Hoeken (2003) reviewed the literature on the prevalence of diagnosed eating disorders in the United States and Western Europe and found consistent rates. An average prevalence rate for anorexia nervosa of 0.3 percent was found for females (aged 11–36). The prevalence rates for bulimia nervosa were 1.0 percent for women (aged 12–44) and 0.1 percent for men of all ages. The authors also concluded that the incidence of anorexia nervosa had increased over the past century until the 1970s. Trends in the prevalence of bulimia nervosa are unclear. Additionally, it is important to note that there is a lack of national data available on the prevalence of binge eating disorders in adolescents.

Substance Use Disorders

Many adolescents use alcohol, illegal drugs, and tobacco. These behaviors, which are discussed in a later section, carry appreciable health risks both during adolescence and extending into adulthood. Additional problems are faced by the subset of substance-using adolescents who develop clinical substance use disorders. These disorders are characterized by a maladaptive pattern of heavy or compulsive use despite ensuing negative consequences (American Psychiatric Association, 2000), and they produce impairment in functioning.

In 2006 more than 2 million adolescents aged 12–17 (8 percent) and 7 million adolescents aged 18–25 (21 percent) were estimated to have abused or been dependent on alcohol or an illicit drug in the past year (Substance Abuse and Mental Health Services Administration, 2007). These data show some variation by gender and race and ethnicity. Males aged 18–25 have a higher prevalence of alcohol and illicit drug abuse or dependence compared with their female counterparts. American Indian and Alaskan Native adolescents aged 12–17 and those aged 18–25 have the highest prevalence of both alcohol and illicit drug abuse or dependence relative to any other racial or ethnic group. Asian adolescents tend to have the lowest rates of both alcohol and illicit drug abuse or dependence (see Table 2-3). Prevalence trends for adolescent substance abuse or dependence are unclear because of differences in study methodologies and sampling characteristics. In 2000, however, 7.7 percent of those aged 12–17 (and 15.4 percent of those aged 18–25) were estimated to have been abusing or dependent on alcohol or illicit drugs in the past year (U.S. Department of Health and Human Services, 2006b).

With respect to tobacco use, in 1991–1993, 28 percent of adolescents aged 12–17 who had smoked during the previous month (9 percent of this population) were reported to be nicotine dependent (Kandel and Chen, 2000). Research has suggested that adolescents experience significantly higher rates of dependence on nicotine than adults at the same level of use (Kandel and Chen, 2000; Rubinstein et al., 2007). The first symptoms of dependence have been seen in adolescents within days or weeks of the onset of only occasional use of tobacco (DiFranza et al., 2000), although individuals vary in this regard, and girls aged 12–13 tend to develop symptoms of dependence more quickly than boys of the same age (DiFranza et al., 2002). Although adolescents may develop symptoms of dependence quickly, a longer time elapses between their first cigarette and the development of a full dependence diagnosis than between their first cigarette and their first dependence symptom. Recent data suggest that 25 percent of adolescents develop nicotine dependence within 23 months of the onset of tobacco use (Kandel et al., 2007). In general, although adolescents who smoke more are more likely to develop tobacco dependence, the relationship between the level of tobacco use and dependence is far from clear: nicotine dependence has been reported among college students who smoke at low levels, while substantial numbers of college students who smoke every day still do not develop a dependence diagnosis (Dierker et al., 2007).

Suicidal Ideation and Suicide Attempts

In 2004, suicide was the third-leading cause of death among adolescents aged 10–19 (National Center for Injury Prevention and Control, 2007). According to the National Vital Statistics System Mortality File, the rate of deaths attributable to suicide in adolescents increases with age. After young adulthood, the rate of suicide drops with increasing age among adults aged 35 and older (U.S. Department of Health and Human Services and Centers for Disease Control and Prevention, 2007). In addition, many adolescents seriously consider suicide without attempting, or attempt but do not complete the act. According to the Youth Risk Behavior Survey, in 2007 about one-sixth of all high school students reported having seriously considered suicide 12 months prior to the survey (Eaton et al., 2008). Half of those students who had seriously considered suicide had actually attempted it (7 percent of all students). The rate of completed suicides was significantly higher among male than female adolescents in high school, although attempts were significantly higher among females. Hispanic female students were significantly more likely to report a suicide attempt than non-Hispanic white or black female students; there were no differences by race and ethnicity among male students. The prevalence of students who reported seriously considering suicide decreased in the 1990s and has remained steady in the first part of the current decade (National Center for Chronic Disease Prevention and Health Promotion and Division of Adolescent and School Health, 2008).

Finding: *Between 10 and 20 percent of adolescents are affected annually by mental disorders, and half of all cases of adult lifetime mental disorders start by age 14. The most common mental health disorder in adolescence is anxiety.*

Sexually Transmitted Infections

In 2003, 47 percent of high school students had ever had sexual intercourse, and 37 percent of sexually active students had not used a condom during their last sexual intercourse (Grunbaum et al., 2004). These and other risky sexual behaviors in adolescence contribute to high rates of sexually transmitted infections (STIs).

Chlamydia, gonorrhea, and syphilis are the most common bacterial causes of STIs. In 2005, non-Hispanic black adolescents had higher rates of chlamydia and gonorrhea than adolescents in other racial and ethnic groups, due in particular to the high rates reported among non-Hispanic black female adolescents (see Table 2-4). In 2005 non-Hispanic black adolescents aged 15–19 had a rate of more than 5,500 cases of chlamydia per 100,000, compared with non-Hispanic white adolescents aged 15–19, who had a rate of 769 cases per 100,000 (Centers for Disease Control and Prevention, 2006b). And non-Hispanic black female adolescents continue to have the highest gonorrhea rates of any group. Females aged 10–19 have higher reported rates of chlamydia and gonorrhea than males in the same age group. Chlamydia rates continue to increase, and although the rate of gonorrhea among adolescents aged 15–19 has decreased in recent years, in 2005 it increased 3.9 percent. It is important to note that higher reported rates of STIs in adolescent females have been attributed to higher rates of utilization of services (i.e., more opportunities to screen), as well as the greater availability of practical screening tests compared with those for males (Centers for Disease Control and Prevention, 2006b).

In 2005, an estimated 1,255 cases of HIV/AIDS were diagnosed among adolescents aged 13–19 (see Table 2-3). Black adolescents are disproportionately affected by HIV/AIDS infection, accounting for almost 70 percent of all new HIV/AIDS diagnoses reported among those aged 13–19 (Centers for Disease Control and Prevention, 2007b). Rates of new diagnoses of HIV/AIDS are higher among male than female adolescents. Between 1998 and 2005, AIDS cases among adolescents aged 13–19 increased by about 75 percent. There are more AIDS cases among male than female adolescents, although this differential has been decreasing over time (Centers for Disease Control and Prevention, 2007b). Information from high school students across the nation indicates that black high school students have a higher prevalence of HIV testing than white or Hispanic high school students; black female students (27 percent) are tested more than black male students (17 percent) (Eaton et al., 2008).

Until recently, there was no known nationally representative survey on the prevalence of genital herpes simplex virus in adolescents. Recent analysis of data from the 2003–2004 National Health and Nutrition Examination Survey (NHANES) indicates that 2 percent of U.S. female adolescents aged 14–19 tested positive for the herpes simplex virus-2 (Forhan, 2008).

The first national surveillance system to measure the prevalence of high-risk types of human papillomavirus (HR-HPV) in U.S. women was established only recently. During 2003–2005, a quarter of female adolescents aged 14–19 were reported to have HR-HPV (Datta, 2006). In addition, recent analysis of the NHANES 2003–2004 data indicates a prevalence of 18 percent of female adolescents (Forhan, 2008). This situation may change dramatically with the introduction of the new HPV vaccine and the recommendation to vaccinate early-adolescent females (Garland et al., 2007; Markowitz et al., 2007; Paavonen et al., 2007).

Finding: Sexually transmitted infections are the most commonly reported infectious diseases in adolescents and continue to increase in this population. Non-Hispanic black adolescents have higher rates of chlamydia and gonorrhea than any other racial or ethnic group.

Oral Health

There is a high prevalence of oral disease among adolescents. Risk factors for oral disease in adolescence mirror those for other diseases and conditions. Risk factors for dental caries include poor eating patterns and poor food choices, coupled with a lack of fluoride use, while those for periodontal disease reflect inadequate personal oral hygiene. The risk for oral and perioral injury is increased by behavior that includes using alcohol and illicit drugs, driving without a seat belt, cycling without a helmet, engaging in contact sports without a mouth guard, and using firearms. Tobacco—both smoked and smokeless—poses a particular risk to oral tissues through direct injury, as well as through systemic effects. Eating disorders are associated with erosion of the teeth and damage to oral soft tissue, while oral sex is linked with oral manifestations of STIs in the form of oral soft-tissue lesions. Finally, pregnancy carries a higher risk of periodontal disease since gingivitis is a common inflammation associated with hormonal changes during pregnancy when other local conditions (poor oral hygiene) are present.

Dental caries The most common dental problem for adolescents is dental caries.[2] During adolescence, the burden of caries grows with increasing age, and this progression continues into early adulthood. Fully 89 percent of those aged 20–39 have experienced caries. Rates of tooth decay among adolescents also increase with age, a progression that likewise continues into adulthood (see Table 2-3) (Beltran-Anguilar et al., 2005; MacKay and Duran, 2007).

In permanent teeth, the prevalence of caries is unevenly distributed among different groups of adolescents. Higher prevalence is reported among Mexican Americans[3] (48 percent of those aged 6–19), compared with blacks and whites of the same age group (about 39 percent). Likewise, prevalence is higher among low-income children (about 48 percent of poor and near-poor children, compared with 36 percent of the nonpoor). A treatment effect bias resulting from higher levels of dental care among white than among black or Mexican American children partially masks estimates

---

[2]Dental caries is a disease that damages the structure of the teeth. Dental cavities and tooth decay are a consequence of dental caries. These three terms are generally used interchangeably.

[3]The NHANES reported information on Mexican American and non-Hispanic black and white populations. Information on other racial and ethnic groups (e.g., Hispanics, Asians) was not reported.

TABLE 2-4 Prevalence of Behavior and Health in Adolescents by Age, Gender, and Race/Ethnicity

	Overall	Male	Female
Risky Driving (%)[a]			
Rode with a driver who had been drinking alcohol			
9th–12th grade	28.5	27.2	29.6
Rarely or never wore a seat belt			
9th–12th grade	10.2	12.5	7.8
Violence			
Weapon carrying (%)[a]			
9th–12th grade	18.5	29.8	7.1
Violent crime victimization[b] (rate per 1,000)			
Ages 12–15	45.3	53.1	34.4
Ages 16–19	45.8	54.0	34.0
Violent crime perpetration[b] (rate per 1,000)			
Ages 12–15	14.7	18.1	11.1
Ages 16–19	17.8	23.4	12.0
Substance Use (%)[c]			
Tobacco use			
Ages 12–17	13.1	14.2	11.9
Binge drinking			
Ages 12–20	18.9	21.1	16.1
Marijuana use			
Ages 12–17	6.8	7.5	6.2
Pregnancy (per 1,000)[d]			
Age 14 or younger[e]	8.6	NA	NA
Ages 15–19[f]	76.4	NA	76.4
Ages 15–17	44.4	NA	44.4
Ages 18–19	125.0	NA	125.0

White-NH	Black-NH	AI/AN-NH	Asian- or A/PI-NH	Hispanic
28.3	24.1	NA	NA	36.1
9.4	13.4	NA	NA	10.6
18.7	16.4	NA	NA	19.0
39.9	59.5	NA	NA	NA
12.3	62.6	NA	NA	NA
11.1	25.4	NA	NA	NA
13.9	41.1	NA	NA	NA
15.7	8.2	26.1	3.1	10.4
22.3	9.1	18.1	7.9	17.9
7.2	7.2	14.9	1.5	6.3
NA	NA	NA	NA	NA
49.0	138.9	NA	NA	135.2
25.1	88.4	NA	NA	85.1
85.3	217.0	NA	NA	210.9

Continued

TABLE 2-4 Continued

Overweight and Physical Activity (%)			
At risk of overweight and overweight[g]			
Ages 12–19	30.9	31.2	30.5
Physical activity[h]			
9th–12th grade	35.8	43.8	27.8

NOTE: A/PI = Asian/Pacific Islander; AI/AN = American Indian/Alaskan Native; NA = not available; NH = non-Hispanic.

[a]Drinking and driving, seat belt use, and weapon carrying are expressed as percentage of students in 9th through 12th grades (MacKay and Duran, 2007).

[b]Prevalence of violent crime victimization and perpetration is expressed as per 1,000 in the age group, 2005. Black and white include both non-Hispanic and Hispanic. Ethnicity data are not broken down by age group and therefore not reported in the table (U.S. Department of Justice, 2006).

[c]Tobacco use is expressed as percent of the population that used any tobacco products at least 1 day in the past 30 days preceding the survey; binge drinking is defined as percent of the population that consumed five or more drinks on the same occasion (i.e., at the same time or within a couple of hours of each other) on at least 1 day in the past 30 days; marijuana use is expressed as percent of the population that used marijuana on at least 1 day in the past 30 days (Substance Abuse and Mental Health Services Administration, 2006).

of disparities in the extent of caries. Nonetheless, Mexican American children demonstrate 17 percent more tooth decay than whites and 29 percent more than blacks (Beltran-Anguilar et al., 2005). The preponderance of *untreated* tooth decay is concentrated in minority populations, with blacks and Mexican Americans aged 6–19 having more untreated caries than whites of the same age (18.1 percent for blacks and 21.8 percent for Mexican Americans versus 10.69 percent for whites). Thus black adolescents have about the same experience with caries but a much lower rate of dental treatment compared with whites, while Mexican American adolescents suffer from both a higher occurrence of caries and lower treatment rates relative to whites. Disparities by gender are much narrower, with females of all ages having slightly higher rates of caries, likely due to higher dental treatment rates.[4] Disparities by income are striking, with 2.4 times more adolescents in or near poverty (less than 100 percent and 100–199 percent of the federal poverty level, respectively) experiencing untreated tooth decay than their more affluent peers.

Because caries is progressive and cumulative, and early experience with

---

[4]This is because dentists employ a lower threshold for counting teeth as having caries relative to the national survey methodology. Thus, dentists may fill teeth that the national survey would not consider as having decay. The filled tooth is counted in the survey as evidence of its having had a cavity.

27.9	36.8	NA	NA	40.7[i]
38.7	29.5	NA	NA	32.9

[d]Pregnancy prevalence is expressed as per 1,000 in the age group.
[e]Ages 14 and under, 2002 (Guttmacher Institute, 2006).
[f]Ages 15–19, 2000 (Ventura et al., 2006).
[g]At risk of overweight and overweight, defined as a body mass index of ≥85th percentile of the sex-specific body mass index-for-age growth chart, is expressed as percentage of the population, 1999–2002 (Hedley et al., 2004).
[h]Students who met currently recommended levels of physical activity in 2005 (percentage of students who were physically active for a total of 60 minutes or more per day on 5 or more of the past 7 days), percentage of the population (Centers for Disease Control and Prevention, 2007c; MacKay and Duran, 2007).
[i]Indicates Mexican American; does not include all Hispanic adolescents

caries predicts later experience, future dental disease among adolescents can be anticipated based on current experience with caries among young children. Historically, rates of caries for all ages have been decreasing; for the first time since the 1970s, however, rates of caries have been increasing substantially among the youngest children.

Periodontal and other soft-tissue diseases A uniquely adolescent variation of common periodontitis, termed "juvenile periodontitis," has a particularly early onset and is especially aggressive (Oh, Eber, and Wang, 2002), with a skewed prevalence by race and ethnicity: 10 percent among African Americans, 5.5 percent among Hispanics, and 1.3 percent among whites aged 13–17 (Albandar, Brown, and Löe, 1997). Another study, for example, found that more than half of late adolescents (58 percent of those aged 18–19) have gingivitis, the precursor to destructive adult periodontitis, but far fewer demonstrate the mild or advanced tissue damage of periodontitis (4.7 percent of those aged 13–21 reportedly have mild periodontitis [Reeves et al., 2006], while 0.5 percent of those aged 18–19 have advanced tissue damage [NHANES III data]). The onset and progression of gingivitis and periodontitis are associated with use of tobacco products of all kinds, diabetes, HIV/AIDS, and a variety of other medical conditions and syndromes. Intraoral and perioral soft-tissue lesions (Oh, Eber, and Wang, 2002) are not unique to adolescents, although some such conditions, such as recurrent labial herpes (fever blisters or cold sores), aphthous stomatitis (canker sores), and angular cheilitis (inflammatory lesions at the corner of the mouth), typically present during adolescence.

Trauma As early as ages 11–13, one in six adolescents have experienced trauma to their front teeth; the prevalence continues to rise to one in five (18.9 percent) at ages 14–17 and one in four thereafter (27.5 percent of those aged 18–35) (NHANES III data, 1988 through 1994). Most soft-tissue trauma is self-healing, but much of the damage induced by oral jewelry (piercings of the tongue, lip, or cheek) causes irreversible destruction of both teeth and periodontal tissues. Reported side effects of oral piercings, for instance, include short-term infection, edema, and hemorrhage, and longer-term fractured teeth, chronic soft-tissue inflammation, injury to gums, and gingival recession (De Moor et al., 2005; Zadik and Sandler, 2007).

> **Finding:** *The most common oral health problem in adolescence is dental caries. Non-Hispanic black adolescents have a higher prevalence of untreated dental caries than non-Hispanic white adolescents.*

BEHAVIOR AND HEALTH

Many unhealthful behaviors initiated during adolescence extend into adulthood and result in significant morbidity and mortality in the short and long terms (Kolbe, Kann, and Collins, 1993). This section reviews the most salient of these behaviors and some of their health-related consequences.

> **Finding:** *Behavior that is unhealthful and/or risky, rather than infectious or chronic diseases, is the leading cause of morbidity among adolescents.*

Risky Driving

As discussed earlier, death rates due to motor vehicle crashes have decreased dramatically since 1970, but continue to be the leading cause of injury death for adolescents aged 10–19. Consumption of alcohol and a lack of seat belt use are often associated with speeding (Juarez et al., 2006)—a lethal combination. A general lack of adequate sleep can also contribute to risky driving.

Alcohol plays a significant role in injury deaths due to motor vehicle crashes. In 2005, almost one-fifth of drivers aged 16–20 involved in fatal motor vehicle crashes were intoxicated, although this proportion was down from one-quarter of drivers aged 15–19 in 1989 (National Highway Traffic Safety Administration, 1989, 2006). In 2007, 29 percent of high school students had ridden in the past month with a driver who had been drinking alcohol, though this was again down from 40 percent in 1991 (Eaton et al., 2008; MacKay and Duran, 2007). While there is no gender variation, Hispanic students were significantly more likely than their non-Hispanic white and black counterparts to ride with a driver who had been drinking (see Table 2-4). Ten percent of 11th- through 12th-grade high school students reported driving after drinking alcohol, a decrease from 17 percent in 1991. Non-Hispanic black 11th- through 12th-grade students were less likely to drive after drinking than non-Hispanic white or Hispanic students. Alcohol use is also an important risk factor for teen drowning deaths and residential fire injuries and deaths.

The most effective means of preventing injury in a crash is use of a seat belt. When properly used, seat belts reduce the risk of injury by 50–60 percent (National Highway Traffic Safety Administration, 2001). As many as 30 percent of adolescents do not wear seat belts, markedly increasing their chances of a fatal outcome in a crash (Glassbrenner, 2003), although one survey revealed that the percentage of high school students (grades 9 through 12) who never or rarely wore seat belts while riding in a car driven by someone else decreased from 26 percent in 1991 to 11 percent in 2007 (Eaton et al., 2008; MacKay and Duran, 2007). While there are no significant differences by race or ethnicity, male high school students are more likely than females not to wear or rarely to wear a seat belt—13 percent versus 8 percent (see Table 2-4).

Sleepiness also contributes to motor vehicle crashes among adolescents. A biological increase in the amount of sleep needed, changing sleep patterns, and social circumstances contribute to a chronic lack of sleep in this population, resulting in more crashes. As reported by Pack and colleagues (1995), the distribution of motor vehicle crashes attributed to drivers who fell asleep at the wheel peaks in the adolescent age range. The effects of this chronic lack of sleep have been compared to alcohol impairment. For example, Pack and colleagues (1995) found that after 17 hours awake, an adolescent's driving performance is impaired to the same extent that it would be with a blood alcohol content of 0.05 percent.

Violence

Violent behavior among adolescents is associated with other high-risk behavior, such as substance abuse and risky sexual activity. In addition to being a public health problem during adolescence, violence among adolescents is the most common precursor of violence in adults. Data from many long-term longitudinal cohort studies indicate that nearly all adults with violent behavior had such behavior during childhood and adolescence (Farrington, 2001; Loeber, Lacourse, and Homish, 2005). Very little adult violence is perpetrated by individuals who had no violent behavior as youths.

Weapon Carrying

Gun carrying in particular is associated with an increased likelihood of fights and other high-risk behavior, such as substance abuse and risky sexual activity (Callahan and Rivara, 1992; Lowry et al., 1998). Access to and ownership of guns increases the likelihood of violent death among adolescents, including both homicide and suicide (Grossman et al., 2005; Kellermann et al., 1992, 1993). In 2005, as many as one in five high school students had carried a weapon to school in the month before being surveyed for the Youth Risk Behavior Survey, increasing their chances of violence and injury. Five percent of high school students reported carrying a gun (MacKay and Duran, 2007; see Table 2-4). The percentage of students who carried a weapon decreased between 1991 and 1999 and remained steady until 2005. Male students were significantly more likely than females to report carrying a gun or other weapon. Seven percent reported carrying a weapon on school property (Eaton et al., 2006). The percentage of high school students carrying a gun or other weapon did not vary significantly by age, race, or ethnicity.

Violent Crime Victimization

In addition to perpetrating violence, adolescents are often its victims. In 2004, approximately 1.6 million adolescents aged 12–19 were victims of violent crime (rape, robbery, and assault) according to the National Crime Victimization Survey (MacKay and Duran, 2007). Crime victimization rates generally increased among adolescents from 1985 through 1995, and then declined between 1995 and 2005 to levels well below those in 1985. The overall increase in violent crime and homicide during the 1980s was due largely to an increase among adolescents, which peaked in the early 1990s and has been related to the crack cocaine epidemic (Blumstein, Rivara, and Rosenfeld, 2000).

Among adolescents of all ages, males are twice as likely as females to be victims of serious crimes (MacKay and Duran, 2007, see Table 2-4). Dating violence also occurs in this age group. One in 11 adolescents have reported being victims of physical dating violence each year, with the frequency being equal among males and females (Black et al., 2006). Similarly, according to the Youth Risk Behavior Survey of high school students, in 2007 almost 10 percent of male and female students reported dating violence. In addition, 8 percent of students reported that they had ever been physically forced to have sexual intercourse; such reports were more common among females (11 percent) than males (4 percent) (Eaton et al., 2008).

There are large racial disparities in violent crime victimization. Black males have the highest rate of homicide victimization of any gender–racial group, with peaks in late adolescence and emerging adulthood. These trends in victimization are also seen in perpetration, with murder rates being highest among black males (U.S. Department of Justice, 2006, see Table 2-4).

Bullying and Fighting

According to the Youth Risk Behavior Survey, in 2007, 35.6 percent of 9th through 12th graders reported being involved in a physical fight in the preceding 12 months, down from 42.5 percent in 1991 (Centers for Disease Control and Prevention, 2006c; Eaton et al., 2008). Approximately 4 percent of these students had been injured in a fight in the prior year. Fighting is a marker for other high-risk behavior in youths, including school failure, substance abuse, weapon carrying, attempted suicide, and risky sexual behavior (Sosin et al., 1995; Swahn and Donovan, 2006; Wright and Fitzpatrick, 2006). In addition, physical fighting between students who are dating appears to be common among both middle and high school students (12 percent) and college students (5.6 percent) (Centers for Disease Control and Prevention, 2006a; DuRant et al., 2007).

Bullying is very common during adolescence, reported to involve as many as 30 percent of students in grades 6–10 either as victims, bullies, or both (Nansel et al., 2001). Bullying is associated with other problems in children, including lower grades and weapon carrying (Glew et al., 2008). Recently, attention has been focused on Internet bullying, reported by 12 percent of 8th graders and 10 percent of 11th graders in a recent survey (Williams and Guerra, 2007). Internet bullying was as common among girls as boys. As with other types of bullying, Internet bullying and harassment are also associated with other high-risk behaviors, such as weapon carrying (Ybarra, Diener-West, and Leaf, 2007).

Substance Use

Substance use, most frequently involving alcohol, tobacco, and marijuana, is common among adolescents. A recent concern is adolescents' misuse of prescription medications, including opiate analgesics, stimulants, and cough medicines (Kuehn, 2007). Adolescents' patterns of substance use can create particular risks for negative consequences. For example, although adolescents drink less frequently than adults, they drink larger quantities. The 2005 National Survey of Drug Use and Health revealed that 19 percent of individuals aged 12–20 consumed five or more drinks per occasion (Substance Abuse and Mental Health Services Administration, 2006). This "binge" pattern places adolescents at risk for drinking-related impairment and for both unintentional and violent injuries, sexual assault, and risky sexual behavior. An appreciable risk for short-term mortality and morbidity from motor vehicle crashes, homicide, and suicide is associated with substance use; for example, underage drinking is responsible for the deaths of approximately 5,000 people below age 21 (National Institute on Alcohol Abuse and Alcoholism, 2006; U.S. Department of Health and Human Services, 2007c). Actions associated with substance use put others at risk as well.

Adolescents may have a particular vulnerability to the negative consequences of substance use,[5] such as the effects of alcohol on cognitive skills and memory (Spear, 2000). Early onset of substance use (before age 15) is associated with a heightened risk for later substance use disorder (Grant and Dawson, 1997, 1998; Robins and Przybeck, 1985). Early onset is also associated with more substance-related problems (Hingson and Kenkel, 2004).

Tobacco Use

Tobacco use is the most common cause of mortality in the United States, accounting for more than 400,000 deaths annually (Mokdad et al., 2004). Nearly all of these deaths occur to people well beyond adolescence, but initiation of smoking occurs primarily among adolescents. By 9th grade, half of children have tried cigarettes, a portion that increases to more than 60 percent by 12th grade (Eaton et al., 2006). Fully 82 percent of adults who currently smoke started smoking before age 18, and virtually no adult smokers started smoking after age 25 (U.S. Department of Health and Human Services, 1994). Adolescent smoking is quite persistent, and the majority of adolescent smokers continue their smoking into young adulthood (Miller, 2005).

In 2005, tobacco use at least once in the preceding month was reported among almost one-fourth of adolescents aged 16–17 (Substance Abuse and Mental Health Services Administration, 2006). The prevalence of tobacco use in adolescents peaked in the late 1990s at 36 percent and recently dipped to its lowest levels since the early 1990s (U.S. Department of Health and Human Services, 2004). Declines in adolescent smoking had been leveling off, but there is mixed information about a new decline in 2007 (Eaton et al., 2008; Johnston et al., 2008). In addition to the health risks faced by

---

[5]These findings come from animal data and have not yet been conclusively established for humans.

adolescents who smoke, it is estimated that in 2000, 18 million youths aged 12–19 were exposed to secondhand smoke (U.S. Department of Health and Human Services, 2006c).

American Indian and Alaskan Native adolescents are more likely to use tobacco than any other racial or ethnic group. Non-Hispanic white and Hispanic adolescents are more likely to use tobacco than non-Hispanic black or Asian adolescents (see Table 2-4). In 2005, 2 percent of high school students were reported to have used smokeless tobacco in the past month and 4 percent to have smoked cigars, a decrease since 1988 (National Institute on Drug Abuse, 1989; Substance Abuse and Mental Health Services Administration, 2006). Gender is not a major factor in the proportion of adolescents using tobacco; however, the prevalence of tobacco use increases with age (Centers for Disease Control and Prevention, 2005). A little over one-quarter of those aged 18–24 reported that they were current smokers (20 percent were daily smokers) (Lawrence et al., 2007).

Tobacco use produces health problems in both adolescence (e.g., less physical fitness, more respiratory illness) and young adulthood, including declines in lung function (U.S. Department of Health and Human Services, 2004). Moreover, adolescent tobacco use creates the risk for serious long-term health consequences in adulthood. Adolescent smoking often persists into adulthood, carrying with it the associated risk of serious adult morbidity and premature death (U.S. Department of Health and Human Services, 2004).

Alcohol Use

More than 60,000 people die annually in the United States from harmful drinking of alcohol (Rivara et al., 2004). These deaths occur because of heavy episodic or binge drinking or high levels of regular drinking. Binge drinking, which, as noted earlier, is especially likely to occur among adolescents, markedly raises the risk of injury, whether intentional or unintentional, and thus directly increases the risk of adolescent morbidity and mortality (Smith, Branas, and Miller, 1999). Most of the consequences of heavy regular drinking are seen during later adulthood and thus do not affect adolescents directly. The one exception is suicide, the risk of which is associated with both binge drinking and moderate to high levels of regular drinking (May et al., 2002).

There is a strong relationship between the age at onset of drinking and the risk of alcohol-related problems in both adolescence and adulthood. The median age of first alcohol use is 15 (DeWit et al., 2000). Alcohol use increases during the teen years, peaks in the early 20s, and decreases thereafter (Casswell, Pledger, and Hooper, 2003; Muthen and Muthen, 2000). The median age at onset for alcohol use disorder is 19–20 (Nelson, Heath, and Kessler, 1998). Early drinking has been associated with a variety of problems, and the risk of these problems increases as age at onset decreases (Hingson, Heeren, and Zakocs, 2001; Hingson et al., 2000, 2002, 2003). More than 40 percent of those who start drinking at age 14 or younger develop alcohol dependence, compared with 10 percent of those who begin drinking at age 20 or older (Hingson, Heeren, and Winter, 2006; Hingson et al., 2003).

In 2005, 28 percent of adolescents aged 12–20 reported drinking alcohol in the past month. Binge drinking was reported by 19 percent of adolescents and heavy alcohol use by 6 percent (Substance Abuse and Mental Health Services Administration, 2006). The prevalence of this behavior increased significantly between ages 12–13 and 18–20. In the late 1990s, the prevalence of current or heavy alcohol use peaked, and it has since decreased below the reported frequency in the early 1990s. Non-Hispanic white adolescents are more likely to binge drink than any other racial or ethnic group. American Indian and Alaskan Native and Hispanic adolescents also have a high prevalence of binge drinking compared with non-Hispanic black and Asian adolescents (aged 12–20). Alcohol use does not vary significantly by gender (see Table 2-4).

Marijuana and Other Illicit Drug Use

Use of drugs other than tobacco and alcohol is an important risky behavior among adolescents. Marijuana is the drug most commonly used by adolescents; according to the Youth Risk Behavior Survey, in 2007 one-fifth of students in high school reported using marijuana one or more times in the past month; almost 40 percent of the students reported having used it one or more times during their life (Eaton et al., 2008). Marijuana use increases with age. In 2005, almost 17 percent of those aged 18–25 reported using marijuana on at least 1 day in the past month, a stark contrast with young adolescents aged 12–17, at almost 7 percent (Substance Abuse and Mental Health Services Administration, 2006, see Table 2-4).

Illicit drug use among high school students has decreased from a peak in the last half of the 1990s (Johnston et al., 2006). This decline has paralleled a change in the attitudes of high school students toward the use of these substances. The majority of adolescents believe that regular use of illicit drugs carries great risk, a belief that extends to regular use of marijuana (Johnston et al., 2006). On the other hand, many fewer adolescents believe that occasional experimentation with illicit drugs poses a great risk of harm. In 2005, almost 8 percent of students in grades 9 to 12 reported using some form of cocaine during their lifetime; 6 percent reported using methamphetamines (Eaton et al., 2006). The prevalence of cocaine use peaked in 1999 and has remained steady, while in 1988, 4 percent of adolescents aged 12–17 reported using amphetamines during their lifetime (National Institute on Drug Abuse, 1989).

Finding: Use of alcohol, tobacco, and illicit drugs and carrying a weapon are adolescent behaviors that pose serious risk.

Pregnancy

In 2002 there were more than 750,000 pregnancies among adolescent girls aged 15–19 (Ventura et al., 2006). This rate represents a 35 percent decrease relative to that in 1990—a decline attributable mainly to a decrease in pregnancy among younger (aged 15–17) compared with older (aged 18–19) adolescents. In 2002 there were approximately 17,000 pregnancies among girls under age 15 (Guttmacher Institute, 2006), representing an even more dramatic decline of 50 percent in this age group between 1990 and 2002. Pregnancy rates in 2002 were more than twice as high among non-Hispanic black and Hispanic adolescents as among non-Hispanic white adolescents (see Table 2-4). Between 1990 and 2002, the pregnancy rate for Hispanic adolescents decreased less dramatically than that for black and non-Hispanic white adolescents; even so, black adolescents continue to have the highest pregnancy rate.

Adolescent childbearing is associated with a number of adverse consequences for adolescent mothers, fathers, and their children. For example, an adolescent mother is less likely than an older mother to complete high school or college, more likely to be a single mother, more likely to have more children sooner on a limited income, and more likely to abuse or neglect the child (Hoffman, 2006). Being the child of adolescent parents carries adverse health and social risks, including low birth weight and prematurity, poverty, school failure, and a greater likelihood of becoming involved in the juvenile justice system (for a boy) or becoming an adolescent mother (for a girl) (Hoffman, 2006).

Birth Rates Among Adolescents

Birth rates among adolescents declined during 1991–2005 to levels that represent a record low; preliminary data for 2005–2006, however, reveal an increased rate for the first time in more than a decade (Federal Interagency Forum on Child and Family Statistics, 2007; Hamilton, Martin, and Ventura, 2007; Ikramullah et al., 2007; Martin et al., 2006). As discussed in the next section, the decline in the teen birth rate has not been driven by more abortions, but by a decrease in the underlying pregnancy rate.

In 2004, the number of births among adolescents aged 10–19 was approximately 422,000 (Martin et al., 2006); births in this age group account for 10 percent of all births each year in the United States. Birth rates among adolescents increase with age. For example, adolescents aged 19 were nine times more likely to give birth than those aged 15. In 2004, there were more than 1 million births to mothers aged 20–24, approximately half of which were second- or higher-order births (Martin et al., 2006). There are substantial racial and ethnic differences in birth rates among adolescents aged 10–19. Hispanic and non-Hispanic black adolescents have the highest rates, followed by American Indian and Alaskan Native adolescents; Asian/Pacific Islander adolescents have the lowest rates (Federal Interagency Forum on Child and Family Statistics, 2007). The birth rate among those aged 20–24 also varies by race and ethnicity. Hispanics in this age group have the highest birth rate, followed by non-Hispanic blacks, American Indians and Alaskan Natives, whites, and Asian/Pacific Islanders (Martin et al., 2006).

Abortion Rates

Paralleling the decline in birth rates, rates of induced abortion among adolescents aged 15–19 declined during 1990–2002 (Ventura et al., 2006). In 2002 there were a reported 21.7 induced abortions per 1,000 adolescents aged 15–19, down approximately 50 percent from the rate in 1990 (Ventura et al., 2006). The rate of induced abortions among adolescents under age 15 decreased 51 percent between 1991 and 2002 (Guttmacher Institute, 2006).

Among adolescents aged 15–19, the reported proportion of pregnancies that ended in abortion was higher among non-Hispanic blacks than among either Hispanic or non-Hispanic whites (Ventura et al., 2006). Rates of induced abortion among adolescents increase with maternal age: 6 percent of all abortions in the United States are to those aged 15–17, while 12 percent are to those aged 18–19 (Jones, Darroch, and Henshaw, 2002).

Fetal Loss Rates

Rates of fetal loss among adolescents declined during 1990–2002 (Guttmacher Institute, 2006; Ventura et al., 2006). In 2002 there were a reported 11.8 losses per 1,000 female adolescents, down approximately 30 percent from the rate in 1990 (Ventura et al., 2006). Rates of fetal loss among adolescents increase with maternal age. Hispanic females aged 19 tend to have higher fetal loss rates than females of other ages and ethnicities.

Finding: Pregnancy rates among adolescents aged 13–19 have decreased since 1990; declines have been seen among all racial and ethnic groups, although the rate of pregnancy among Hispanic adolescents has been decreasing less dramatically. Pregnancy rates among Hispanic and non-Hispanic black adolescents continue to be twice as high as those among non-Hispanic white adolescents.

Unhealthful and Risky Eating Behavior

Eating behavior during adolescence has lifelong implications for health and well-being. Overweight and obese adolescents are more likely to be overweight and obese adults, who in turn are more likely to have diabetes and cardiovascular disease. In addition, overweight and obese adolescents are more likely to have decreased self-esteem and depression that persist into adulthood.

Overweight and Obesity

More than 10 million adolescents (31 percent) aged 12–19 were considered at risk of being overweight and overweight[6] in 1999–2002 (Hedley et al., 2004, see Table 2-4). More than 17 percent of adolescents in this age group were considered overweight in 2004 (MacKay and Duran, 2007), a percentage that had more than tripled since 1980 (MacKay and Duran, 2007). Given that obesity is a condition that develops over time, it is relevant to note that in 2001, 22 percent of those aged 19–26 were considered obese.[7] Among this group, the prevalence of extreme obesity—individuals with a body mass index ≥40—was more than 4 percent overall (Gordon-Larsen et al., 2004).

The percentage of adolescents who are overweight varies by race or ethnicity and gender. During 2001–2004, non-Hispanic black female adolescents and Mexican American adolescents (both genders) were more likely to be overweight than non-Hispanic white adolescents (both genders) aged 12–19. Information on other racial and ethnic groups, including Hispanics, Asians, and other populations, is unavailable. The proportion of overweight adolescents does not vary significantly according to economic status (MacKay and Duran, 2007).

Adolescents aged 10–17 in urban areas are somewhat less likely than those in rural areas to be overweight—14.2 percent versus more than 17 percent (Maternal and Child Health Bureau, 2005b). One of the most noticeable differences by location occurs among adolescents aged 12–14:

---

[6]At risk of being overweight is defined as having a body mass index (kg/m^2) between the 85th and 94th percentiles, while overweight is defined as having a body mass index greater than or equal to the 95th percentile, based on gender and age, from the 2000 CDC growth charts.

[7]Obesity is defined in adults over age 18 as having a body mass index (in kg/m^2) of ≥30.

13.3 percent in this age group who live in urban areas are overweight, compared with 18.7 percent in rural areas (Maternal and Child Health Bureau, 2005b).

Overweight and obesity have serious health consequences for adolescents, increasing the risk of high cholesterol, hypertension, diabetes, and the metabolic syndrome (Dietz, 1998). There is substantial evidence from longitudinal studies that, as noted above, being overweight or obese during childhood and extending into adolescence is associated with a markedly higher probability of being overweight or obese as an adult (Deshmukh-Taskar et al., 2006; U.S. Department of Health and Human Services, 2007b; Whitaker et al., 1997). For example, in the Bogalusa Heart Study, 59 percent of males and 69 percent of females aged 15–17 who were at risk of being overweight (body mass index between the 85th and 94th percentiles) were overweight as adults. Among those who were overweight as adolescents, nearly 90 percent were obese as adults (Freedman et al., 2005b). Obesity in childhood and adolescence was more likely to lead to obesity in adulthood among blacks than among whites (Freedman et al., 2005a). Being overweight during childhood and adolescence also increases the likelihood of hypertension as an adult (Field, Cook, and Gillman, 2005).

Nutrition

According to the U.S. Department of Agriculture's Nationwide Food Consumption Survey, in the 1970s the diet of U.S. adolescents was lower than recommended (National Research Council, 1989) in energy intake; vitamin B_6; calcium; iron; dietary fiber; and sometimes vitamin C, folic acid, thiamin, and riboflavin (U.S. Congress and Office of Technology Assessment, 1991). Adolescents also were reported to consume excessive fat, cholesterol, sodium, and low-nutrient foods. More recent data indicate substantial increases in adolescent calorie (energy) and carbohydrate intake since the 1970s (Institute of Medicine, 2006b). For example, an increase of at least 100 calories per day has been noted for adolescents, who consume about double the suggested limit of added sugars in their diet (Enns, Mickle, and Goldman, 2003). Additionally, the data still show excessive intake of low-nutrient foods, total fat, saturated fat, and sodium relative to what is recommended (i.e., the Dietary Reference Intakes) (Institute of Medicine, 2006a,b). In 2003, 78 percent of adolescents participating in a national survey had not eaten five or more servings of fruits and vegetables a day during the 7 preceding days (Grunbaum et al., 2004). Adolescent females in particular are reported to consume inadequate amounts of iron.

Other Risky Eating Behavior

Risky eating behavior includes not eating for 24 hours or more and vomiting or taking laxatives. In 2007 the Youth Risk Behavior Survey found that 12 percent of high school students (9th through 12th grades) had not eaten for 24 hours or more in the 30 days prior to the survey—a steady prevalence since 1999 (Eaton et al., 2008; MacKay and Duran, 2007). More than 4 percent of students reported vomiting or taking a laxative; the prevalence of this behavior peaked in 2003 and subsequently decreased back to levels reported in 1997. Female students were more than twice as likely as males to report this risky eating behavior. This behavior does not vary by age or race or ethnicity.

Finding: The percentage of overweight adolescents has more than tripled since 1980, with more than 17 percent of adolescents aged 12–19 being considered overweight.

Physical Activity

Currently, only one-third of adults and two-thirds of children and younger adolescents engage in regular leisure-time physical activity (Barnes and Schoenborn, 2003; Duke, Huhman, and Heitzler, 2003). There is evidence that levels of physical activity during adolescence are directly related to those in adulthood, although this relationship is only moderately strong (Hallal et al., 2006). While the exercise patterns established during adolescence can carry over into adulthood, a myriad of other factors are influential as well.

Physical activity during adolescence is important for bone health in adulthood (Hallal et al., 2006). Moreover, physical inactivity is associated with an increased risk of death, as well as a host of diseases, including diabetes, obesity, cardiovascular disease, and other chronic illnesses.

Various national studies have quantified the amount of physical activity in which adolescents participate. However, the definitions used for physical activity have varied throughout the last two decades, making it difficult to compare results and describe trends accurately over time. For example, in 2007, 35 percent of adolescents in grades 9 through 12 reported meeting current recommendations for the level of physical activity (Eaton et al., 2008). In 1985, 59 percent of 5th through 12th graders reported engaging in appropriate physical activity (Ross and Gilbert, 1985). Although these data reveal a decrease in adequate physical activity over time, the two studies used different definitions of physical activity, and therefore no accurate conclusion can be drawn.[8] On the other hand, a national survey that used the same definition (different from the above two) of physical activity from 1999 through 2005, a 6-year time frame, found that in 2005, 69 percent of students had participated in currently recommended levels (20 minutes of vigorous physical activity on 3 or more of the past 7 days and/or at least 30 minutes of moderate activity five or more times in the past week)—a percentage that had remained steady since 1999 (Centers for Disease Control and Prevention, 2007c; MacKay and Duran, 2007).

Although the prevalence and trend over time in participation in physical activity are difficult to describe accurately, studies reveal disparities among the adolescent population by gender and race or ethnicity. Participation in physical activity at the current recommended level was found to be substantially more likely among male than female students, but did not vary greatly by age. Non-Hispanic white students were more likely than non-Hispanic black students to have met the recommended level. Non-Hispanic white and Hispanic students were more likely than non-Hispanic black students to participate in moderate to vigorous physical activity (Centers for Disease Control and Prevention, 2007c; MacKay and Duran, 2007).

Adolescents aged 10–17 in rural areas are more likely than those in urban areas to participate in regular physical activity (3 or more days a week). Parents of girls aged 10–17 in urban areas report the lowest percentage of regular physical activity (Maternal and Child Health Bureau, 2005b).

HEALTH OF SPECIFIC SUBPOPULATIONS

The health status of adolescents can be characterized by the health conditions and behaviors discussed above. Not reflected in these data, however, is the fact that some groups of adolescents have particularly high rates of comorbid diseases, health conditions, or risky behaviors. As well, some groups of adolescents may face disparities or biases in the delivery of health services, as underscored by the Institute of Medicine (2003) report *Unequal Treatment: Confronting Racial and Ethnic Disparities in Health Care*. These adolescents face special challenges, and highlighting their health status underscores the complex services and settings that need to be encompassed by a health system that is responsive to all adolescents. As described in *Losing Generations: Adolescents in High Risk Situations*, a report of the National Research Council (1993), these at-risk populations have had to confront negative aspects of the social environment that

---

[8]Appropriate or currently recommended physical activity was defined in 2007 as being physically active for a total of 60 minutes or more per day on 5 or more of the past 7 days, and in 1985 was defined as engaging in activity requiring 60 percent or greater of an individual's cardiovascular capacity at least three times per week for at least 20 minutes.

decrease their opportunities for a successful transition through adolescence to adulthood.

Minority, Low-Income, and Rural Adolescents

Minority adolescents, those in low-income families, and those who live in rural areas experience particular disparities in health status and therefore face additional challenges in accessing needed health services:

- The racial and ethnic makeup of adolescents in the United States is becoming more diverse (see Chapter 1). By 2050, it is estimated that more than 53 percent of adolescents aged 10–19 will be members of racial or ethnic minority groups (U.S. Census Bureau, 2007).
- Adolescents who are in low-income families (income below $19,971 for a family of four in 2005) make up 16 percent of the adolescent population aged 10–17, while an additional 20 percent of adolescents live in near-poor families (income up to $37,619 for a family of four) (MacKay and Duran, 2007).
- Of U.S. adolescents aged 12–17, 19 percent, or 4.6 million, live in rural areas (nonmetropolitan counties including no city with a population of greater than 10,000) (Fields, 2003). The population of rural adolescents increased from 1990 to 2002 (U.S. Census Bureau, 1992, 2003).

When available, information on the disparities in health status (i.e., mortality, morbidity, and health-related behavior) experienced by these specific groups of adolescents is presented throughout this chapter. It should be noted, however, that while some data exist on the health of low-income adolescents, these data are limited given that many of these adolescents are uninsured and not receiving consistent health services whereby their health status can be tracked. Additionally, it is often difficult to separate the effects of race and ethnicity from those of socioeconomic status. Without better data on these most vulnerable adolescents, understanding their specific health needs is problematic.

Adolescents in the Foster Care System[9]

In 2005, there were 3.3 million complaints to child protection agencies alleging child abuse and neglect (child maltreatment), involving 6 million

---

[9]The available literature included in this section encompasses both children and adolescents (ages 8 and older, usually up to age 17) and thus is not specific to the adolescent population only; the text therefore refers to "children and adolescents" in discussing these data.

children and adolescents. As a result of the initial screening of those complaints, 3.6 million children and adolescents were referred for investigation by child protection authorities as the victims of child maltreatment. Those investigations substantiated that 900,000 children and adolescents were the victims of child maltreatment in 2005 (Children's Bureau, Administration for Children and Families, and U.S. Department of Health and Human Services, 2007). On any given day in 2005, it is estimated that 514,000 children and adolescents lived in foster care to ensure their safety; approximately half were aged 8 or older (Children's Bureau, Administration for Children and Families, and U.S. Department of Health and Human Services, 2007).

Children and adolescents in foster care have significantly more health problems than those in the general population (Hansen, Kagle, and Black, 2004). These problems include asthma, anemia, recurrent ear infections, and neurological abnormalities such as seizure disorders (Halfon, Mendonca, and Berkowitz, 1995). A significant number frequently experience upper respiratory infections, dermatological disorders, dental caries, and malnutrition (Silver, Haecker, and Forkey, 1999). In New York City, Chicago, Baltimore, and Canada, children in foster care have been found to have higher rates of vision, hearing, growth, and dental problems than other children (Barbell and Freundlich, 2001; Moffat et al., 1985; Swire and Kavaler, 1977; White, Benedict, and Jaffe, 1987). An estimated four in five also have a multitude of chronic health problems (Barton, 1999; Halfon, Mendonca, and Berkowitz, 1995; National Research Council and Institute of Medicine, 2004). Compared with other children and adolescents from the same socioeconomic background, those in foster care have much higher rates of serious emotional and behavioral problems, chronic physical disabilities, birth defects, and developmental delays (Committee on Early Childhood, Adoption, and Dependent Care and American Academy of Pediatrics, 2002).

Up to 80 percent of children and adolescents entering foster care have mental health problems (Simms, Dubowitz, and Szilagyi, 2000), as compared with 18–22 percent of children in the general population (Roberts, Attkisson, and Rosenblatt, 1998). One-third have at least one mental health diagnosis—most commonly post-traumatic stress disorder, alcohol abuse, substance abuse, or major depression. It has been reported that adolescents who have been in the foster care system have higher rates of illicit drug use than those who have never been in foster care (Substance Abuse and Mental Health Services Administration, 2005b). Males are more likely than females to be diagnosed with recent alcohol or substance abuse, while females are more likely to be diagnosed with recent depression (Leslie et al., 2000).

Approximately 60 percent of preschool-age children in foster care experience developmental delays (Inkeles and Halfon, 2002). In addition, it has been found that foster children tend to have more physical or mental health conditions that negatively impact school performance and psychosocial functioning (Kortenkamp and Ehrele, 2002).

Not only are these findings a concern as regards the immediate well-being of these children, but it has been reported that a disproportionate number of former foster children have mental disorders as adults (Casey Family Programs, 2005). Approximately half of adults who were placed in foster care as children have one or more mental health problems in adulthood, and 25 percent suffer from post-traumatic stress disorder (Pecora et al., 2005).

Homeless Adolescents

It has been estimated that there are between 1.3 million and 2 million homeless adolescents in the United States (Cauce et al., 1998; Hammer, Finkelhor, and Sedlak, 2002; Patel and Greydanus, 2002). This population is split almost evenly between males and females, and around 70 percent comprises adolescents aged 15–17 (Hammer, Finkelhor, and Sedlak, 2002). The precise number of homeless adolescents is difficult to determine, however, since homelessness is a dynamic status, with youths often migrating between staying with family and friends, in shelters, and on the street. Moreover, it is difficult to locate and count individuals who have no permanent address.

Collecting information on the health status of homeless adolescents is a particular challenge. With a population that is as transient and diverse as homeless adolescents, it is nearly impossible to find a large, randomly selected sample; collect data on these individuals over time; and develop a study with external and internal validity. Thus, much of the available literature in this area has serious limitations (Robertson and Toro, 1999). Nonetheless, the growing body of knowledge suggests that homeless adolescents are a sizable population, and that they face unique and significant health challenges.

Three major factors influence the physical and mental health of homeless adolescents: (1) homeless youths are more likely to come from troubled backgrounds (Cauce et al., 2000); (2) the challenges and stresses of living on the streets lead to high-risk behavior and a heightened danger of victimization; and (3) these individuals face multiple barriers to accessing health care.

Most homeless adolescents have already grappled with substantial health issues in their lives even before leaving home. They are more likely than other adolescents to have experienced sexual and physical abuse (Cauce et al., 2000; Haley et al., 2004; Rew, Taylor-Seehafer, and Fitzgerald, 2001), to come from homes where parents abuse alcohol or drugs (Cauce et al., 1998), and to suffer from mental health disorders (Rohde et al., 2001). Whether adolescents run away or are thrown out of their home, these issues are often a precipitating factor; self-reported reasons for becoming homeless include physical and sexual abuse, violence at home, drug use by a family member, and neglect (Cauce et al., 1998). In addition to triggering homelessness, these difficult life experiences can increase the chances that an individual will adopt risky behaviors, suffer from depression, and abuse drugs and alcohol (Rew, Taylor-Seehafer, and Fitzgerald, 2001; Stein, Leslie, and Nyamathi, 2002).

Abuse

The prevalence of physical and sexual abuse among homeless adolescents is significantly higher than is the case among the general population. It is estimated that 12.3 of every 1,000 children in the United States are victims of abuse (Childhelp, 2006), but studies of homeless adolescents indicate a much higher frequency: approximately half of homeless girls have been sexually abused (Haley et al., 2004; Rew, Fouladi, and Yockey, 2002; Wenzel et al., 2006) and around 20 percent of boys (Cauce et al., 1998, 2000), and physical abuse for both ranges up to 70 percent (Bao, Whitbeck, and Hoyt, 2000; Cauce et al., 2000). Physical and sexual abuse are among the most common reasons for leaving home (Andres-Lemay, Jamieson, and MacMillan, 2005; Cauce et al., 1998), and once on the streets, abused adolescents are at higher risk of further victimization (Craig and Hodson, 1998). Compared with other homeless adolescents, girls who have been abused are more likely to become pregnant (Haley et al., 2004), to contract an STI, and to experience psychological distress and depression (Stein, Leslie, and Nyamathi, 2002; Wenzel et al., 2006). Abused children of both genders are more likely to use alcohol and drugs, to consider or attempt suicide (Rew, Taylor-Seehafer, and Fitzgerald, 2001), to resort to violent and antisocial behavior (Moore, 2005), to participate in survival sex[10] (Greene, Ennett, and Ringwalt, 1999), and to be sexually or physically assaulted on the streets (Cauce et al., 2000; MacLean, Embry, and Cauce, 1999).

Sexual Activity

For homeless adolescents, sexual activity starts early—their median age of first consensual sex is around 13 (Beech et al., 2003; Cauce et al., 1998), as opposed to approximately 17 for the general population (Guttmacher Institute, 2002). Sexual activity among homeless adolescents may be con-

---

[10]Survival sex can be defined as the "selling of sex to meet subsistence needs," including "shelter, food, drugs, or money" (Greene, Ennett, and Ringwalt, 1999, p. 1406).

sensual, or it may be manipulated, coerced, or forced. In addition to rape (Cauce et al., 1998) and involuntary sex while drunk or high (Rosenthal and Mallett, 2003), survival sex is a pervasive phenomenon in this population (Greene, Ennett, and Ringwalt, 1999; Van Leeuwen et al., 2004; Weber et al., 2004). One large, national study found that 27.5 percent of street youths and 9.5 percent of youths living in shelters had engaged in survival sex (Greene, Ennett, and Ringwalt, 1999). Other studies indicate similar numbers, ranging from 11 percent to more than 30 percent (Beech et al., 2003; Haley et al., 2004; Van Leeuwen et al., 2004). Although adolescents adopt this strategy to survive on the streets, the practice places them at higher risk of victimization, pregnancy, STIs, and sexual and physical assault.

Whether sex among homeless adolescents is voluntary or involuntary, it is likely to be unsafe. Although knowledge and attitudes about safe sex practices vary widely among different subpopulations of homeless adolescents, studies show inconsistent use of condoms both with clients and with casual or main sex partners (Haley et al., 2004; Wagner et al., 2001). Homeless adolescents may be less likely to practice safe sex because they lack access to condoms or are under the influence of alcohol or drugs, or because of the semicoercive nature of survival sex (Tyler et al., 2000). In addition, because most safe sex campaigns target school-based youths, street youths have less access to information about safe sex practices (Beech et al., 2003).

Unsafe sexual practices have serious consequences, including high rates of STIs and unintended pregnancy. Rates of STIs among homeless adolescents are far higher than among their nonhomeless peers (Boivin et al., 2005). Studies of homeless adolescents have found rates of HIV infection ranging as high as 16 percent among certain subpopulations (Beech et al., 2003; Lalota et al., 2005), with one study showing a median rate in four major cities of 2.3 percent (Robertson, 1996). It is estimated that the risk of contracting HIV is 6 to 12 times higher for a homeless than for a nonhomeless adolescent (Rotheram-Borus et al., 2003). The prevalence of other STIs is similarly troubling: rates of hepatitis B, hepatitis C, gonorrhea, syphilis, and chlamydia are all significantly higher than in the general adolescent population (Beech et al., 2003; Rew, Fouladi, and Yockey, 2002; Wagner et al., 2001); overall, between 17 and 28 percent of homeless adolescents have self-reported a history of STIs (Halcon and Lifson, 2004). There is even evidence to suggest a dose-response relationship between running away and STIs: a 2007 study showed that for every one unit increase in running away, there was a correlated 3 percent increase in the likelihood of having an STI (Tyler et al., 2007).

Homeless adolescent girls are at particular risk of the consequences of unsafe sexual practices. They are far more likely than homeless boys to be infected with an STI (Tyler et al., 2007), and are far more likely than their nonhomeless counterparts to become pregnant. More than half report having been pregnant at least once (Halcon and Lifson, 2004), although there is some question whether this number is accurate or is inflated because of malnourished girls mistaking amennorhea for pregnancy (Cauce et al., 1998). Many of these pregnancies end in miscarriage or abortion (Halcon and Lifson, 2004), and girls report knowing of friends who have tried drugs or abuse to self-induce abortion (Ensign, 2000). Homeless girls who are pregnant lack access to medical care and good nutrition and are more likely to use alcohol or drugs, resulting in poor health outcomes for both mother and child (Little et al., 2007).

Drug and Alcohol Use

The prevalence of drug and alcohol use among homeless adolescents is staggeringly high. In many cases, substance use starts before the adolescent leaves home (Rew, Taylor-Seehafer, and Fitzgerald, 2001); however, there exists a "continuum of risk" of substance use, with street youths using the most, nonhomeless youths the least, and shelter-based youths falling in between (Feldmann and Middleman, 2003). In addition to the health effects directly associated with drug and alcohol use, substance dependence can lead to secondary health risks, such as intravenous drug–related HIV and hepatitis exposure, the trading of unsafe sex for drugs, and a heightened danger of sexual or physical victimization (Rosenthal and Mallett, 2003).

Homeless adolescents start using substances early—one study indicates that a majority begin using alcohol, marijuana, and cocaine by age 12 (Rew, Taylor-Seehafer, and Fitzgerald, 2001). They use a wide variety of substances, including alcohol, marijuana, cocaine, methamphetamines, ecstasy, heroin, crack, hallucinogens, and ketamine. Exact rates of use are difficult to ascertain, but most studies suggest that homeless adolescents use at far higher rates than their nonhomeless peers (Thompson, 2004). More than 50 percent of homeless adolescents use alcohol, and more than a third consume in excess of 15 drinks a week (Lifson and Halcon, 2001; Van Leeuwen et al., 2004). Marijuana is one of the most frequently used drugs, at rates of up to 75 percent, and more than a third of homeless adolescents use marijuana at least three times a week (Lifson and Halcon, 2001; Van Leeuwen et al., 2004). Use of intravenous drugs, with its concomitant risk of HIV and hepatitis, is cause for serious concern. Rates of use of these drugs range from 15 percent to more than 30 percent (Feldmann and Middleman, 2003; Lifson and Halcon, 2001), and studies indicate that homelessness is associated with initiating and continuing the injection of drugs (Roy et al., 2003; Steensma et al., 2005).

Mental Health

The prevalence of mental health disorders in homeless adolescents is considerably higher than in the general adolescent population (Boivin et al., 2005; Unger et al., 1997). In this population, depression, dysthymia, internalizing and externalizing disorders, and dissociative symptoms are common diagnoses, and suicide is one of the leading causes of death (Boivin et al., 2005; Cauce et al., 2000; MacLean, Embry, and Cauce, 1999; Tyler, Cauce, and Whitbeck, 2004). Some of these mental health disorders exist before homelessness, and they may, in fact, play a role in an adolescent's leaving or being kicked out of the home (Rohde et al., 2001). Other mental health problems, however, are the direct consequence of life on the streets. Many homeless adolescents are dealing with a history of abuse, substance abuse issues, a feeling of being trapped or helpless, and daily survival—all of which render mental health disorders practically inevitable (Kidd, 2006; Thompson et al., 2007; Tyler, Cauce, and Whitbeck, 2004).

Many studies note the link between stressful situations and the development of mental health disorders in homeless adolescents. Rew (2002) asserts that simply surviving in stressful environments makes homeless adolescents particularly vulnerable to psychological problems. Thompson and colleagues (2007) identify post-traumatic stress disorder as a consequence of exposure to street life. Tyler and Cauce (2002) observe that when homeless youths, who lack resources and support, experience stressors, they may turn to dissociative behavior in order to cope. Unger and colleagues (1998) find an association between stressful life events and depressive symptoms in homeless adolescents. Away from home, adolescents must deal with finding food and shelter, facing the risk of criminal and sexual victimization, and adapting to the culture of street life. These pressures are likely to contribute to emotional distress and mental health disorders, particularly when coupled with a lack of resources, support, and mental health care services.

In addition to the stress of living on the streets, two other factors commonly faced by homeless adolescents are highly correlated with mental health disorders: a history of physical, emotional, and sexual abuse, and current substance abuse issues. Youths with a history of abuse are far more likely to be depressed (Feldmann and Middleman, 2003; Stein, Leslie, Nyamathi, 2002), to display dissociative symptoms (Tyler, Cauce, and Whitbeck, 2004), to self-mutilate (Tyler et al., 2003), and to be suicidal (Unger et al., 1997). Among homeless adolescents, abuse of drugs and alcohol is associated with suicide (Rohde et al., 2001; Unger et al., 1997), self-injurious behavior, depression, and low self-esteem (Unger et al., 1997).

Regardless of when or how mental health disorders arise, it is evident that they are widespread in this population and that they have serious consequences for the affected individuals. One study found that two-thirds of its sample had symptoms that matched the criteria listed in the *Diagnostic and Statistical Manual*, Third Edition Revised (DSM III-R),[11] for such a disorder (Cauce et al., 2000). Highly prevalent disorders included depression, mania, post-traumatic stress disorder, and schizophrenia (Cauce et al., 2000). Another study found that 12.2 percent of its sample had a DSM, Fourth Edition (DSM-IV), diagnosis of major depression, and 6.5 percent had been diagnosed with dysthymia. Homeless adolescents themselves report high rates of mental health disorders: 44 percent in one study reported feeling "depressed or sad often" (Feldmann and Middleman, 2003), and in another study, 32 percent "perceived a need for help with mental health problems" (Solorio et al., 2006). Unfortunately, these adolescents often resort to hurting themselves. Self-injurious behavior and self-mutilation are widespread among homeless adolescents (Tyler et al., 2003; Unger et al., 1997). As noted, suicide is among the leading causes of death for homeless adolescents (Boivin et al., 2005; Roy et al., 2004); moreover, studies have found suicide attempt rates ranging from 18 to 53 percent, and suicide ideation rates of 28 to 62 percent (Yoder et al., 2008).

In sum, homeless adolescents are at acute risk of developing mental health disorders because of both their family history and their everyday life. With a lack of resources, support, and mental health care, these disorders can have life-or-death consequences.

Homeless Adolescents Who Are Lesbian, Gay, Bisexual, or Transgender

Within the population of homeless adolescents, those who are lesbian, gay, bisexual, or transgender (LGBT)[12] are at an even greater risk of poor physical and mental health and more likely to engage in risky behaviors. (The health risks faced by LGBT adolescents generally are discussed in detail in a later section.) LGBT youths make up a sizable proportion of homeless adolescents. Numbers vary widely, but an analysis of the available literature performed by the National Gay and Lesbian Task Force suggests that between 20 and 40 percent of homeless youths are LGBT (Ray, 2006). Being LGBT increases the likelihood of becoming homeless: "coming out" can be a trigger for leaving home, whether because of verbal or physical disputes with parents or parents kicking the youths out (Ray, 2006; Rew, Fouladi, and Yockey, 2002). Once homeless, LGBT youths are more likely

---

[11]*The Diagnostic and Statistical Manual of Mental Disorders* is the U.S. standard diagnostic tool for mental disorders of the American Psychiatric Association (http://www.psychiatryonline.com/).

[12]The group referred to as "lesbian, gay, bisexual, and transgender" sometimes also encompasses the term "questioning" and is commonly referred to by the acronym LGBT (or GLBT) or LGBTQ (or GLBTQ). For the purposes of this report, the identifier "lesbian, gay, bisexual, and transgender" or LGBT is used.

than other homeless youths to engage in a multitude of practices associated with health problems, including substance abuse, survival sex, and risky sex.

Multiple factors are involved in LGBT youths' increased health risks. Homeless LGBT youths are more likely to have been abused as children, more likely to abuse substances, and more likely to have mental health disorders relative to other homeless youths (Noell and Ochs, 2001; Rew et al., 2005; Whitbeck et al., 2004). When these factors are compounded by a lack of familial support, the increased threat of victimization, and the social stigma and discrimination faced by all LGBT youths, homeless LGBT adolescents are at a profound risk for poor mental and physical health outcomes. LGBT homeless adolescents are far more likely than their heterosexual counterparts to engage in survival sex (Gaetz, 2004; Weber et al., 2004); they are more likely to engage in risky sexual behavior (Cochran et al., 2002); and their higher incidence of STIs, including HIV, reflects this difference (Rew et al., 2005). LGBT homeless adolescents abuse alcohol and drugs at greater rates than their heterosexual peers (Noell and Ochs, 2001; Van Leeuwen et al., 2004), putting them at greater risk of associated comorbidities, including mental health disorders and disease related to the use of intravenous drugs. LGBT status among homeless adolescents is correlated with higher rates of depression (Noell and Ochs, 2001) and other mental health disorders (Cochran et al., 2002; Whitbeck et al., 2004), increasing the chances of considered or attempted suicide (Gibson, 1989). Finally, LGBT homeless adolescents are at greater risk of victimization on the streets: according to one study, they "reported an average of 7.4 more perpetrators of sexual victimization than did heterosexual youths" (Cochran et al., 2002, p. 774). LGBT homeless adolescents must contend with both the unique issues of being a sexual minority and the stresses of street life, and these multiple factors amplify and exacerbate their risk of poor mental and physical health.

Adolescents in Families That Have Recently Immigrated

The dramatic change in the racial and ethnic makeup of the United States since the decennial census in 1990 has been fueled by immigration at levels unseen since the early 1900s (Schmidley, 2001), as well as by high birth rates among immigrant women, largely of Hispanic origin (Sutton and Mathews, 2006). Over the 10-year period from 1990 to 2000, the proportion of children in the United States living in immigrant families rose from 15 to 20 percent (Hernandez, 2004). Children living in immigrant households may themselves be foreign born, or may be U.S. citizens with one or two foreign-born parents. Of all children under age 18 living in households in 2005, 20 percent were of Hispanic origin, 4 percent were Asian, and a total of 4 percent were foreign born. Four of five children of immigrants are U.S. citizens, and three of five children of immigrants have at least one parent who is a noncitizen (Capps et al., 2004). However, citizenship status decreases with increasing age. Nearly 2.5 million adolescents aged 10–19 are not U.S. citizens, compared with fewer than 1 million children aged 0–9 (U.S. Census Bureau, 2005). As will be described, the mere fact that a child or adolescent lives in an immigrant family has an impact on his or her health and health care.

Children and adolescents in immigrant families may be located along the three traditional migrant streams in the United States or in major urban centers, but they increasingly reside in nontraditional immigrant centers, described as "new Latino destinations . . . from Wilmington to West Palm Beach, from Little Rock to Las Vegas" and marked by rapid population change from 1990 to 2000 (Suro and Singer, 2002, p. 5). The likelihood that these children are foreign born, being either legalized residents or undocumented immigrants, rises with their age, recognizing that most immigrant families are of mixed status, with one or two noncitizen parents and younger children that are likely to be U.S. citizens (Capps et al., 2004). In addition to a higher likelihood of living in poverty, overcrowded housing, and linguistic and social isolation, these adolescents are less likely to have graduated from high school at age 19 (with Mexican, Central American, Dominican, Indochinese, and Haitian immigrant children being least likely among all racial and ethnic groups) (Hernandez, 2004). They are also less likely to have access to family supports through federal benefits such as the Temporary Assistance for Needy Families program or food stamps because of ineligibility due to their immigration status (Capps et al., 2004).

A subset of the children in immigrant families live in the families of migrant or seasonal workers, where the very nature of that work and the situation in which they live place their health at additional risk. In the 2001–2002 school year, nearly 875,000 students aged 3–21 were eligible for services in the Migrant Education Program. Although the vast majority of these students were Hispanic (89 percent), there were white, black, Asian, and American Indian/Alaskan Native children in migrant families as well. In 2001–2002, more than 190,000 of these students were in grades 7–12 (U.S. Department of Education, 2006). Knowledge of health risks to the children of migrant and seasonal agricultural workers has existed for more than 30 years. These risks range from environmental factors such as increased exposure to lead (Osband and Tobin, 1972) and nutritional deficiencies (Berman, 2003), to infectious hazards related to close living quarters and poor sanitation (Gwyther and Jenkins, 1998), to injuries associated with the agricultural milieu (Wilk, 1993) in which these children live. Higher infant mortality rates (Slesinger, Christenson, and Cautley, 1986) and poor oral health (Castiglia, 1997; Flores et al., 2002) have also been seen in these families, and agricultural workers continue to have the highest worker fatality rates in the nation (U.S. Bureau of Labor Statistics, 2007).

Unfortunately, results of more recent research using participatory methods show that this burden of risk is compounded by the fact that children of agricultural workers have high levels of unmet health needs—far above, for instance, those of their nonmigrant Hispanic or Mexican American contemporaries (Weathers et al., 2003). Although this research and a subsequent study by the same group did not focus specifically on adolescents, a lack of transportation and not knowing where to go for health services were the two main reasons identified for the most recent unmet medical need (Weathers et al., 2003), factors that would presumably apply to adolescents either within a migrant family or, even more so, on their own in the agricultural environment.

The health status of immigrant children and adolescents has received increased emphasis in the literature recently as more attention has been paid to the overall health status of racial and ethnic minority children, particularly Latinos, in the United States. However, much remains to be learned. What has been and continues to be well described is the "healthy immigrant effect," which denotes direct relationships between lower acculturation (by a variety of surrogate measures) and lower rates of obesity and mental disorders in adults and better neonatal outcomes (Flores and Brotanek, 2005). Concerning risky and health-protective behaviors among adolescents, lower acculturation has been found to be associated with both later onset and lower rate of sexual intercourse (Adam et al., 2005), less alcohol use, less cigarette use, and increased likelihood of eating breakfast (Ebin et al., 2001). It appears, however, that this protective effect on health status and health behaviors wanes with the amount of time an adolescent lives in the United States and is nearly gone by the third generation (National Research Council and Institute of Medicine, 1998). Furthermore, there is much heterogeneity among immigrant adolescents, including within racial and ethnic subgroups. Factors such as country of origin and language spoken, as well as length of time in the United States, have a significant impact in research seeking to tease out the best measure of acculturation and its most accurate correlation with health status and health risk (Yu et al., 2003). Tremendous public health gains would be realized with enhanced understanding of this link between acculturation and health (Flores and Brotanek, 2005).

Lesbian, Gay, Bisexual, and Transgender Adolescents

LGBT adolescents face the typical issues that all adolescents encounter as they transition to adulthood; however, they have unique needs due to the social stigma that results from the minority status of their sexual orientation and gender identity (Perrin, 2002). Many of these adolescents endure rejection, ridicule, harassment, social isolation, and discrimination; some fail to find support within their families or communities to help them cope with these challenges. For some adolescents, this stigma may induce psychosocial stress that can lead to increased risky behavior and possibly poorer health outcomes due to a lack of access to appropriate health services.

Researchers face numerous challenges in estimating the prevalence of homosexuality in the general population of adolescents or adults, including difficulties in identifying representative sample populations and measuring sexual minority status. Most prevalence estimates are likely underestimates, in part because of the societal stigmatization of homosexual orientation (Stronski Huwiler and Remafedi, 1998). The use of differing methods for measuring sexual orientation (self-identified sexual orientation, romantic attraction, or sexual activity) has made comparisons among studies problematic at best (Friedman and Downey, 1994). As well, existing data may disproportionately reflect the experience of LGBT adolescents who are participating in more risky behavior, since those adolescents who participate less in such behavior may not have health issues that result in their appearing in health settings where the data are collected, or may be less public about their sexual orientation. Although the prevalence data discussed below are limited by these methodological issues, they nonetheless represent a starting point for understanding the impact of the healthy development of LGBT adolescents on the health of the overall U.S. adult population.

In a national population-based survey of junior high and high school students, 7 percent reported having same-sex romantic attractions or relationships (Russell and Joyner, 2001). In another national study, adolescent children of participants in the Nurses Health Study II were asked to identify themselves on a spectrum of sexuality, from completely heterosexual to completely homosexual.[13] One percent of the adolescents described themselves as homosexual or bisexual, 5 percent as mostly heterosexual, and 2 percent as unsure (Austin et al., 2004a). Finally, in a statewide representative sample of 7th through 12th graders in Minnesota,[14] 1.1 percent of students identified themselves as homosexual or bisexual, while 4.5 percent reported same-sex sexual attractions. The proportion of students reporting that they were unsure of their sexual orientation declined with age: 25 percent of 12-year-olds compared with 5 percent of 18-year-olds (Remafedi et

---

[13]The Growing Up Today Study surveyed 16,882 children of women from the ongoing Nurses Health Study II. Youths were asked to identify themselves as completely heterosexual, mostly heterosexual, bisexual, mostly homosexual, completely homosexual, or not sure. Those reporting mostly homosexual, completely homosexual, and bisexual were combined to create an LGB category.

[14]The 1987 Minnesota Adolescent Health Survey included 34,706 students. It asked about sexual orientation and about the sex of individuals involved in their sexual fantasies, attractions, and experiences.

al., 1992). Among the adult population, estimates of homosexuality range from 3 to 10 percent, although a larger proportion report ever having same-sex attractions or behavior (Fay et al., 1989; Friedman and Downey, 1994; Seidman and Rieder, 1994; Sell, Wells, and Wypij, 1995; Stronski Huwiler and Remafedi, 1998).

A plethora of studies have examined health-related behavior and outcomes for LGB[15] adolescents (Kourany, 1987; Lemp et al., 1994; Noell and Ochs, 2001; Safren and Heimberg, 1999). However, many of these studies are based on nonrepresentative, convenience, or community samples (Russell, 2003). Several statewide school-based surveys and two large national surveys provide limited data on the differences between LGB and heterosexual adolescents with respect to a variety of health-related behaviors and outcomes (Austin et al., 2004b; Garofalo et al., 1998; Robin et al., 2002; Saewyc et al., 1998; Udry and Chantala, 2002). The rest of this section details these data in the areas of suicide, substance abuse and smoking, eating disorders, sexual activity and STIs, violence, and psychosocial stressors. This is followed by a discussion of special issues for transgender teens.

Suicide

State and national random samples of high school students demonstrate a higher rate of suicide attempts among LGB compared with heterosexual adolescents. In a study using representative data from the Vermont and Massachusetts Youth Risk Behavior Survey (YRBS),[16] students who reported sexual experiences with members of both sexes were five times more likely to report serious suicide attempts (controlling for age, gender, and incidence of forced sex) than those who reported sexual experiences with members of the same sex only. This difference in risk did not exist for students with same-sex sexual experiences compared with those with opposite-sex sexual experiences (Robin et al., 2002). In a representative sample from the Minnesota Adolescent Health Survey, after controlling for demographic factors, those boys identifying themselves as homosexual or bisexual were seven times more likely to attempt suicide than heterosexual males (Remafedi et al., 1998; Robin et al., 2002). In data from both the

---

[15] In most cases, the data presented do not include an explicit focus on transgender adolescents, and therefore the acronym LGB is used. A separate discussion of transgender adolescents follows this section.

[16] The 1995 and 1997 YRBS from Massachusetts (n = 4,159 and n = 3,982, respectively) and Vermont (n = 5,987 and n = 8,636, respectively) surveyed 9th- through 12th-grade students. In Massachusetts, the surveys asked students about the sex of individuals with whom they had had sexual contact and their own sexual orientation (heterosexual, gay/lesbian, bisexual, not sure). In Vermont, students were asked only the sex of those with whom they had had sexual contact (male, female, both).

U.S. National Longitudinal Study of Adolescent Health (Add Health)[17] and the Massachusetts YRBS, sexual orientation was an independent predictor of suicide attempts; LGB adolescents were twice as likely to attempt suicide, after controlling for such mediating factors as substance abuse, violence, victimization, and depression (Russell and Joyner, 2001; Udry and Chantala, 2002).

Substance Abuse and Smoking

Adolescents who report having sexual contact with, attractions to, or relationships with individuals of both sexes are at higher risk for substance use than their peers reporting sexual contact with, attractions to, and relationships with the opposite sex only. State and national data indicate that these adolescents are more likely to report marijuana use, binge drinking, getting drunk, drinking alone, and illicit drug use than their heterosexual peers (Robin et al., 2002; Russell, Driscoll, and Truong, 2002). Rates of substance use for adolescents reporting same-sex sexual attractions and behavior are comparable to the rates for their heterosexual peers. A similar pattern exists for tobacco use. In Add Health, although there were no differences in tobacco use between adolescents with same-sex and opposite-sex attractions, adolescents reporting attractions to both sexes smoked more cigarettes than those reporting attractions only to the opposite sex. In the Massachusetts YRBS, adolescents describing themselves as LGB were more likely to smoke cigarettes than heterosexual adolescents; however, this study did not analyze smoking rates for homosexual and bisexual adolescents separately (Garofalo et al., 1998; Russell, Driscoll, and Truong, 2002).

Eating Disorders

Data from the Growing Up Today Study show that health risk behaviors related to eating and body image disorders are less likely among self-identified lesbian girls than among heterosexual girls, while the opposite is true for self-identified gay versus heterosexual boys. Lesbian and bisexual girls are happier with their bodies and less likely to report trying to look like images of women in the media, whereas gay and bisexual boys are more concerned with trying to look like images of men in the media and more likely to binge eat (Austin et al., 2004b).

---

[17]This study surveyed 11,940 students using an audio computer-aided interview and asked about the sex of the individuals to whom they had been attracted or with whom they had had sexual relationships.

Sexual Activity and Sexually Transmitted Infections

Risky sexual behavior puts all adolescents at risk for STIs, including HIV/AIDS. LGB adolescents report more unprotected sex, earlier age at initiation of sexual intercourse, and more sexual partners than heterosexual adolescents (Garofalo et al., 1998). Anal intercourse without a condom puts gay and bisexual male adolescents at high risk for HIV/AIDS, hepatitis B, and HPV anal carcinoma, as well as other STIs (Makadon, 2006). In addition, unprotected anal or oral sex increases the risk for transmission of hepatitis A (Garofalo and Harper, 2003). Lesbian adolescents are also more likely to engage in risky sexual behavior and may experience higher rates of negative health outcomes compared with heterosexual girls. In the Massachusetts YRBS, self-identified lesbian and bisexual girls who had had sexual intercourse were more likely to report unprotected sex with a male and had more pregnancies than heterosexual girls who had had sexual intercourse (Carlson et al., 1995). This behavior poses an increased risk for STIs, HIV/AIDS, and unintended pregnancy. In working to improve these sexual health outcomes for LGB adolescents, it is important to recognize that it is sexual activity, not sexual orientation, that puts adolescents at increased risk of these outcomes (Garofalo and Katz, 2001; Perrin, 2002).

Violence

LGB adolescents face a disproportionate risk for violence as a result of their sexual minority status. Those who report same-sex attractions have higher rates of being threatened with a weapon, being in a physical fight in the previous 12 months, being forced to have sex in the previous 12 months, and missing school because of fear for their own safety (Robin et al., 2002; Russell, Franz, and Driscoll, 2001).

Psychosocial Stressors

LGB adolescents must endure the emotional stress related to social isolation and fear of discovery, which itself can lead to peer rejection, loss of friends, school failure, and discrimination (Kreiss and Patterson, 1997). They must decide whether to disclose their sexual orientation or even questions about their sexual orientation to others. Disclosure can result in family conflict and rejection, which in some cases can lead to homelessness (Kreiss and Patterson, 1997; Perrin, 2002). As discussed above, homeless teens face a number of other risks, including survival sex, poverty, poor access to health services, and victimization (Kruks, 1991).

Special Issues for Transgender Teens

The term transgender denotes individuals who have persistent and distressing discomfort with their biological sex (White, 1998). In DSM-IV, these individuals are considered to have gender identity disorder, a diagnosis that requires evidence of a strong and persistent cross-gender identification (the desire to be or the insistence that one is of the other sex) and persistent discomfort about one's phenotypic sex. There must be evidence of clinically significant distress or impairment in functioning without a concurrent intersex condition (American Psychiatric Association, 2000). Transgender adolescents may be romantically attracted to males, females, or members of both sexes; gender identity does not confer or assume any particular sexual orientation.

While there are no U.S. national or state-based representative data on transgenderism in adolescents, convenience and other nonrepresentative samples have revealed that these adolescents often suffer from depression, suicide attempts, risky sexual behavior, violence, HIV infection, and homelessness (Clements-Nolle et al., 2001; Garofalo et al., 2006; Lombardi et al., 2001). Transgender individuals frequently encounter extreme social prejudice because of their gender-atypical behavior, causing them even greater psychological and emotional distress (Lombardi, 2001).

Adolescents in the Juvenile Justice System

According to the then acting U.S. Surgeon General, Rear Admiral Kenneth Moritsugu:

> On an average day, approximately 100,000 young people are housed in juvenile justice residential facilities and about one-half million are on court-ordered community supervision. An additional 100,000 young people are on informal probation supervision. These young people are medically underserved in the community; they are underinsured and are less likely to have a medical home. (Office of Juvenile Justice and Delinquency Prevention, 2007b)

In 2005, there were 2.1 million juvenile (adolescents under age 18) arrests, a substantial decline from the number in 1996 (Office of Juvenile Justice and Delinquency Prevention, 2007a). Approximately 16 percent of these arrests were for substance use–related crimes (including drug abuse and liquor law violations, driving under the influence, and drunkenness). In 2005, females accounted for 29 percent of all juvenile arrests; this percentage increased in the 1990s. There are more racial and ethnic minority than white adolescents in juvenile justice residential settings (American Academy of Pediatrics Committee on Adolescence, 2001). Further analysis of the adolescent population in residential settings reveals that 62 percent are minorities, 85 percent are males, and a majority lack adequate health insurance (Sickmund, Sladky, and Kang, 2004). Of those arrested, however, most do not end up at trial, and of those whose cases are adjudicated, two-thirds are sentenced to probation (National Center for Juvenile Justice, 2007), allowing for community-based interventions.

Adolescents who come in contact with the justice system and are detained or incarcerated in correctional facilities have a variety of medical and emotional disorders and, as noted, are generally medically underserved (American Academy of Pediatrics Committee on Adolescence, 2001). According to the American Academy of Pediatrics Committee on Adolescence (2001), these youths not only enter the system with preexisting health problems, but also develop acute problems linked to their arrest and their stay in the detention or correctional facility. Thus they show greater rates of physical and emotional problems such as substance abuse, STIs, unplanned pregnancies, and psychiatric disorders upon entry (American Academy of Pediatrics Committee on Adolescence, 2001); an elevated risk of suicide during their incarceration (Gallagher and Dobrin, 2006; Roberts and Bender, 2006); and post-traumatic stress disorder upon both entry and release (Mahoney et al., 2004; National Center for Mental Health and Juvenile Justice, 2007) (see the discussion below). This is particularly true for juvenile offenders transferred into the adult criminal justice system and held in adult jails or correctional facilities (Woolard et al., 2005). Moreover, within facilities, girls are more likely than boys to be sexually victimized and to die while incarcerated (Physicians for Human Rights, 2007).

Mental Health and Substance Abuse Problems

Most adolescents held in custody meet diagnostic criteria for some mental or substance abuse disorder, and a substantial percentage meet criteria for both. It is estimated, for example, that 65–70 percent of adolescents in the juvenile justice system have a mental disorder, and for approximately 20 percent, this disorder is serious (Skowyra and Cocozza, 2006; Teplin et al., 2002). The National Center for Addiction and Substance Abuse found that a majority of the juvenile justice population was affected by addiction and substance abuse disorders. The center's 2004 report concluded that four of every five, or 1.9 million out of 2.4 million, juvenile arrests involved offenders who were under the influence of alcohol or drugs at the time of the offense, tested positive for drugs, were arrested for an alcohol- or drug-related offense, or were admitted for substance abuse. In addition to use of alcohol and illegal drugs, there are high rates of cigarette smoking among this population, necessitating smoking cessation interventions. One study also found that 63 percent of detained juveniles assessed as having a substance abuse disorder also had at least one comorbid mental health diagnosis (Hussey et al., 2005), including ADHD, conduct disorder, posttraumatic stress disorder, depression, and oppositional defiant disorder (Clark and Gehshan, 2006).

Oral Health

Although mental health, substance abuse, and other medical conditions within this population have received significant attention, much less consideration has been given to oral health concerns. Although there are no national prevalence data on this issue for the juvenile justice system, a survey in Washington State found that 65.9 percent of adolescents in its juvenile justice system reported dental problems (Anderson and Farrow, 1998).

Sexually Transmitted Infections

Adolescents in the juvenile justice system have particularly elevated rates of STIs. A recent review (Golzari, Hunt, and Anoshiravani, 2006) found prevalence rates of up to 18–22 percent, depending on whether a specific individual disease or a general category of "any" STI was considered.

Other Medical Problems

Feinstein and colleagues (1998) report that 10 percent of adolescents admitted to detention had significant medical problems other than substance abuse or STIs. Common among these problems were asthma, orthopedic problems, and otolaryngologic conditions. Yet only one-third of adolescents in detention had a regular provider of medical care, and just 20 percent had a private physician. With growing numbers of females in the justice system, gynecological and prenatal care is also required (American Academy of Pediatrics Committee on Adolescence, 2001).

Risk of Victimization Within Facilities

The National Commission on Correctional Health Care (1998) noted that juveniles in adult correctional facilities are particularly vulnerable to victimization, and stated that the incarceration of adolescents in adult facilities is "detrimental to [their] health and developmental well-being." This conclusion is further supported by Woolard and colleagues (2005) and other researchers (Bishop et al., 1996; Committee on Adolescence, 2001; Forst, Fagan, and Scott, 1989; Steinberg, Chung, and Little, 2004), who have found that adolescents in adult prisons are a particularly vulnerable population, at risk for physical and emotional abuse, suicide, and death.

Finding: Certain subpopulations of adolescents defined by selected demographic characteristics and other circumstances—such as those who are poor or members of a racial or ethnic minority; in the foster care system; homeless; in a family that has recently immigrated to the United States; lesbian, gay, bisexual, or transgender; or in the juvenile justice system—have higher rates of chronic health problems and may engage in more risky behavior relative to the overall adolescent population.

SUMMARY

Most adolescents are healthy as defined by traditional measures of mortality, morbidity, and use of health services. Even though these traditional indicators give reason for optimism, behavioral indicators of health status continue to show little improvement in the overall well-being of adolescents. The health problems of adolescents are primarily behavioral and environmental in origin, dominated by interpersonal violence, motor vehicle crashes, substance (including tobacco and alcohol) use and abuse, problems associated with risky sexual behavior, risky eating behavior, inadequate physical activity, and mental disorders. These behaviors not only affect adolescents' immediate health, but also have a significant impact on their health as adults. It is important as well to provide health services that are attentive and responsive to the needs of specific subpopulations of adolescents with certain characteristics, such as being low-income, a racial/ethnic minority, in the foster care system, homeless, living in an immigrant family, LGBT, or in the juvenile justice system, since evidence shows that these young people often have higher rates of chronic health problems, may engage in more risky behavior, and may live in social environments that place them at greater risk relative to the overall adolescent population. Looking at these data, the committee is struck by the need for a focus on prevention; on behavioral health issues; on mental health issues; on oral health issues; and on disparities in health status that derive from income, race, and special circumstances. Available health services for adolescents and the extent to which they respond to these needs are explored in subsequent chapters.

REFERENCES

Adam, M., McGuire, J., Walsh, M., Basta, J., and LeCroy, C. (2005). Acculturation as a predictor of the onset of sexual intercourse among Hispanic and white teens. *Archives of Pediatrics and Adolescent Medicine, 159,* 261–265.

Akinbami, L. J. (2006). The state of childhood asthma, United States, 1980–2005. *Vital Health Statistics, 381,* 1–24.

Albandar, J. J., Brown, L. J., and Löe, H. (1997). Clinical features of early-onset periodontitis. *Journal of the American Dental Association, 128*, 1393–1399.

American Academy of Pediatrics Committee on Adolescence. (2001). Health care for children and adolescents in the juvenile correctional care system. *Pediatrics, 107*, 799–803.

American Psychiatric Association. (2000). *Diagnostic and Statistical Manual of Mental Disorders*, Text Revision, 4th ed. Washington, DC: American Psychiatric Association.

Anderson, B., and Farrow, J. A. (1998). Incarcerated adolescents in Washington State. *Adolescent Health, 22*, 363–367.

Anderson, R., Dearwater, S. R., Olson, T., Aaron, D. J., Kriska, A. M., and LaPorte, R. E. (1994). The role of socioeconomic status and injury morbidity in adolescents. *Archives of Pediatric and Adolescent Medicine, 148*, 245–249.

Andres-Lemay, V. J., Jamieson, E., and MacMillan, H. L. (2005). Child abuse, psychiatric disorder, and running away in a community sample of women. *Canadian Journal of Psychiatry, 50*, 684–689.

Austin, S. B., Ziyadeh, N., Fisher, L. B., Kahn, J. A., Colditz, G. A., and Frazier, A. L. (2004a). Sexual orientation and tobacco use in a cohort study of U.S. adolescent girls and boys. *Archives of Pediatrics and Adolescent Medicine, 158*, 317–322.

Austin, S. B., Ziyadeh, N., Kahn, J. A., Camargo, C. A., Jr., Colditz, G. A., and Field, A. E. (2004b). Sexual orientation, weight concerns, and eating-disordered behaviors in adolescent girls and boys. *Journal of the American Academy of Child and Adolescent Psychiatry, 43*, 1115–1123.

Bao, W. N., Whitbeck, L. B., and Hoyt, D. R. (2000). Abuse, support, and depression among homeless and runaway adolescents. *Journal of Health and Social Behavior, 41*, 408–420.

Barbell, K., and Freundlich, M. (2001). *Foster Care Today*. Available: www.casey.org [June 18, 2007].

Barnes, P. M., and Schoenborn, C. A. (2003). *Physical Activity among Adults: United States, 2000*. Hyattsville, MD: National Center for Health Statistics.

Barton, S. J. (1999). Promoting family-centered care with foster families. *Pediatric Nursing, 25*, 57–60.

Beech, B. M., Myers, L., Beech, D. J., and Kernick, N. S. (2003). Human immunodeficiency syndrome and Hepatitis B and C infections among homeless adolescents. *Seminars in Pediatric Infectious Diseases, 14*, 12–19.

Beltran-Anguilar, E. D., Barker, L. K., Canto, M. T., Dye, B. A., Gooch, B. F., Griffin, S. O., Hyman, J., Jaramillo, F., Kingman, A., Nowjack-Raymer, R., Selwitz, R. H., and Wu, T. (2005). Surveillance for dental caries, dental sealants, tooth retention, edentulism, and enamel fluorosis—United States, 1988–1994 and 1999–2002. *Morbidity and Mortality Weekly Report Surveillance Summaries, 54*, 1–44.

Berman, S. (2003). Health care research on migrant farm worker children: Why has it not had a higher priority? *Pediatrics, 111*, 1106–1107.

Bethell, C., Read, D., Blumberg, J. S., and Newacheck, W. P. (2008). What is the prevalence of children with special health care needs? Toward an understanding of variations in findings and methods across three national durveys. *Maternal and Child Health, 12*(1), 1–14.

Bishop, D. M., Frazier, C. E., Lanza-Kaduce, L., and Winner, L. (1996). The transfer of juveniles to criminal court: Does it make a difference? *Crime and Delinquency, 42*, 171–191.

Black, M. C., Noonan, R., Legg, M., Eaton, D., and Breiding, M. J. (2006). Physical dating violence among high school students—United States, 2003. *Morbidity and Mortality Weekly Report, 55*(19), 532–535.

Bleyer, A., O'Leary, M., Barr, R., and Ries, L. A. G. (Eds.). (2006). *Cancer Epidemiology in Older Adolescents and Young Adults 15 to 29 Years of Age, Including SEER Incidence and Survival: 1975-2000* (NIH Publication No. 06-5767). Bethesda, MD: National Cancer Institute.

Bloom, B., Dey, A. N., and Freeman, G. (2006). Summary health statistics for U.S. children: National Health Interview Survey, 2005. *Vital Health and Statistics, 10*(231), 1–84.

Blumstein, A., Rivara, F. P., and Rosenfeld, R. (2000). The rise and decline of homicide—and why. *Annual Reviews of Public Health, 21,* 505–541.

Boivin, J. F., Roy, E., Haley, N., and Galbaud du Fort, G. (2005). The health of street youth: A Canadian perspective. *Canadian Journal of Public Health, 96,* 432–437.

Callahan, C. M., and Rivara, F. P. (1992). Urban high school youth and handguns. A school-based survey. *Journal of the American Medical Association, 267,* 3038–3042.

Capps, R., Fix, M., Ost, J., Reardon-Anderson, J., and Passel, J. (2004). *The Health and Well-Being of Young Children of Immigrants.* Washington, DC: The Urban Institute.

Carlson, E., Resnick, M., Bearinger, L., and Blum, R. (1995). Clinical and research poster presentations at the Annual Meeting of the Society for Adolescent Medicine: Heterosexual behaviors and pregnancy among non-heterosexual adolescent girls [Abstract]. *Journal of Adolescent Health, 16,* 161.

Casey Family Programs (2005). *Improving Family Foster Care: Findings from the Northwest Foster Care Alumni Study.* Available: www.casey.org [June 18, 2007].

Casswell, S., Pledger, M., and Hooper, R. (2003). Socioeconomic status and drinking patterns in young adults. *Addiction, 98,* 601–610.

Castiglia, P. (1997). Health needs of migrant children. *Journal of Pediatric Health Care, 11,* 280–282.

Cauce, A. M., Paradise, M., Embry, L., Morgan, C., Theofelis, J., Heger, J., and Wagner, V. (1998). Homeless youth in Seattle: Youth characteristics, mental health needs, and intensive case management. In M. Epstein, K. Kutash, and A. Duchnowski (Eds.), *Outcomes for Children and Youth with Emotional and Behavioral Disorders and their Families: Programs and Evaluation Best Practices* (pp. 611–632). Austin, TX: PRO-ED.

Cauce, A. M., Paradise, M., Ginzler, J. A., Embry, L., Morgan, C. J., Lohr, Y., and Theofelis, J. (2000). The characteristics and mental health of homeless adolescents: Age and gender differences. *Journal of Emotional and Behavioral Disorders, 8,* 230–239.

Centers for Disease Control and Prevention. (2005). Tobacco use, access, and exposure to tobacco in media among middle and high school students—United States, 2004. *Morbidity and Mortality Weekly Report, 54,* 297–301.

Centers for Disease Control and Prevention. (2006a). Physical dating violence among high school students—United States, 2003. *Morbidity and Mortality Weekly Reports, 55,* 532–535.

Centers for Disease Control and Prevention. (2006b). *Sexually Transmitted Disease Surveillance, 2005.* Atlanta, GA: Division of Sexually Transmitted Disease Prevention.

Centers for Disease Control and Prevention. (2006c). *YRBSS Trend Fact Sheets, 1991-2005: Violence.* Available: http://www.cdc.gov/Healthyyouth/yrbs/trends.htm [February 29, 2008].

Centers for Disease Control and Prevention. (2007a). *Diabetes Problems.* Available: http://www.cdc.gov/diabetes/consumer/diabproblems.htm [March 19, 2008].

Centers for Disease Control and Prevention. (2007b). *HIV/AIDS Surveillance in Adolescents and Young Adults (through 2005).* Available: http://www.cdc.gov/hiv/topics/surveillance/resources/slides/adolescents/ [August 7, 2007].

Centers for Disease Control and Prevention. (2007c). *Youth Online: Comprehensive Results Youth Risk Behavior Survey.* Available: http://www.cdc.gov/healthyyouth/physicalactivity/ [August 8, 2007].

Chen, K. W., Killeya-Jones, L. A., and Vega, W. A. (2005). Prevalence and co-occurrence of psychiatric symptom clusters in the U.S. adolescent population using DISC predictive scales. *Clinical Practice and Epidemiology in Mental Health, 1,* 22.

Child and Adolescent Health Measurement Initiative. (2008). *2005/2006 National Survey of Children with Special Health Needs.* Available: www.cshcndata.org [February 20, 2008].

Childhelp. (2006). *National Child Abuse Statistics.* Available: http://www.childhelp.org/resources/learning-center/statistics [March 28, 2008].

Children's Bureau, Administration for Children and Families, and U.S. Department of Health and Human Services. (2007). *Trends in Foster Care and Adoption FY 2000–FY 2005.* Available: http://www.acf.hhs.gov/programs/cb/stats_research/afcars/trends.htm [June 18, 2007].

Clark, K., and Gehshan, S. (2006). *Meeting the Health Needs of Youth Involved in the Juvenile Justice System.* Portland, ME: National Academy for State Health Policy.

Clements-Nolle, K., Marx, R., Guzman, R., and Katz, M. (2001). HIV prevalence, risk behaviors, health care use, and mental health status of transgender persons: Implications for public health intervention. *American Journal of Public Health, 91,* 915–921.

Cochran, B. N., Stewart, A. J., Ginzler, J. A., and Cauce, A. M. (2002). Challenges faced by homeless sexual minorities: Comparison of gay, lesbian, bisexual, and transgender homeless adolescents with their heterosexual counterparts. *American Journal of Public Health, 92*(5), 773–777.

Cohen, P., Cohen, J., Kasen, S. Velez, C. N., Hartmark, C., Johnson, J., Rojas, M., Brook, J., and Streuning, E. L. (1993). An epidemiological study of disorders in late childhood and adolescence, I: Age and gender-specific prevalence. *Journal of Child Psychology and Psychiatry, 34,* 851–867.

Committee on Adolescence. (2001). American Academy of Pediatrics: Health care for children and adolescent in the juvenile correctional care system. *Pediatrics, 107,* 799–803.

Committee on Early Childhood, Adoption, and Dependent Care and American Academy of Pediatrics. (2002). Health care of young children in foster care. *Pediatrics, 109,* 536–541.

Costello, E. J. (1999). Commentary on "Prevalence and impact of parent-reported disabling mental health conditions among U.S. children." *Journal of the American Academy of Child and Adolescent Psychiatry, 38,* 610–613.

Costello, E. J., Angold, A., Burns, B., Stangl, D., Tweed, D., Erkanli, A., and Worthman, C. (1996). The Great Smoky Mountains Study of Youth: Goals, design, methods, and prevalence of DSM-III-R disorders. *Archives of General Psychiatry, 53,* 1129–1136.

Costello, E. J., Mustillo, S., Erkanli, A., Keeler, G., and Angold, A. (2003). Prevalence and development of psychiatric disorders in childhood and adolescence. *Archives of General Psychiatry, 60,* 837–844.

Craig, T. K., and Hodson, S. (1998). Homeless youth in London: I. Childhood antecedents and psychiatric disorder. *Psychological Medicine, 28*(6), 1379–1388.

Datta, D. (2006). *HPV Surveillance in Family Planning Settings.* Presented at the National Title X Grantee Meeting, September, Phoenix, AZ. Available: http://www.ent-s-t.com/OFP_TitleX_Meeting/presentations/N-Deblina%20Day%201%20Plenary%201130am%20b.ppt [September 10, 2007].

De Moor, R. J., De Witte, A. M., Delmé, K. I., De Bruyne, M. A., Hommez, G. M., and Goyvaerts, D. (2005). Dental and oral complications of lip and tongue piercings. *British Dental Journal, 199,* 506–509.

Deshmukh-Taskar, P., Nicklas, T. A., Morales, M., Yang, S. J., Zakeri, I., and Berenson, G. S. (2006). Tracking of overweight status from childhood to young adulthood: The Bogalusa Heart Study. *European Journal of Clinical Nutrition, 60,* 48–57.

DeWit, D. J., Adlaf, E. M., Offord, D. R., and Ogborne, A. C. (2000). Age at first alcohol use: A risk factor for the development of alcohol disorders. *American Journal of Psychiatry, 157,* 745–750.
Dierker, L. C., Donny, E., Tiffany, S., Colby, S. M., Perrine, N., Clayton, R. R., and Tobacco Etiology Research Network. (2007). The association between cigarette smoking and DSM-IV nicotine dependence among first year college students. *Drug and Alcohol Dependence, 86,* 106–114.
Dietz, W. H. (1998). Health consequences of obesity in youth: Childhood predictors of adult disease. *Pediatrics, 101*(3 Pt. 2), 518–525.
DiFranza, J. R., Rigotti, N. A., McNeill, A. D., Ockene, J. K., Savageau, J. A., St Cyr, D., and Coleman, M. (2000). Initial symptoms of nicotine dependence in adolescents. *Tobacco Control, 9,* 313–319.
DiFranza, J. R., Savageau, J. A., Rigotti, N. A., Fletcher, K., Ockene, J. K., McNeill, A. D., Coleman, M., and Wood, C. (2002). Development of symptoms of tobacco dependence in youths: 30-month follow up data from the DANDY study. *Tobacco Control, 11,* 228–235.
Duke, J., Huhman, M., and Heitzler, C. (2003). Physical activity levels among children aged 9–13 years: United States, 2002. *Morbidity and Mortality Weekly Report, 52,* 785–788.
Duncan, G. E. (2006). Prevalence of diabetes and impaired fasting glucose levels among U.S. adolescents. National Health and Nutrition Examination Survey, 1999–2002. *Archives of Pediatric and Adolescent Medicine, 160,* 523–528.
DuRant, R., Champion, H., Wolfson, M., Omli, M., McCoy, T., D'Agostino, R. B., Jr., Wagoner, K., and Mitra, A. (2007). Date fighting experiences among college students: Are they associated with other health-risk behaviors? *Journal of the American College of Health, 55,* 291–296.
Eaton, D. K., Kann, L., Kinchen, S., Ross, J., Hawkins, J., Harris, W. A., Lowry, R., McManus, T., Chyen, D., Shanklin, S., Lim, C., Grunbaum, J. A., and Wechsler, H. (2006). Youth risk behavior surveillance—United States, 2005. *Morbidity and Mortality Weekly Report, 55*(SS-5), 1–108.
Eaton, D. K., Kann, L., Kinchen, S., Shanklin, S., Ross, J., Hawkins, J., Harris, W. A., Lowry, R., McManus, T., Chyen, D., Lim, C., Brener, N. D., and Wechsler, H. (2008). Youth risk behavior surveillance—United States, 2007. *Morbidity and Mortality Weekly Report, 57*(SS-4), 1–131.
Ebin, V. J., Sneed, C. D., Morisky, D. E., Rotheram-Borus, M. J., Magnusson, A. M., and Malotte, C. K. (2001). Acculturation and interrelationships between problem and health-promoting behaviors among Latino adolescents. *Journal of Adolescent Health, 28,* 62–72.
Enns, C. W., Mickle, S. J., and Goldman, J. D. (2003). Trends in food and nutrient intakes by adolescents in the United States. *Family Economics and Nutrition Reviews, 15,* 15–27.
Ensign, J. (2000). Reproductive health of homeless adolescent women in Seattle, Washington, USA. *Women and Health, 31*(2–3), 133–151.
Fagot-Campagna, A., Saaddine, J. B., Flegal, K. M., and Beckles, G. L. (2001). Diabetes, impaired fasting glucose, and elevated HbA1c in U.S. adolescents: The Third National Health and Nutrition Examination Survey. *Diabetes Care, 24,* 834–837.
Farrington, D. P. (2001). The causes and prevention of violence. In J. Shepherd (Ed.), *Violence in Health Care* (pp. 1–27). Oxford: Oxford University Press.
Fay, R. E., Turner, C. F., Klassen, A. D., and Gagnon, J. H. (1989). Prevalence and patterns of same-gender sexual contact among men. *Science, 243,* 338–348.
Federal Interagency Forum on Child and Family Statistics. (2007). *America's Children: Key National Indicators of Well-Being, 2007.* Washington, DC: U.S. Government Printing Office.

Feinstein, R., Lampkin, A., Lorish, C., Klerman, L., and Maisiakj, R. (1998). Medical status of adolescents at the time of admission to a juvenile detention center. *Journal of Adolescent Health, 22,* 190–196.

Feldmann, J., and Middleman, A. B. (2003). Homeless adolescents: Common clinical concerns. *Seminars in Pediatric Infectious Diseases, 14*(1), 6–11.

Field, A. E., Cook, N. R., and Gillman, M. W. (2005). Weight status in childhood as a predictor of becoming overweight or hypertensive in early adulthood. *Obesity Research, 13,* 163–169.

Fields, J. (2003). Children's living arrangements and characteristics: March 2002. *Current Population Reports, P20-547,* June.

Flores, G., and Brotanek, J. (2005). The healthy immigrant effect: A greater understanding might help us improve the health of all children. *Archives of Pediatrics and Adolescent Medicine, 159,* 295–297.

Flores, G., Fuentes-Afflick, E., Barbot, O., Carter-Pokras, O., Claudio, L., Lara, M., McLaurin, J., Pachter, L., Gomez, F. R., Mendoza, F., Valdez, B., Villaruel, A., Zambrana, R., Greenberg, R., and Weitzman, M. (2002). The health of Latino children: Urgent priorities, unanswered questions, and a research agenda. *Journal of the American Medical Association, 288,* 82–90.

Forhan, S. E. (2008). *Prevalence of Sexually Transmitted Infections and Bacterial Vaginosis among Female Adolescents in the United States: Data from the National Health and Nutrition Examination Survey (NHANES) 2003–2004.* Presentation at the 2008 National STD Prevention Conference, March, Chicago, IL.

Forst, J., Fagan, J., and Scott, T. V. (1989). Youth in prison and training schools: Perceptions and consequences of the treatment-custody dichotomy. *Juvenile and Family Court Journal, 40,* 1–4.

Frank, R. G., and Glied, S. (2006). The population with mental illness. In R. G. Frank and S. Glied (Eds.), *Better But Not Well: Mental Health Policy in the United States Since 1950* (pp. 8–25). Baltimore, MD: The Johns Hopkins University Press.

Freedman, D. S., Khan, L. K., Serdula, M. K., Dietz, W. H., Srinivasan, S. R., and Berenson, G. S. (2005a). Racial differences in the tracking of childhood BMI to adulthood. *Obesity Research, 13,* 928–935.

Freedman, D. S., Khan, L. K., Serdula, M. K., Dietz, W. H., Srinivasan, S. R., and Berenson, G. S. (2005b). The relation of childhood BMI to adult adiposity: The Bogalusa Heart Study. *Pediatrics, 115,* 22–27.

Friedman, R. C., and Downey, J. I. (1994). Homosexuality. *New England Journal of Medicine, 331,* 923–930.

Gaetz, S. (2004). Safe streets for whom? Homeless youth, social exclusion, and criminal victimization. *Canadian Journal of Criminology and Criminal Justice, 46*(4), 423–455.

Gallagher, C., and Dobrin, A. (2006). Deaths in juvenile justice residential facilities. *Journal of Adolescent Health, 38,* 662–668.

Garland, S. M., Hernandez-Avila, M., Wheeler, C. M., Perez, G., Harper, D. M., Leodolter, S., Tang, G. W., Ferris, D. G., Steben, M., Bryan, J., Taddeo, F. J., Railkar, R., Esser, M. T., Sings, H. L., Nelson, M., Boslego, J., Sattler, C., Barr, E., Koutsky, L. A., and Females United to Unilaterally Reduce Endo/Ectocervical Disease Investigators. (2007). Quadrivalent vaccine against human papillomavirus to prevent anogenital diseases. *New England Journal of Medicine, 356,* 1928–1943.

Garofalo, R., and Harper, G. W. (2003). Not all adolescents are the same: Addressing the unique needs of gay and bisexual male youth. *Adolescent Medicine State of the Art Reviews, 14,* 595–611.

Garofalo, R., and Katz, E. (2001). Health care issues of gay and lesbian youth. *Current Opinion in Pediatrics, 13,* 298–302.

Garofalo, R., Wolf, R. C., Kessel, S., Palfrey, S. J., and DuRant, R. H. (1998). The association between health risk behaviors and sexual orientation among a school-based sample of adolescents. *Pediatrics, 101,* 895–902.

Garofalo, R., Deleon, J., Osmer, E., Doll, M., and Harper, G. W. (2006). Overlooked, misunderstood and at-risk: Exploring the lives and HIV risk of ethnic minority male-to-female transgender youth. *Journal of Adolescent Health, 38,* 230–236.

Gibson, P. (1989). *Gay Male and Lesbian Youth Suicide.* Report of the Secretary's Task Force on Youth Suicide. Rockville, MD: U.S. Department of Health and Human Services.

Gjelsvik, A., Zierler, S., and Blume, J. (2004). Homicide risk across race and class: A small-area analysis in Massachusetts and Rhode Island. *Journal of Urban Health, 81,* 702–718.

Glassbrenner, D. (2003). *Safety Belt Use in 2002—Demographic Characteristics.* Washington, DC: National Highway Traffic Safety Administration.

Glew, G. M., Fan, M. Y., Katon, W., and Rivara F. P. (2008). Bullying and school safety. *Journal of Pediatrics, 152,* 123–128.

Golzari, M., Hunt, S., and Anoshiravani, A. (2006). The health status of youth in juvenile detention facilities. *Journal of Adolescent Health, 38,* 776–782.

Gordon-Larsen, P., Adair, L. S., Nelson, M. C., and Popkin, B. M. (2004). Five-year obesity incidence in the transition period between adolescence and adulthood: The National Longitudinal Study of Adolescent Health. *American Journal of Clinical Nutrition, 80,* 569–575.

Gortmaker, S. L., and Sappenfield, W. (1984). Chronic childhood disorders: Prevalence and impact. *Pediatric Clinics of North America, 31,* 3–18.

Grant, B. F., and Dawson, D. A. (1997). Age of onset of alcohol use and its association with DSM-IV alcohol abuse and dependence: Results from the National Longitudinal Alcohol Epidemiologic Survey. *Journal of Substance Abuse, 9,* 103–110.

Grant, B. F., and Dawson, D. A. (1998). Age of onset of drug use and its association with DSM-IV drug abuse and dependence: Results from the National Longitudinal Alcohol Epidemiologic Survey. *Journal of Substance Abuse, 10,* 163–173.

Greene, J. M., Ennett, S. T., and Ringwalt, C. L. (1999). Prevalence and correlates of survival sex among runaway and homeless youth. *American Journal of Public Health, 89,* 1406–1409.

Grossman, D. C., Mueller, B. A., Riedy, C., Dowd, M. D., Villaveces, A., Prodzinski, J., Nakagawara, J., Howard, J., Thiersch, N., and Harruff, R. (2005). Gun storage practices and risk of youth suicide and unintentional firearm injuries. *Journal of the American Medical Association, 293,* 707–714.

Grunbaum, J. A., Kann, L., Kinchen, S., Ross, J., Hawkins, J., Lowry, R., Harris, W. A., McManus, T., Chyen, D., and Collins, J. (2004). Youth Risk Behavior Surveillance—United States, 2003. *Morbidity and Mortality Weekly Report: Surveillance Summaries, 53*(SS-02), 1–96.

Guttmacher Institute. (2002). *In Their Own Right: Addressing the Sexual and Reproductive Health Needs of American Men.* New York: Alan Guttmacher Institute.

Guttmacher Institute. (2006). *U.S. Teenage Pregnancy Statistics National and State Trends by Race and Ethnicity.* New York: Alan Guttmacher Institute.

Gwyther, M., and Jenkins, M. (1998). Migrant farmworker children: Health status, barriers to care, and nursing innovations in health care delivery. *Journal of Pediatric Health Care 12,* 60–66.

Halcon, L. L., and Lifson, A. R. (2004). Prevalence and predictors of sexual risks among homeless youth. *Journal of Youth and Adolescence, 33*(1), 71–80.

Haley, N., Roy, E., Leclerc, P., Boudreau, J. F., and Boivin, J. F. (2004). Characteristics of adolescent street youth with a history of pregnancy. *Journal of Pediatric and Adolescent Gynecology, 17*(5), 313–320.

Halfon, N., Mendonca, A., and Berkowitz, G. (1995). Health status of children in foster care: The experience of the center for the vulnerable child. *Archives of Pediatrics and Medicine, 149,* 386–392.

Hallal, P. C., Victora, C. G., Azevedo, M. R., and Wells, J. C. (2006). Adolescent physical activity and health: A systematic review. *Sports Medicine, 36,* 1019–1030.

Hamilton, B. E., Martin, J. A., and Ventura, S. J. (2007). Births: Preliminary data for 2006. *National Vital Statistics Reports, 56*(7). Hyattsville, MD: National Center for Health Statistics.

Hammer, H., Finkelhor, D., and Sedlak, A. J. (2002). *Runaway/thrownaway children: National estimates and characteristics.* Washington, DC: U.S. Department of Justice. Available: http://www.ncjrs.gov/html/ojjdp/nismart/04/ [September 26, 2008].

Hansen, R. L., Kagle, J. D., and Black, J. E. (2004). Comparing the health status of low income children in and out of foster care. *Child Welfare, 83,* 376–380.

Hedley, A. A., Ogden, C. L., Johnson, C. L., Carroll, M. D., Curtin, L. R., and Flegal, K. M. (2004). Prevalence of overweight and obesity among U.S. children, adolescents, and adults, 1999–2002. *Journal of the American Medical Association, 291,* 2847–2850.

Hernandez, D. J. (2004). Demographic change and the life circumstances of immigrant families. *The Future of Children, 14,* 17–47.

Hingson, R. W., and Kenkel, D. (2004). Social health and economic consequences of underage drinking. In National Research Council, *Reducing Underage Drinking: A Collective Responsibility* (pp. 351–382). Washington, DC: The National Academies Press.

Hingson, R. W., Heeren, T., Jamanka, A., and Howland, J. (2000). Age of drinking onset and unintentional injury involvement after drinking. *Journal of the American Medical Association, 284,* 1527–1533.

Hingson, R. W., Heeren, T., and Zakocs, R. (2001). Age of drinking onset and involvement in physical fights after drinking. *Pediatrics, 108,* 872–877.

Hingson, R. W., Heeren, T., Levenson, S., Jamanka, A., and Voas, R. (2002). Age of drinking onset, driving after drinking, and involvement in alcohol related motor-vehicle crashes. *Accident Analysis and Prevention, 34,* 85–92.

Hingson, R. W., Heeren, T., Zakocs, R., Winter, M., and Wechsler, H. (2003). Age of first intoxication, heavy drinking, driving after drinking and risk of unintentional injury among U.S. college students. *Journal of Studies on Alcohol, 64,* 23–31.

Hingson, R. W., Heeren, T., and Winter, M. R. (2006). Age of alcohol-dependence onset: Associations with severity of dependence and seeking treatment. *Pediatrics, 118,* e755–e763.

Hoek, H. W., and van Hoeken, D. (2003). Review of the prevalence and incidence of eating disorders. *International Journal of Eating Disorders, 34,* 383–396.

Hoffman, S. D. (2006). *By the Numbers: The Public Costs of Teen Childbearing.* Washington, DC: National Campaign to Prevent Teen Pregnancy.

Hussey, D., Drinkard, A., Murphy, M., and Ols, K. (2005). *Year-One Outcomes from the Cuyahoga County Strengthening Communities Youth (SCY) Project.* Poster presentation at the 2005 Joint Meeting on Adolescent Treatment Effectiveness. Washington, DC: Substance Abuse and Mental Health Services Administration, Center for Substance Abuse Treatment.

Ikramullah, E., Schelar, E., Manlove, J., and Moore, K. A. (2007). *Facts at a Glance: June 2007.* Washington, DC: Child Trends.

Inkeles, M., and Halfon, N. (2002). *Medicaid and Financing of Health Care for Children in Foster Care: Findings from a National Survey.* Los Angeles: UCLA Center for Healthier Children, Families and Communities.

Institute of Medicine. (2003). *Unequal Treatment: Confronting Racial and Ethnic Disparities in Health Care.* Washington, DC: The National Academies Press.

Institute of Medicine. (2006a). *Dietary Reference Intakes. The Essential Guide to Nutrient Requirements.* Washington, DC: The National Academies Press.
Institute of Medicine. (2006b). *Food Marketing to Children and Youth. Threat or Opportunity?* J. M. McGinnis, J. A. Gootman, and V. I. Kraak, (Eds.). Washington, DC: The National Academies Press.
Johnston, L. D., O'Malley, P. M., Bachman, J. G., and Schulenberg, J. E. (2006). *Monitoring the Future National Survey on Drug Use, 1975–2005. Volume I, Secondary School Students.* Bethesda, MD: National Institute on Drug Abuse.
Johnston, L. D., O'Malley, P. M., Bachman, J. G., and Schulenberg, J. E. (2008). *Monitoring the Future National Results on Adolescent Drug Use: Overview of Key Findings, 2007.* (NIH Publication No. 08-6418.) Bethesda, MD: National Institute on Drug Abuse.
Jones, R. K., Darroch, J. E., and Henshaw, S. K. (2002). Patterns in the socioeconomic characteristics of women obtaining abortions in 2000–2001. *Perspectives on Sexual and Reproductive Health, 34,* 226–235.
Juarez, P., Schlundt, D. G., Goldzweig, I., and Stinson, N., Jr. (2006). A conceptual framework for reducing risky teen driving behaviors among minority youth. *Injury Prevention,* 12(Suppl. 1), i49–i55.
Kandel, D. B., and Chen, K. (2000). Extent of smoking and nicotine dependence in the United States: 1991–1993. *Nicotine and Tobacco Research, 2,* 263–274.
Kandel, D. B., Hu, M. C., Griesler, P. C., and Schaffran, C. (2007). On the development of nicotine dependence in adolescence. *Drug and Alcohol Dependence, 86,* 26–39.
Kashani, J. H., Daniel, A. E., Sulzberger, L. A., Rosemberg, T. K., and Reid, J. C. (1987). Conduct disordered adolescents from a community sample. *Canadian Journal of Psychiatry, 32,* 756–760.
Kataoka, S. H., Zhang, L., and Wells, K. B. (2002). Unmet need for mental health among U.S. children: Variation by ethnicity and insurance status. *American Journal of Psychiatry, 159,* 1548–1555.
Kellermann, A. L., Rivara, F. P., Somes, G., Reay, D. T., Francisco, J., Banton, J. G., Prodzinski, J., Fligner, C., and Hackman, B. B. (1992). Suicide in the home in relation to gun ownership. *New England Journal of Medicine, 327,* 467–472.
Kellermann, A. L., Rivara, F. P., Rushforth, N. B., Banton, J. G., Reay, D. T., Francisco, J. T., Locci, A. B., Prodzinski, J., Hackman, B. B., and Somes, G. (1993). Gun ownership as a risk factor for homicide in the home. *New England Journal of Medicine, 329,* 1084–1091.
Kessler, R. C., and Walters, E. E. (1998). Epidemiology of DSM-III-R major depression and minor depression among adolescents and young adults in The National Comorbidity Survey. *Depression and Anxiety, 7,* 3–14.
Kessler, R. C., Berglund, P., Demler, O., Jin, R., Merikangas, K., and Walters, E. (2005). Lifetime prevalence and age-of-onset distributions of DSM-IV disorders in the National Comorbidity Survey Replication. *Archives of General Psychiatry, 62,* 593–602.
Kidd, S. A. (2006). Factors precipitating suicidality among homeless youth: A quantitative follow-up. *Youth and Society, 37*(4), 393–422.
Kolbe, L. J., Kann, L., and Collins, J. L. (1993). Overview of the Youth Risk Behavior Surveillance System. *Public Health Reports, 108*(Suppl. 1), 2–10.
Kortenkamp, K., and Ehrele, J. (2002). *The Well-Being of Children Involved in the Child Welfare System: A National Overview.* Washington, DC: Urban Institute.
Kourany, R. F. (1987). Suicide among homosexual adolescents. *Journal of Homosexuality, 13,* 111–117.
Kreiss, J. L., and Patterson, D. L. (1997). Psychosocial issues in primary care of lesbian, gay, bisexual, and transgender youth. *Journal of Pediatric Health Care, 11,* 266–274.

Kruks, G. (1991). Gay and lesbian homeless/street youth: Special issues and concerns. *Journal of Adolescent Health, 12,* 515–518.
Kubik, M., Lytle, L., Birnbaum, A., Murray, D., and Perry, C. (2003). Prevalence and correlates of depressive symptoms in young adolescents. *American Journal of Health Behavior, 27,* 546–553.
Kuehn, B. (2007). Many teens abusing medications. *Journal of the American Medical Association, 297,* 578–579.
Lahey, B. B., Miller, T. L., Gordon, R. A., and Riley, A. W. (1999). Developmental Epidemiology of the Disruptive Behavior Disorders. *Handbook of the Disruptive Behavior Disorders.* New York: Plenum Press.
Lalota, M., Kwan, B. W., Waters, M., Hernandez, L. E., and Liberti, T. M. (2005). The Miami, Florida, young men's survey: HIV prevalence and risk behaviors among urban young men who have sex with men who have ever run away. *Journal of Urban Health, 82*(2), 327–338.
Lawrence, D., Fagan, P., Backinger, C. L., Gibson, J. T., and Hartman, A. (2007). Cigarette smoking patterns among young adults aged 18–24 years in the United States. *Nicotine and Tobacco Research, 9,* 687–697.
Lemp, G. F., Hirozawa, A. M., Givertz, D., Nieri, G. N., Anderson, L., Lindegren, M. L., Janssen, R. S., and Katz, M. (1994). Seroprevalence of HIV and risk behaviors among young homosexual and bisexual men. The San Francisco/Berkeley Young Men's Survey. *Journal of the American Medical Association, 272,* 449–454.
Leslie, L. K., Landsverk, J., Ezzet-Lofstrom, R., Tschann, J. M., Slymen, D. S., and Garland, A. (2000). Children in foster care: Factors influencing mental health services utilization. *Child Abuse and Neglect, 24,* 465–476.
Lifson, A. R., and Halcon, L. L. (2001). Substance abuse and high-risk needle-related behaviors among homeless youth in Minneapolis: Implications for prevention. *Journal of Urban Health, 78*(4), 690–698.
Little, M., Gorman, A., Dzendoletas, D., and Moravac, C. (2007). Caring for the most vulnerable: A collaborative approach to supporting pregnant homeless youth. *Nursing for Women's Health, 11*(5), 458–466.
Loeber, R., Burke, J. D., Lahey, B. B., Winters, A., and Zera, M. (2000). Oppositional defiant and conduct disorder: A review of the past 10 years, part I. *Journal of the American Academy of Child and Adolescent Psychiatry, 39,* 1468–1484.
Loeber, R., Lacourse, E., and Homish, D. L. (2005). Homicide, violence and developmental trajectories. In R. E. Tremblay, W. W. Hartup, and J. Archer (Eds.), *Developmental Origins of Aggression* (pp. 202–219). New York: Guilford Press.
Lombardi, E. L. (2001). Enhancing transgender health care. *American Journal of Public Health, 91,* 869–872.
Lombardi, E. L., Wilchins, R. A., Priesing, D., and Malouf, D. (2001). Gender violence: Transgender experiences with violence and discrimination. *Journal of Homosexuality, 42,* 89–101.
Lowry, R., Powell, K. E., Kann, L., Collins, J. L., and Kolbe, L. J. (1998). Weapon-carrying, physical fighting, and fight-related injury among U.S. adolescents. *American Journal of Preventive Medicine, 14,* 122–129.
MacKay, A. P., and Duran, C. (2007). *Adolescent Health in the United States, 2007.* Hyattsville, MD: National Center for Health Statistics.
MacLean, M. G., Embry, L. E., and Cauce, A. M. (1999). Homeless adolescents' paths to separation from family: Comparison of family characteristics, psychology adjustment, and victimization. *Journal of Community Psychology, 27*(2), 179–187.

Mahoney, K., Ford, J., Ko, S., and Siegfried, C. (2004). *Trauma-Focused Interventions for Youth in the Juvenile Justice System*. Los Angeles: National Child Traumatic Stress Network, Juvenile Justice Working Group.

Makadon, H. (2006). Improving health care for the lesbian and gay communities. *New England Journal of Medicine, 354,* 895–897.

Markowitz, L. E., Dunne, E. F., Saraiya, M., Lawson, H. W., Chesson, H., and Unger, E. R. (2007). Quadrivalent human papillomavirus vaccine. Recommendations of the Advisory Committee on Immunization Practices (ACIP). *Morbidity and Mortality Weekly Report, 56,* RR-2.

Martin, J. A., Hamilton, B. E., Sutton, P. D., Ventura, S. J., Menacker, F., and Kirmeyer, S. (2006). Births: Final data for 2004. *National Vital Statistics Reports, 55*(1), 1–101.

Maternal and Child Health Bureau. (2005a). *The Health and Well-Being of Children: A Portrait of States and the Nation, 2005.* Rockville, MD: U.S. Department of Health and Human Services, Health Resources and Services Administration.

Maternal and Child Health Bureau. (2005b). *The Health and Well-Being of Children in Rural Areas: A Portrait of the Nation, 2005.* Rockville, MD: U.S. Department of Health and Human Services, Health Resources and Services Administration.

May, P. A., Van Winkle, N. W., Williams, M. B., McFeeley, P. J., DeBruyn, L. M., and Serna, P. (2002). Alcohol and suicide death among American Indians of New Mexico: 1980–1998. *Suicide and Life-Threatening Behavior, 32,* 240–255.

McCracken, M., Jiles, R., and Michels Blanck, H. (2007, April). Health behaviors of the young adult U.S. population: Behavioral Risk Factor Surveillance System, 2003. *Prevention Chronic Disease, 4,* A25. Available: http://www.pubmedcentral.nih.gov/picrender.fcgi?artid=1893124&blobtype=pdf [September 10, 2007].

McGinnis, J. M., and Foege, W. H. (1993). Actual causes of death in the United States. *Journal of the American Medical Association, 270,* 2207–2212.

McPherson, M., Arango, P., Fox, H., Lauver, C., McManus, M., Newacheck, P., Perrin, J., Shonkoff, J., and Strickland, B. (1998). A new definition of children with special health care needs. *Pediatrics, 102,* 137–140.

Miller, D. (2005). *Adolescent Cigarette Smoking: A Longitudinal Analysis through Young Adulthood.* NCES 2005-333. Washington, DC: National Center for Education Statistics.

Moffat, M., Peddie, M., Stulginskas, J., Pless, I., and Steinmetz, N. (1985). Health care delivery to foster children: A study. *Health and Social Work, 10,* 129–137.

Mokdad, A. H., Marks, J. S., Stroup, D. F., and Gerberding, J. L. (2004). Actual causes of death in the United States, 2000. *Journal of the American Medical Association, 291,* 1238–1245.

Moore, J. (2005). *Unaccompanied and Homeless Youth Review of Literature (1995–2005).* Greensboro, NC: National Center for Homeless Education.

Muthen, B. O., and Muthen, L. K. (2000). The development of heavy drinking and alcohol-related problems from ages 18 to 37 in a U.S. national sample. *Journal of Studies on Alcohol, 61,* 290–300.

Nansel, T. R., Overpeck, M., Pilla, R. S., Ruan, W. J., Simons-Morton, B., and Scheidt, P. (2001). Bullying behaviors among US youth: Prevalence and association with psychosocial adjustment. *Journal of the American Medical Association, 285,* 2094–2100.

National Cancer Institute. (2008). *Fast Stats: All Cancer Sites.* [Data file]. Available: http://seer.cancer.gov/faststats/sites.php?site=All%20Cancer%20Sites&stat=Prevalence [March 19, 2008].

National Center for Chronic Disease Prevention and Health Promotion and Division of Adolescent and School Health. (2008). *Trends in the Prevalence of Suicide-Related Behaviors.* Available: http://www.yrbs07_us_suicide_related_behaviors_trend[1].pdf.

National Center for Health Statistics. (2007). *Health Data for All Ages, 2003–2005*. Available: http://www.cdc.gov/nchs/health_data_for_all_ages.htm [August 2, 2007].

National Center for Injury Prevention and Control. (2007). *Leading Causes of Death and Fatal Injury Reports* [2004 data]. Available: http://www.cdc.gov/ncipc/wisqars/ [July 30, 2007].

National Center for Juvenile Justice. (2007). *Frequently Asked Questions: Crime Statistics*. Available: http://ncjj.servehttp.com/NCJJWebsite/faq/crimestats.htm [October 17, 2007].

National Center for Mental Health and Juvenile Justice. (2007). *Blueprint for Change: A Comprehensive Model for the Identification and Treatment of Youth with Mental Health Needs in Contact with the Juvenile Justice System*. Available: www.ncmhjj.com/blueprint/cornerstones/treatment_actions.shtml [June 7, 2007].

National Commission on Correctional Health Care. (1998). *Position Statement: Health Services to Adolescents in Adult Correctional Facilities*. Available: http://www.ncchc.org/resources/statements/adolescents.html [November 12, 2007].

National Highway Traffic Safety Administration. (1989). *Drunk Driving Facts*. Washington, DC: National Center for Statistics and Analysis, U.S. Department of Transportation.

National Highway Traffic Safety Administration. (2001). *Motor Vehicle Traffic Crash Fatality and Injury Estimates for 2000*. Washington, DC: U.S. National Highway Transportation Safety Administration.

National Highway Traffic Safety Administration. (2006). *Alcohol-Related Fatalities and Alcohol Involvement among Drivers and Motorcycle Operators in 2005*. DOT HS 810 644. Washington, DC: National Highway Traffic Safety Administration.

National Institute on Alcohol Abuse and Alcoholism. (2006). Underage drinking. Why do adolescents drink, what are the risks, and how can underage drinking be prevented? *Alcohol Alert, 67*, January.

National Institute on Drug Abuse. (1989). *National Household Survey on Drug Abuse: Main Findings 1988*. Oakland, CA: Third Party.

National Research Council. (1989). *Recommended Dietary Allowances*. 10th ed. Washington, DC: National Academy Press.

National Research Council. (1993). *Losing Generations: Adolescents in High-Risk Settings*. Washington, DC: National Academy Press.

National Research Council and Institute of Medicine. (1998). *From Generation to Generation: The Health and Well-Being of Immigrant Families*. Washington, DC: National Academy Press.

National Research Council and Institute of Medicine. (2004). *Children's Health, the Nation's Wealth: Assessing and Improving Child Health*. Washington, DC: The National Academies Press.

Nelson, C. B., Heath, A. C., and Kessler, R. C. (1998). Temporal progression of alcohol dependence symptoms in the U.S. household population: Results from the National Comorbidity Survey. *Journal of Consulting and Clinical Psychology, 66*, 474–483.

Newacheck, P. W., and Taylor, W. R. (1992). Childhood chronic illness: Prevalence, severity, and impact. *American Journal of Public Health, 82*, 364–371.

Nock, M. K., Kazdin, A. E., Hirpiri, E., and Kessler, R. (2006). Prevalence, subtypes, and correlates of DSM-IV conduct disorder in the National Comorbidity Survey Replication. *Psychology Medicine, 36*, 699–710.

Noell, J. W., and Ochs, L. M. (2001). Relationship of sexual orientation to substance use, suicidal ideation, suicide attempts, and other factors in a population of homeless adolescents. *Journal of Adolescent Health, 29*, 31–36.

Office of Juvenile Justice and Delinquency Prevention. (2007a). *Law Enforcement and Juvenile Crime. Juvenile Arrests*. Available: http://ojjdp.ncjrs.org/ojstatbb/crime/qa05101. asp?qaDate=2005 [October 17, 2007].

Office of Juvenile Justice and Delinquency Prevention. (2007b). *News @ a Glance*. Washington, DC: U.S. Department of Justice. Available: http://www.ncjrs.gov/html/ojjdp/news_at_glance/217676/topstory.html [June 7, 2007].

Oh, T. J., Eber, R., and Wang, H. L. (2002). Periodontal diseases in the child and adolescent. *Journal of Clinical Periodontology, 29*, 400–410.

Osband, M., and Tobin, J. (1972). Lead paint exposure in migrant labor camps. *Pediatrics, 49*, 604–606.

Paavonen, J., Jenkins, D., Bosch, F. X., Naud, P., Salmerón, J., Wheeler, C. M., Chow, S. N., Apter, D. L., Kitchener, H. C., Castellsague, X., de Carvalho, N. S., Skinner, S. R., Harper, D. M., Hedrick, J. A., Jaisamrarn, U., Limson, G. A., Dionne, M., Quint, W., Spiessens, B., Peeters, P., Struyf, F., Wieting, S. L., Lehtinen, M. O., Dubin, G., and HPV PATRICIA Study Group. (2007). Efficacy of a prophylactic adjuvanted bivalent L1 virus-like-particle vaccine against infection with human papillomavirus types 16 and 18 in young women: An interim analysis of a phase III double-blind, randomised controlled trial. *Lancet, 369*, 2161–2170.

Pack, A. I., Pack, A. M., Rodgman, E., Cucchiara, A., Dinges, D. F., and Schwab, C. W. (1995). Characteristics of crashes attributed to the driver having fallen asleep. *Accident Analysis and Prevention, 27*, 769–775.

Park, M. J., Mulye, T. P., Adams, S. H., Brindis, C. D., and Irwin, C. E., Jr. (2006). The health status of young adults in the United States. *Journal of Adolescent Health, 39*, 305–317.

Park, M. J., Brindis, C. D., Chang, F., and Irwin, C. E., Jr. (2008). A midcourse review of Healthy People 2010: 21 critical objectives for adolescents and young adults. *Journal of Adolescent Health, 42*, 329–334.

Patel, D. R., and Greydanus, D. E. (2002). Homeless adolescents in the United States: An overview for pediatricians. *International Pediatrics, 17*(2), 71–75.

Pecora, P., Kessler, R., Williams, J., O'Brien, K., Downs, A. C., and English, D. (2005). *Improving Family Foster Care: Findings from the Northwest Foster Care Alumni Study*. Available: www.casey.org/NR/rdonlyres/4E1E7C77-7624-4260-A253-892C5A6CB9E1/923/CaseyAlumniStudyupdated082006.pdf [June 18, 2007].

Perrin, E. (2002). *Sexual Orientation in Child and Adolescent Health Care*. New York: Kluwer Academic/Plenum Press.

Perrin, J. M., Bloom, S. R., and Gortmaker, S. L. (2007). The increase of childhood chronic conditions in the United States. *Journal of the American Medical Association, 297*, 2755–2759.

Physicians for Humans Rights. (2007). *Unique Needs of Girls in the Juvenile Justice System*. Cambridge, MA: Physicians for Human Rights.

Ray, N. (2006). *Lesbian, Gay, Bisexual and Transgender Youth: An Epidemic of Homelessness*. New York, National Gay and Lesbian Task Force Policy Institute and the National Coalition for the Homeless.

Reeves, A. F., Rees, J. M., Schiff, M., and Hujoel, P. (2006). Total body weight and waist circumference associated with chronic periodontitis among adolescents in the United States. *Archives of Pediatric Adolescent Medicine, 160*, 894–899.

Remafedi, G., Resnick, M., Blum, R., and Harris, L. (1992). Demography of sexual orientation in adolescents. *Pediatrics, 89*, 714–721.

Remafedi, G., French, S., Story, M., Resnick, M. D., and Blum, R. (1998). The relationship between suicide risk and sexual orientation: Results of a population-based study. *American Journal of Public Health, 88*, 57–60.

Rew, L. (2002). Characteristics and health care needs of homeless adolescents. *Nursing Clinics of North America, 37*(3), 423–431.

Rew, L., Taylor-Seehafer, M., and Fitzgerald, M. L. (2001). Sexual abuse, alcohol and other drug use, and suicidal behaviors in homeless adolescents. *Issues in Comprehensive Pediatric Nursing, 24*(4), 225–240.

Rew, L., Fouladi, R. T., and Yockey, R. D. (2002). Sexual health practices of homeless youth. *Journal of Nursing Scholarship, 34*(2), 139–145.

Rew, L., Whittaker, T. A., Taylor-Seehafer, M. A., and Smith, L. R. (2005). Sexual health risks and protective resources in gay, lesbian, bisexual, and heterosexual homeless youth. *Journal for Specialists in Pediatric Nursing, 10*(1), 11–19.

Rivara, F. P., Garrison, M. M., Ebel, B., McCarty, C. A., and Christakis, D. A. (2004). Mortality attributable to harmful drinking in the United States, 2000. *Journal of Studies on Alcohol, 65*, 530–536.

Roberts, A., and Bender, K. (2006). Juvenile offender suicide: Prevalence, risk factors, assessment, and crisis intervention protocols. *International Journal of Emergency Mental Health, 8*, 255–265.

Roberts, R. E., Roberts, C. R., and Chen, Y. R. (1997). Ethnocultural differences in prevalence of adolescent depression. *American Journal of Community Psychology, 25*, 95–110.

Roberts, R. E., Attkisson, C. C., and Rosenblatt, A. (1998). Prevalence of psychopathology among children and adolescents. *American Journal of Psychiatry, 155*, 715–725.

Roberts, R. E., Roberts, C. R., and Xing, Y. (2007). Rates of DSM-IV psychiatric disorders among adolescents in a large metropolitan area. *Journal of Psychiatric Research, 41*, 959–967.

Robertson, M. J. (1996). *Homeless Youth on Their Own.* Berkeley, CA: Alcohol Research Group.

Robertson, M. J., and Toro, P. A. (1999). *Homeless Youth: Research, Intervention, and Policy.* Washington, DC: U.S. Department of Housing and Urban Development and U.S. Department of Health and Human Services.

Robin, L., Brener, N. D., Donahue, S. F., Hack, T., Hale, K., and Goodenow, C. (2002). Associations between health risk behaviors and opposite-, same-, and both-sex sexual partners in representative samples of Vermont and Massachusetts high school students. *Archives of Pediatrics and Adolescent Medicine, 156*, 349–355.

Robins, L. N., and Przybeck, T. R. (1985). Age of onset of drug use as a factor in drug and other disorders. In C. L. Jones and R. J. Battjes (Eds.), *Etiology of Drug Abuse: Implications for Prevention* (pp. 178–192) (NIDA Research Monograph 56). Rockville, MD: National Institute on Drug Abuse.

Rohde, P., Noell, J., Ochs, L., and Seeley, J. R. (2001). Depression, suicidal ideation and STD-related risk in homeless older adolescents. *Journal of Adolescence, 24*(4), 447–460.

Rosenthal, D., and Mallett, S. (2003). Involuntary sex experienced by homeless young people: A public health problem. *Psychological Reports, 93*(3 II), 1195–1196.

Ross, J. G., and Gilbert, G. G. (1985). The National Youth and Fitness Study: A summary of findings. *Journal of Physical Education, 1*, 45–50.

Rotheram-Borus, M. J., Song, J., Gwadz, M., Lee, M., Van Rossem, R., and Koopman, C. (2003). Reductions in HIV risk among runaway youth. *Prevention Science, 4*(3), 173–187.

Roy, E., Haley, N., Leclerc, P., Cedras, L., Blais, L., and Boivin, J.-F. (2003). Drug injection among street youths in Montreal: Predictors of initiation. *Journal of Urban Health, 80*(1), 92–105.

Roy, E., Haley, N., Leclerc, P., Sochanski, B., Boudreau, J.-F., and Boivin, J.-F. (2004). Mortality in a cohort of street youth in Montreal. *Journal of the American Medical Association, 292*(5), 569–574.

Rubinstein, M. L., Thompson, P. J., Benowitz, N. L., Shiffman, S., and Moscicki, A. B. (2007). Cotinine levels in relation to smoking behavior and addiction in young adolescent smokers. *Nicotine and Tobacco Research, 9,* 129–135.

Rudd, R. A., and Moorman, J. E. (2007). Asthma incidence: Data from the National Health Interview Survey, 1980–1996. *Journal of Asthma, 44,* 65–70.

Russell, S. T. (2003). Sexual minority youth and suicide risk. *American Behavioral Scientist, 46,* 1241–1257.

Russell, S. T., and Joyner, K. (2001). Adolescent sexual orientation and suicide risk: Evidence from a national study. *American Journal of Public Health, 91,* 1276–1281.

Russell, S. T., Franz, B. T., and Driscoll, A. K. (2001). Same-sex romantic attraction and experiences of violence in adolescence. *American Journal of Public Health, 91,* 903–906.

Russell, S. T., Driscoll, A. K., and Truong, N. (2002). Adolescent same-sex romantic attractions and relationships: Implications for substance use and abuse. *American Journal of Public Health, 92,* 198–202.

Saewyc, E. M., Bearinger, L. H., Heinz, P. A., Blum, R. W., and Resnick, M. D. (1998). Gender differences in health and risk behaviors among bisexual and homosexual adolescents. *Journal of Adolescent Health, 23,* 181–188.

Safren, S. A., and Heimberg, R. G. (1999). Depression, hopelessness, suicidality, and related factors in sexual minority and heterosexual adolescents. *Journal of Consulting and Clinical Psychology, 67,* 859–866.

Schmidley, A. (2001). *Profile of the Foreign-Born Population in the United States: 2000.* Washington, DC: U.S. Census Bureau.

SEARCH for Diabetes in Youth Study Group. (2006). The burden of diabetes mellitus among U.S. youth: Prevalence estimates from the SEARCH for Diabetes in Youth Study. *Pediatrics, 118,* 1510–1518.

Seidman, S. N., and Rieder, R. O. (1994). A review of sexual behavior in the United States. *American Journal of Psychiatry, 151,* 330–341.

Sell, R. L., Wells, J. A., and Wypij, D. (1995). The prevalence of homosexual behavior and attraction in the United States, the United Kingdom, and France: Results of national population-based samples. *Archives of Sexual Behavior, 24,* 235–248.

Shaffer, D., Fisher, P., Dulcan, M. K., Davies, M., Piacentini, J., Schwab-Stone, M. E., Lahey, B. B., Bourdon, K., Jensen, P. S., Bird, H. R., Canino, G., and Regier, D. A. (1996). The NIMH Diagnostic Interview Schedule for Children Version 2.3 (DISC-2.3): Description, acceptability, prevalence rates, and performance in the MECA study. *Journal of the American Academy of Child and Adolescent Psychiatry, 35,* 865–877.

Sickmund, M., Sladky, T. J., and Kang, W. (2004). *Census of Juveniles in Residential Placement Databook.* Available: http://ojjdp.ncjrs.org/ojstatbb/cjrp/ [October 17, 2007].

Silver, J. A., Haecker, T., and Forkey, H. C. (1999). Health care for young children in foster care. In J. A. Silver, B. J. Amster, and T. Haecker (Eds.), *Young Children and Foster Care: A Guide for Professionals* (pp. 161–193). Baltimore, MD: Brookes.

Simms, M. D., Dubowitz, H., and Szilagyi, M. A. (2000). Health care needs of children in foster care system. *Pediatrics, 106,* 909–918.

Skowyra, K., and Cocozza, J. (2006). *Blueprint for Change: A Comprehensive Model for the Identification and Treatment of Youth with Mental Health Needs in Contact with the Juvenile Justice System: Executive Summary.* Delmar, NY: The National Center for Mental Health and Juvenile Justice Policy Research Associates and the Office of Juvenile Justice and Delinquency Prevention.

Slesinger, D., Christenson, B., and Cautley, E. (1986). Health and mortality of migrant farm children. *Social Science and Medicine, 23,* 65–74.

Smith, G. S., Branas, C. C., and Miller, T. R. (1999). Fatal nontraffic injuries involving alcohol: A metaanalysis. *Annals of Emergency Medicine, 33,* 659–668.

Solorio, M. R., Milburn, N. G., Andersen, R. M., Trifskin, S., and Rodriguez, M. A. (2006). Emotional distress and mental health service use among urban homeless adolescents. *Journal of Behavioral Health Services and Research*, 33(4), 381–393.

Sosin, D. M., Koepsell, T. D., Rivara, F. P., and Mercy, J. A. (1995). Fighting as a marker for multiple problem behaviors in adolescents. *Journal of Adolescent Health*, 16, 209–215.

Spear, L. P. (2000). The adolescent brain and age-related behavioral manifestations. *Neuroscience and Biobehavioral Reviews*, 24, 417–463.

Steensma, C., Boivin, J. F., Blais, L., and Roy, E. (2005). Cessation of injecting drug use among street-based youth. *Journal of Urban Health*, 82(4), 622–637.

Stein, J. A., Leslie, M. B., and Nyamathi, A. (2002). Relative contributions of parent substance use and childhood maltreatment to chronic homelessness, depression, and substance abuse problems among homeless women: Mediating roles of self-esteem and abuse in adulthood. *Child Abuse and Neglect*, 26(10), 1011–1027.

Steinberg, L., Chung, H. L., and Little, M. (2004). Reentry of young offenders from the justice system: A developmental perspective. *Youth Violence and Juvenile Justice*, 2, 21–38.

Stronski Huwiler, S. M., and Remafedi, G. (1998). Adolescent homosexuality. *Advances in Pediatrics*, 45, 107–144.

Substance Abuse and Mental Health Services Administration. (2005a). Adolescents with co-occurring psychiatric disorders: 2003. *The DSASIS Report, December 23*. Available: http://www.oas.samhsa.gov/2k5/youthMH/youthMH.htm [August 31, 2007].

Substance Abuse and Mental Health Services Administration. (2005b). *The NSDUH Report: Substance Use and Need for Treatment among Youths Who Have Been in Foster Care*. Washington, DC: Substance Abuse and Mental Health Services Administration, Office of Applied Studies.

Substance Abuse and Mental Health Services Administration. (2006). *Results from the 2005 National Survey on Drug Use and Health: National Findings*. Office of Applied Studies, NSDUH Series H-30, DHHS Publication No. SMA 06-4194. Rockville, MD: U.S. Department of Health and Human Services. Available: http://oas.samhsa.gov/nsduh/2k5nsduh/2k5Results.pdf [November 9, 2007].

Substance Abuse and Mental Health Services Administration. (2007). *Results from the 2006 National Survey on Drug Use and Health: National Findings*. SMA 07-4293. Rockville, MD: Office of Applied Studies, U.S. Department of Health and Human Services.

Suro, R., and Singer, A. (2002). *Latino Growth in Metropolitan America: Changing Patterns, New Locations*. Washington, DC: The Brookings Institution Center on Urban & Metropolitan Policy and The Pew Hispanic Center.

Sutton, P., and Mathews, T. (2006). *Birth and Fertility Rates by Hispanic Origin Subgroups: United States, 1990 and 2000*. Hyattsville, MD: National Center for Health Statistics.

Swahn, M. H., and Donovan, J. E. (2006). Alcohol and violence: Comparison of the psychosocial correlates of adolescent involvement in alcohol-related physical fighting versus other physical fighting. *Addictive Behaviors*, 31, 2014–2029.

Swire, M., and Kavaler, F. (1977). The health status of foster children. *Child Welfare*, 56, 635–653.

Teplin, L. A., Abram, K. M., McClelland, G. M., Dulcan, M. K., and Mericle, A. A. (2002). Psychiatric disorders in youth in juvenile detention. *Archives of General Psychiatry*, 59, 1133–1143.

Thompson, S. J. (2004). Risk/protective factors associated with substance use among runaway/homeless youth utilizing emergency shelter services nationwide. *Substance Abuse*, 25(3), 13–26.

Thompson, S. J., Maccio, E. M., Desselle, S. K., and Zittel-Palamara, K. (2007). Predictors of posttraumatic stress symptoms among runaway youth utilizing two service sectors. *Journal of Traumatic Stress*, 20(4), 553–563.

Tyler, K. A., and Cauce, A. M. (2002). Perpetrators of early physical and sexual abuse among homeless and runaway adolescents. *Child Abuse & Neglect*, 26(12), 1261–1274.
Tyler, K. A., Whitbeck, L. B., Hoyt, D. R., and Yoder, K. A. (2000). Predictors of self-reported sexually transmitted diseases among homeless and runaway adolescents. *Journal of Sex Research*, 37(4), 369–377.
Tyler, K. A., Whitbeck, L. B., Hoyt, D. R., and Johnson, K. D. (2003). Self-mutilation and homeless youth: The role of family abuse, street experiences, and mental disorders. *Journal of Research on Adolescence*, 13(4), 457–474.
Tyler, K. A., Cauce, A. M., and Whitbeck, L. (2004). Family risk factors and prevalence of dissociative symptoms among homeless and runaway youth. *Child Abuse and Neglect*, 28(3), 355–366.
Tyler, K. A., Whitbeck, L. B., Chen, X., and Johnson, K. (2007). Sexual health of homeless youth: Prevalence and correlates of sexually transmissible infections. *Sexual Health*, 4(1), 57–61.
Udry, J. R., and Chantala, K. (2002). Risk assessment of adolescents with same-sex relationships. *Journal of Adolescent Health*, 31, 84–92.
Unger, J. B., Kipke, M. D., Simon, T. R., Montgomery, S. B., and Johnson, C. J. (1997). Homeless youths and young adults in Los Angeles: Prevalence of mental health problems and the relationship between mental health and substance abuse disorders. *American Journal of Community Psychology*, 25(3), 371–394.
Unger, J. B., Kipke, M. D., Simon, T. R., Johnson, C. J., Montgomery, S. B., and Iverson, E. (1998). Stress, coping, and social support among homeless youth. *Journal of Adolescent Research*, 13(2), 134–157.
U.S. Bureau of Labor Statistics. (2007). *News: National Census of Fatal Occupational Injuries in 2006*. Washington, DC: U.S. Department of Labor.
U.S. Census Bureau. (1992). *1990 Census of Population: General Population Characteristics, United States* (CP-1-1). Available: http://www.census.gov/prod/cen1990/cp1/cp-1-1.pdf [August 13, 2007].
U.S. Census Bureau. (2003). *American FactFinder, Census 1990 Summary Tape File 1* [tabulated data]. Washington, DC: U.S. Census Bureau.
U.S. Census Bureau. (2005). *Foreign-Born Population of the United States Current Population Survey—March 2004, Table 1.1a*. Available: http://www.census.gov/population/www/socdemo/foreign/ppl-176.html [May 22, 2008].
U.S. Census Bureau. (2007). *U.S. Interim Projections by Age, Sex, Race, and Hispanic Origin*. Available: http://www.census.gov/ipc/www/usinterimproj/ [November 6, 2007].
U.S. Congress and Office of Technology Assessment. (1991). *Adolescent Health*. OTA-H-466, 467, and 468. Washington, DC: U.S. Government Printing Office.
U.S. Department of Education. (2006). *Migrant Education Program Annual Report: Eligibility, Participation, Services (2001–02) and Achievement (2002–03)*. Washington, DC: Office of the Planning, Education and Policy Development, Policy and Program Studies Service.
U.S. Department of Health and Human Services. (1994). *Preventing Tobacco Use among Young People: A Report of the Surgeon General*. Atlanta, GA: U.S. Department of Health and Human Services, Public Health Service, Centers for Disease Control and Prevention, National Center for Chronic Disease Prevention and Health Promotion, Office on Smoking and Health.
U.S. Department of Health and Human Services. (1999). *Mental Health: A Report of the Surgeon General*. Rockville, MD: U.S. Department of Health and Human Services.
U.S. Department of Health and Human Services. (2000). *Healthy People 2010* (2nd ed.). Washington, DC: U.S. Government Printing Office.

U.S. Department of Health and Human Services. (2004). *The Health Consequences of Smoking: A Report of the Surgeon General.* Washington, DC: Centers for Disease Control and Prevention, National Center for Chronic Disease Prevention and Health Promotion, Office on Smoking and Health.

U.S. Department of Health and Human Services. (2006a). *Midcourse Review. Healthy People 2010.* Available: http://www.healthypeople.gov/data/midcourse/html/default.htm#FocusAreas [November 9, 2007].

U.S. Department of Health and Human Services. (2006b). *Results from the 2005 National Survey on Drug Use and Health: Detailed Tables.* Rockville, MD: Substance Abuse and Mental Health Services Administration, Office of Applied Studies. Available: http://www.oas.samhsa.gov/nsduh/2k5nsduh/tabs/2k5TabsCover.pdf [August 31, 2007].

U.S. Department of Health and Human Services (2006c). *The Health Consequences of Involuntary Exposure to Tobacco Smoke: A Report of the Surgeon General.* Atlanta, GA: U.S. Department of Health and Human Services, Centers for Disease Control and Prevention, Coordinating Center for Health Promotion, National Center for Chronic Disease Prevention and Health Promotion, Office on Smoking and Health.

U.S. Department of Health and Human Services. (2007a). *21 Critical Health Objectives for Adolescents and Young Adults.* Available: http://www.cdc.gov/HealthyYouth/AdolescentHealth/NationalInitiative/pdf/21objectives.pdf [October 17, 2007].

U.S. Department of Health and Human Services. (2007b). *The Surgeon General's Call to Action to Prevent and Decrease Overweight and Obesity.* Available: http://www.surgeongeneral.gov/topics/obesity/calltoaction/fact_adolescents.htm [February 6, 2007].

U.S. Department of Health and Human Services. (2007c). *The Surgeon General's Call to Action to Prevent and Reduce Underage Drinking.* U.S. Department of Health and Human Services, Office of the Surgeon General.

U.S. Department of Health and Human Services and Centers for Disease Control and Prevention. (2007). *Health Data for All Ages* [Data tables]. Available: http://www.cdc.gov/nchs/health_data_for_all_ages.htm [October 17, 2007].

U.S. Department of Justice. (2006). *Criminal Victimization in the United States, 2005: Statistical Tables.* Bureau of Justice Statistics. Available: http://www.ojp.usdoj.gov/bjs/pub/pdf/cvus05.pdf [October 2, 2007].

Van Leeuwen, J. M., Hopfer, C., Hooks, S., White, R., Petersen, J., and Pirkopf, J. (2004). A snapshot of substance abuse among homeless and runaway youth in Denver, Colorado. *Journal of Community Health, 29*(3), 217–229.

Ventura, S. J., Abma, J. C., Mosher, W. E., and Henshaw, S. K. (2006). *Recent Trends in Teenage Pregnancy in the United States, 1990–2002.* Health E-stats. Hyattsville, MD: National Center for Health Statistics.

Wagner, L. S., Carlin, P. L., Cauce, A. M., and Tenner, A. (2001). A snapshot of homeless youth in Seattle: Their characteristics, behaviors and beliefs about HIV protective strategies. *Journal of Community Health, 26*(3), 219–232.

Weathers, A., Minkovitz, C., O'Campo, P., and Disener-West, M. (2003). Health services use by children of migratory agricultural workers: Exploring the role of need for care. *Pediatrics, 111,* 956–963.

Weber, A. E., Boivin, J. F., Blais, L., Haley, N., and Roy, E. (2004). Predictors of initiation into prostitution among female street youths. *Journal of Urban Health, 81*(4), 584–595.

Wenzel, S. L., Hambarsoomian, K., D'Amico, E. J., Ellison, M., and Tucker, J. S. (2006). Victimization and health among indigent young women in the transition to adulthood: A portrait of need. *Journal of Adolescent Health, 38*(5), 536–543.

Whitaker, R. C., Wright, J. A., Pepe, M. S., Seidel, K. D., and Dietz, W. H. (1997). Predicting obesity in young adulthood from childhood and parental obesity. *New England Journal of Medicine, 337,* 869–873.

Whitbeck, L. B., Chen, X., Hoyt, D. R., Tyler, K. A., and Johnson, K. D. (2004). Mental disorder, subsistence strategies, and victimization among gay, lesbian, and bisexual homeless and runaway adolescents. *Journal of Sex Research, 41*(4), 329–342.

White, J. (1998). Transgender medicine: Issues and definitions. *Journal of Gay and Lesbian Medical Association, 2,* 1–3.

White, R., Benedict, M., and Jaffe, S. (1987). Foster child health care supervision. *Child Welfare, 66,* 387–398.

Wilk, V. (1993). Health hazards to children in agriculture. *American Journal of Industrial Medicine, 24,* 283–290.

Williams, K. R., and Guerra, N. G. (2007). Prevalence and predictors of Internet bullying. *Journal of Adolescent Health, 41,* S14–S21.

Wise, P. H. (2004). The transformation of child health in the United States. *Health Affairs, 23,* 9–25.

Woolard, J. L., Odgers, C., Lanza-Kaduce, L., and Daglis, H. (2005). Juveniles within adult correctional settings: Legal pathways and developmental considerations. *International Journal of Forensic Mental Health, 4,* 1–18.

Wright, D. R., and Fitzpatrick, K. M. (2006). Violence and minority youth: The effects of risk and asset factors on fighting among African American children and adolescents. *Adolescence, 41,* 251–262.

Ybarra, M. L., Diener-West, M., and Leaf, P. J. (2007). Examining the overlap in Internet harassment and school bullying. Implications for school intervention. *Journal of Adolescent Health, 41,* S42–S50.

Yoder, K., Longley, S., Whitbeck, L., and Hoyt, D. (2008). A dimensional model of psychopathology among homeless adolescents: Suicidality, internalizing, and externalizing disorders. *Journal of Abnormal Child Psychology, 36*(1), 95–104.

Yu, S. M., Huang, Z. J., Schwalberg, R., Overpeck, M., and Kogan, M. D. (2003). Acculturation, and the health and well-being of US immigrant adolescents. *Journal of Adolescent Health, 33,* 479–488.

Zadik, Y., and Sandler, Y. (2007). Periodontal attachment loss due to applying force by tongue piercing. *Journal of the California Dental Association, 35,* 551–553.

3

Current Adolescent Health Services, Settings, and Providers

SUMMARY

A Systems Perspective

- Five objectives identified by the World Health Organization provide a basis for assessing the quality of current and future systems of health services for adolescents: accessibility, acceptability, appropriateness, effectiveness, and equity.

Primary Care Services

- Evidence shows that while private office-based primary care services are available to most adolescents, those services depend significantly on fee-based reimbursement and are not:
  - accessible to adolescents who are uninsured or underinsured.
  - offered in acceptable settings that foster open communication of sensitive behaviors or health conditions.
  - provided by personnel who are skilled in addressing health conditions and behaviors that are appropriate for this stage of development.
  - effective at fostering health promotion or addressing risky behaviors that are prevalent among adolescents, such as substance use and unsafe sexual activity.

- Evidence shows that safety-net health services for adolescents are
  - accessible to many adolescents who are uninsured or do not find private office-based services acceptable for their needs.
  - frequently more acceptable to adolescents who are uncomfortable with private office-based primary care providers, especially when they can establish relationships with providers who are sensitive to their needs and promote open communication.
  - sometimes able to offer a more appropriate mix of skills and counseling services that address risky behaviors.
  - able to provide effective disease prevention and health promotion services while also addressing issues related to risky behavior. However, such centers often can become unstable during times of fiscal uncertainty and may experience frequent personnel transitions. They also face unique challenges associated with financing of prevention and health promotion services that cannot be reimbursed.
  - important mechanisms for resolving the disparities and inequities that exist within private office-based primary care.

Specialty Care Services

- Evidence shows that specialty care services for the adolescent population are not accessible to most adolescents. Existing specialty services in the areas of mental health, sexual and reproductive health, oral health, and substance use treatment and prevention are generally insufficient to meet the needs of many adolescents. While evidence-based therapies are available in a number of these areas, they are not integrated into many practice settings.
- Even when specialty services are accessible, many adolescents do not find them acceptable because of concerns about disclosure of treatment in sensitive areas (such as substance use or sexual health).
- Many specialty providers lack appropriate training to address the needs of adolescent patients, and certification programs for treating adolescents are frequently unavailable in many specialty areas.
- The lack of appropriate specialty services that are suitable for adolescents means that effective treatment is often delayed, care is of limited duration, and services are poorly reimbursed.
- Limitations in the quality of or access to specialty services are especially prevalent among at-risk adolescents in whom problems

in the above areas frequently co-occur, contributing to health care inequities and disparities.

Prevention and Health Promotion

- Routine screening for risk factors and unhealthful behaviors that emerge during adolescence is not available or accessible for most adolescents.
- Many health care providers who treat adolescents fail to adhere to recommended prevention guidelines, to screen for appropriate risk factors and unhealthful behaviors that emerge during adolescence, and to provide effective counseling that would reduce risks and foster health promotion.

Racial and Ethnic Disparities

- Disparities and biases affect the quality of health services for adolescents and deserve serious consideration in any efforts to improve access to appropriate services and reduce inequities in the health system.

Confidential Services

- Evidence shows that health services that are confidential increase the acceptability of services and the willingness of adolescents to seek them, especially for issues related to sexual behavior, reproductive health, mental health, and substance use.
- Existing state and federal policies generally protect the confidentiality of adolescents' health information when they are legally allowed to consent to their own care.

This chapter introduces a framework for examining the strengths and limitations of current health system approaches for adolescents. This framework comprises five major objectives—accessibility, acceptability, appropriateness, effectiveness, and equity—that serve as criteria for assessing the use, adequacy, and quality of adolescent health services. The chapter then reviews the current array of mainstream and safety-net primary care services, as well as specialty services, that respond to the adolescent health needs identified in Chapter 2; a brief discussion of inpatient hospital services for adolescents is also presented. This review is followed by a discussion of what is known about adolescents' use of health services.

The chapter then considers how *context matters*—that is, how such factors such as income, race and ethnicity, and community affect access to and utilization of adolescent health services. Next is a discussion of consent and confidentiality and their influence on the acceptability of health services to adolescents. The chapter ends with a summary of the gaps between adolescents' health service needs and the services and settings that exist to address those needs.

This chapter deals with several important issues: the overall inadequacy of preventive screening, counseling, and health education for adolescents, which are crucial to high-quality care for this population; the value of having health services available in diverse locations; the lack of an integrated health system that recognizes and reflects the particular needs and interests of adolescents; and the importance of confidentiality and privacy of visits between adolescents and providers. Chapter 4 responds to the findings presented in this chapter by exploring elements of improved health services within an adolescent health system that would be more accessible, acceptable, appropriate, effective, and equitable relative to adolescents' current health status, health service needs, and population variations.

OBJECTIVES OF HEALTH SERVICES FOR ADOLESCENTS

An array of studies has emerged describing the types of health services frequently used by adolescents in the United States and other countries, as well as gaps between the nature of these services and the health needs of adolescents, as identified in Chapter 2 (Chung et al., 2006; Tylee et al., 2007; U.S. Congress and Office of Technology Assessment, 1991). While evidence is insufficient to indicate that any one particular setting or practice structure meets the complex needs of all U.S. adolescents better than others, a variety of national and international organizations studying both adolescents and health care providers (Donovan et al., 1997; Ford et al., 1997; Ginsburg et al., 1995; Kang et al., 2003; Veit et al., 1996) have (1) defined critical elements of health services that would improve adolescents' access to appropriate services, (2) highlighted design elements that would improve the quality of those services, and (3) identified ways to foster patient–provider relationships that can lead to better health for adolescents. This research from various sources and the experiences of adolescents and health care providers, health organizations, and research centers have directed attention to the importance of designing primary care services that can attract and engage adolescents, create opportunities to discuss sensitive health and behavioral issues, and offer high-quality health services as well as guidance on both disease prevention and health promotion.

Through a series of reports and consultations, the World Health Organization focused attention on the importance of adolescent-friendly health services (Brabin, 2002; Tylee et al., 2007; World Health Organization, 1999, 2001). These activities led to a general consensus on five objectives that promote responsive adolescent health services:

- **Accessible.** Policies and procedures ensure that services are broadly accessible.
- **Acceptable.** Policies and procedures consider culture and relationships and the climate of engagement.
- **Appropriate.** Health services fulfill the needs of all young people.
- **Effective.** Health services reflect evidence-based standards of care and professional guidelines.
- **Equitable.** Policies and procedures do not restrict the provision of and eligibility for services.

These objectives provided the committee with a valuable framework for assessing the use, adequacy, and quality of adolescent health services; comparing and contrasting the extent to which different services, settings, and providers address the health needs of young people in the United States; identifying the gaps that keep services from meeting these objectives; and recommending ways to fill those gaps. Using such a framework is superior to relying solely on process measures, such as rates of utilization, professional licensure standards, or anecdotal reports of institutional reputations. This framework could be used to inform future local, state, and national assessments of adolescent health and health services, and to monitor progress toward achievement of the 21 Critical Health Objectives for adolescents and young adults (a subset of the Healthy People 2010 goals, as described in Chapter 2 [U.S. Department of Health and Human Services, 2007]), as well as the oral health objectives for adolescents (U.S. Department of Health and Human Services, 2000). It and the framework of behavioral and contextual characteristics presented in Chapter 1 complement each other and together help to provide a more comprehensive picture of the features of the health system that should be improved to provide adolescents with high-quality care and thus improve their health status, addressing the health needs of all adolescents while also attending to the needs of specific, often underserved, subpopulations and high-risk groups.

The committee compared the five WHO objectives with the fundamental aims for the health system set forth by the Institute of Medicine (IOM, 2001) as described in Box 3-1. Table 3-1 summarizes this comparison and illustrates that while there is considerable overlap between the two frameworks, there are important differences that merit consideration. The IOM framework reflects concerns about how to improve quality and reduce inefficiencies in services received by patients who have access to health care providers, especially those who need specialty care for chronic conditions

> **BOX 3-1**
> **Characteristics of Two Frameworks for**
> **Delivering Health Services**
>
> **World Health Organization Framework for Delivering Adolescent-Friendly Health Services (as summarized by Tylee et al., 2007)**
>
> - *Accessible*—Policies and procedures ensure that services are broadly accessible.
> - *Acceptable*—Policies and procedures consider culture and relationships and the climate of engagement.
> - *Appropriate*—Health services fulfill the needs of all young people.
> - *Effective*—Health services reflect evidence-based standards of care and professional guidelines.
> - *Equitable*—Policies and procedures do not restrict the provision of and eligibility for services.
>
> **Institute of Medicine Framework for Delivering Quality Health Services (as set forth in Institute of Medicine, 2001)**
>
> - *Efficient*—Services are designed to reduce unnecessary time and costs.
> - *Timely*—Waiting times between assessment and treatment are reduced.
> - *Patient-centered*—Services are sensitive to the needs and preferences of the patient.
> - *Equitable*—Services do not reflect disparities within the general population.
> - *Effective*—Services reflect accepted standards of clinical care.
> - *Safe*—Protocols are in place to reduce medical errors and foster quality assurance.

(such as diabetes or eating disorders, which generally involve coordination of multiple specialty services). By contrast, the WHO framework is focused on how to improve access to and engagement with appropriate primary care services. Since all adolescents need to interact with primary care providers and fewer need specialty services, the WHO framework offers a more appropriate conceptual design for an analysis of the adolescent health system.

With the WHO framework in mind, the committee reviewed components of the current adolescent health system—adolescent health services, the settings where these services are delivered, how services are delivered in these settings, and by whom. The committee considered the extent to which these services are accessible, acceptable, appropriate, effective, and equitable.

Health services for adolescents in the United States are delivered through two sectors: primary care and specialty care. Each sector involves

TABLE 3-1 Comparison of Criteria of the Institute of Medicine and World Health Organization Frameworks for Delivering Health Services

	IOM Framework					
	Efficient	Timely	Patient-Centered	Equitable	Effective	Safe
WHO Framework						
Accessible		X				
Acceptable			X			
Appropriate			X			
Effective					X	X
Equitable				X		

NOTES: IOM = Institute of Medicine; WHO = World Health Organization.
SOURCES: Institute of Medicine (2001); Tylee et al. (2007).

multiple providers and institutions, and some providers work with specific subpopulations of youths. Primary care programs strive to meet the basic health needs of all adolescents, including routine checkups, immunizations, anticipatory guidance, and screening and assessment for disorders and risk factors. Specialty care programs serve adolescents with specific health needs (for example, those with chronic illnesses such as diabetes or asthma, those with eating disorders, those needing reproductive health services or treatment for sexually transmitted infections [STIs], those with clinical mental health needs, or those with substance use disorders). In some situations, specialty health services may be offered through primary care settings, and primary care services may sometimes be available within specialty clinics. Examples include the primary care services offered by Planned Parenthood clinics (which specialize in reproductive health care), as well as mental health services that are offered within certain types of community health or hospital-affiliated primary care clinics.

Assessing the relative merits of various care settings requires close attention to the nature of their interactions and their experience with different health conditions and subpopulations of adolescents. It also requires consensus on the criteria that should be applied in weighing the strengths and limitations of particular service settings.

The adolescent health system shares the same basic problems as those embedded in the organization of adult health services: the lack of communication, collaboration, and system-level planning among various private and public health services, settings, and providers (Institute of Medicine, 2003). As noted in the IOM (2003) report, the vast array of clinicians, hospitals, other health care facilities, insurance plans, and purchasers operate in various configurations of groups, networks, and independent practices that are collectively termed "the health care delivery system." However, this phrase suggests an order, integration, and accountability that do not exist, and whose absence results in barriers to and gaps in care. In some areas, such as the organization of mental health services for adolescents, the system of services is in substantial disarray because of financial barriers, eligibility gaps, the limited availability of providers, and concerns about confidentiality and privacy that impede smooth transitions across health service settings.

Finding:

- *Five objectives identified by the World Health Organization provide a basis for assessing the quality of current and future systems of health services for adolescents: accessibility, acceptability, appropriateness, effectiveness, and equity.*

PRIMARY CARE SERVICES

Traditional primary care encompasses provider-based services offered in private practices, such as pediatric, family medicine, and dental offices, as well as safety-net programs that include community health centers or hospital-affiliated primary care services. School-based health centers are also generally considered part of the primary care sector. Some primary care settings are structured to serve the health needs of specific populations with unique profiles (such as those who are homeless or runaways; those who are involved in the foster care or juvenile justice system; or those who are lesbian, gay, bisexual, or transgender[1] [LGBT]).

Private Office-Based Care

The majority of adolescents have private insurance through family plans offered by one or both parents' employers. These adolescents commonly receive their primary medical care from private provider offices, usually a pediatrician, family physician, general internist, or nurse practitioner, or for older female adolescents, a gynecologist. Adolescents with public insurance (such as Medicaid or the State Children's Health Insurance Program [SCHIP]) also routinely interact with provider offices in the private or public sectors that accept their insurance plans.

Private office-based primary care services frequently cover the following: health maintenance or well-care visits (the scope of which is often guided by local school board policies), basic diagnostic tests (such as height, weight, and blood pressure), vision and hearing screening, and brief consultation on health concerns or health promotion. The administration of recommended vaccines may or may not be included in an annual office visit, depending on local school requirements, state programs for free vaccines, insurance coverage, and reimbursement practices.

Significant variations frequently occur in private and public health plans that limit or influence the nature and duration of services eligible for reimbursement in private office-based primary care settings. For example, traditional plans allow reimbursement for health maintenance visits, laboratory tests, care for certain categories of acute and chronic medical conditions, and prescription medications. They generally do not cover extended or periodic counseling services beyond the brief contact associated with a health maintenance visit, nor do they reimburse many of the counseling or case management expenses associated with treatment of a number of

---

[1]The group referred to as "lesbian, gay, bisexual, and transgender" sometimes also encompasses the term "questioning" and is commonly referred to by the acronym LGBT (or GLBT) or LGBTQ (or GLBTQ). For the purposes of this report, the identifier "lesbian, gay, bisexual, and transgender" or LGBT is used.

behavioral problems, such as anorexia or bulimia, substance use, sexual or reproductive health practices, trauma, or behavioral or emotional problems that fail to meet the threshold criteria for a clinical disorder (Fox, Limb, and McManus, 2007; Fox, McManus, and Reichman, 2003; see Chapter 6 for more detail).

A review of several studies found that 70 percent of adolescent morbidity and mortality involves consequences from such behavior as unsafe sexual activity, violence, substance use, tobacco use, poor nutritional habits, risky driving, and inadequate physical activity (National Research Council, 1999). Yet even though this age group is at significant risk for the onset of many health conditions that may persist into adulthood, only a minority of adolescents receive developmental or psychosocial services through routine assessment (Chung et al., 2006). While clinician surveys indicate that most private providers perform routine surveillance for risky behaviors, diet, and exercise, fewer than half of adolescents responded affirmatively to survey items asking whether they had spoken with their provider about sexual activity, other risk behaviors, STIs, diet, exercise, and emotional health (Bethell, Klein, and Peck, 2001; Chung et al., 2006; Ellen et al., 1998; Halpern-Felsher et al., 2000; Millstein and Marcell, 2003; Millstein, Igra, and Gans, 1996).

Several factors account for the lack of appropriate private office-based health services for adolescents that are tailored to their behavioral and developmental needs. For example, insurance reimbursements are often inadequate to compensate for the time it takes to offer adequate health promotion or disease prevention services for adolescents (McManus, Shejavali, and Fox, 2003; O'Connor, Johnson, and Brown, 2000). This and other finance issues are discussed in more detail in Chapter 6.

Another challenge involves the nature and skills of the workforce that is available to address the health needs of adolescents. According to the National Medical Ambulatory Survey and the National Hospital Ambulatory Medical Care Survey, 40 percent of health visits for adolescents aged 11–14 were to pediatricians during 1994–2003. As adolescents matured and reached adulthood, they encountered a more diverse array of providers, moving from pediatricians to family physicians, internal medicine physicians, and gynecologists. For example, among females and males aged 18–21, only 4 percent and 7 percent, respectively, had met with pediatricians. For the two age groups, 22 percent and 29 percent of visits, respectively, were to family physicians. Half of female and 70 percent of male health maintenance visits in the older age group were to family physicians. After age 18, females were more likely to visit obstetricians/gynecologists than any other type of physician (Rand et al., 2007).

In some cases, adolescents are able to interact with a specialist in adolescent medicine in a private office-based primary care setting. An adolescent medicine specialist has received extensive training in the particular health conditions and concerns of adolescents, as discussed later in this chapter and further in Chapter 5. These specialists may be more prepared than other practitioners to address multiple health problems faced by adolescents, identify specific behavioral disorders, and offer guidance on health promotion and disease prevention. But access to adolescent specialists is severely limited, since these practitioners are commonly available only in academic health centers. According to one recent estimate, just 466 certificates in adolescent medicine were issued from 1996 to 2005 (for a population of about 40 million people aged 10–19), compared with 2,839 certificates issued in geriatric medicine during the same period (Hoffman, 2007).

In addition to difficulties associated with insurance conditions and the shortage of specialists, opportunities to engage adolescents in discussions pertinent to their particular needs and circumstances and to monitor their general health status are severely constrained by a lack of continuity with a clinician or place of care, a lack of privacy, a lack of clinical awareness or skill, racial and ethnic barriers, language-related barriers, clinician and patient gender-related barriers, and a lack of time to provide comprehensive preventive care even if adolescents attend their recommended visits (Chung et al., 2006). In their review of the literature, Chung and colleagues (2006) found that fulfilling only the most conservative (i.e., evidence- and cost/benefit-based) counseling recommendations of the U.S. Preventive Care Task Force would take an average clinician nearly 40 minutes per adolescent per year. Both national surveys of pediatricians and case studies have found that insurance reimbursements are inadequate to cover the necessary time (McManus, Shejavali, and Fox, 2003; O'Connor, Johnson, and Brown, 2000).

Several group plans and managed care organizations have recognized the importance of offering primary care services tailored to the needs of adolescents. These plans and organizations tend to provide greater opportunity for adolescents and their parents to engage with providers who are specially equipped to address their concerns and are skilled in discussing sensitive health issues, such as pubertal changes, sexual activity, behavioral and mental health conditions, and substance use.

More commonly, however, providers in private office-based primary care settings believe they are inadequately trained in adolescent health, and they are uncomfortable with discussing sensitive health issues of particular concern to adolescents and their families (as discussed further in Chapter 5). Moreover, few of these providers are aware of the Guidelines for Adolescent Preventive Services (discussed in Chapter 4) or the Healthy People 2010 objectives for adolescents and young adults (described in Chapter 2) (American Medical Association, 1997; U.S. Department of Health and Human Services, 2007). They fail to recognize the importance of incorporating health promotion and disease prevention as a fundamental part of routine health services for adolescents. Most providers practice in environments that fail to encourage adolescents to ask health questions, express their health concerns, or explore disease prevention strategies that might prepare them to address significant risks and vulnerabilities that often emerge in adolescence (such as the use of tobacco, alcohol, and drugs; sexual activity; risky driving; and violent behavior) (Klein and Wilson, 2002).

One study of ambulatory care for children in different settings found that few medical practitioners are able to provide comprehensive, coordinated, or sensitive health services tailored to adolescent needs (Mangione-Smith et al., 2007). Likewise, adolescent disease prevention services received the lowest score for quality among clinical services for children and youths (as measured by eight indicators): 4.5 percent as compared with 92 percent for treatment of upper respiratory tract infections and 85.3 percent for treatment of allergic rhinitis (Mangione-Smith et al., 2007).

In summary, while many adolescents have access to private office-based primary care services, such services are not suited to the particular behavioral and developmental needs of this stage of life. The lack of reimbursement for counseling and case management services, as well as the diversity of health care providers who are involved in the care of adolescents, creates unique challenges that affect both the availability and acceptability of prevention and health promotion services. Even when effective services are available, they are frequently not integrated into routine primary care settings.

Furthermore, few centers are specifically focused on the primary care needs of special subpopulations of adolescents, such as those who are in the foster care system, in families that have recently immigrated, or LGBT. The lack of quality private office-based primary care services for these groups creates service gaps that constitute basic disparities and inequities in the health care system. These special subpopulations rely on safety-net centers for their health care, as discussed in the following section.

Findings:

- *Evidence shows that while private office-based primary care services are available to many adolescents, those services depend significantly on fee-based reimbursement and are not:*
  - *accessible to adolescents who are uninsured or underinsured.*
  - *offered in acceptable settings that foster open communication of sensitive behaviors or health conditions.*

- *provided by personnel who are skilled in addressing health conditions and behaviors that are appropriate for this stage of development.*
- *effective at fostering health promotion or addressing risky behaviors that are prevalent among adolescents, such as substance use and unsafe sexual activity.*

Safety-Net Primary Care Services

Many adolescents are uninsured or underinsured and are therefore ineligible to receive primary care services from private office-based providers. Other adolescents may not have an established relationship with a primary care provider or may be concerned about the confidentiality of visits with their primary care provider. These young people often rely on safety-net providers, defined as "those providers that organize and deliver a significant level of health care and other health-related services to uninsured, Medicaid, and other vulnerable patients" (Institute of Medicine, 2000, p. 21). Core safety-net providers have two distinguishing characteristics: (1) they have a legal mandate or explicit mission to "maintain an 'open door,' offering access to services to patients regardless of their ability to pay; and (2) a substantial share of their patient mix is uninsured, Medicaid, and other vulnerable patients" (Institute of Medicine, 2000, pp. 3–4).

As noted in earlier IOM studies, the safety net consists of public hospital systems; academic health centers; community health centers or clinics funded by federal, state, and local public health agencies; and local health departments. An additional feature of the safety net for adolescents is the presence of school-based health centers. The organization and delivery of safety-net services vary widely from state to state and community to community.

A literature review presented at a workshop convened in January 2007 as part of this study revealed that many reports focused on improving services and outcomes for adolescents frequently omit safety-net health services (see, for example, National Research Council and Institute of Medicine, 2002). Studies of the quality of adolescent safety-net health services vary in methodological rigor; randomized studies are rare; extensive variations exist in populations, settings, topics, and time; single-site studies predominate; and a meta-analysis or synthesis of essential components is not possible given the quality of the available research (Dougherty, 2007). Overall, the review presented in the study workshop was striking in revealing the absence or low quality of the existing evidence on safety-net sites of care for adolescents (see Table 3-2).

TABLE 3-2 Studies Evaluating the Delivery of Adolescent Health Services in School-Based and Community Health Centers

Site/System	Study Design
School-Based Health Centers	
Effectiveness	
Britto et al. (2001)	2-year comparison with control schools (within state)
Crespo and Shaler (2000)	3-year national comparison with other school-based health centers
Culligan (2002)	Survey of adolescent users of school-based health centers statewide
Guo et al. (2005)	2-year comparison with control schools (within a metropolitan area)
Key, Washington, and Hulsey (2002)	Retrospective 3-year comparison with adolescents not enrolled in center, but in the same school
Kisker and Brown (1996)	Comparison with national sample in other urban areas
Mental health programs	
Armbruster and Lichtman (1999)	Comparison with community clinic services
Chatterji et al. (2004)	Estimate of costs of a mental health screening and treatment program; implemented all students
Slade (2002)	Comparison with services in other settings; population-based survey
Comprehensive pregnancy programs	
Barnet, Duggan, and Devoe (2003)	Comparison with a hospital-based pregnancy program
Disease management programs	
Anderson et al. (2004)	Nonrandomized controlled comparison with other schools without disease management program
Quality	
Center for Reproductive Health Research Policy (n.d.)	Comparison of countywide program with schools without centers
Gance-Cleveland, Costin, and Degenstein (2003)	Comparison of quality standards in centers (statewide)
Kalafat and Illback (1998)	Evaluation of programs (statewide)

Populations	Findings
Middle and high school students	Increased receipt of needed health care among users of school center
Middle and high school students	Increased enrollment and continued high utilization among users of school center
Middle and high school students	Improved health knowledge and reported health behavior among users of school center
Elementary and middle school students with asthma	Lower risk of asthma-related hospitalization and emergency department utilization among users of school center
General population aged 10–15	Decrease in emergency department utilization among users of school center
High school students	Increased access to health services and improved health knowledge among users of school center
Children and adolescents aged 5–18	Comparable improvement on Children's Global Assessment Scale and Global Assessment of Function
Middle school students, mostly Hispanic, low-income	Baseline cost of implementation for 2 years, societal perspective
Students in grades 7–12	Increased utilization of mental health counseling services in school-based program
Primarily pregnant African American adolescents	Lower risk of low-birthweight infants in school-based program
Children and adolescents, low-income	Lower emergency department utilization and hospitalization, less follow-up for asthma among users of school center
Elementary, middle, high school students	Increased receipt of needed health care in schools with centers; provided a baseline for further evaluation
Elementary, middle, high school students	Mixed results; set baseline goals for improvement
Elementary, middle, high school students	Qualitative associations to provide a baseline for further evaluation

Continued

TABLE 3-2 Continued

Site/System	Study Design
Community Health Centers	
Lieberman (1974)	Evaluation of quality
Orso (1979)	Utilization data of center calculated using city population census data
Shields et al. (2002)	Retrospective with comparison (hospital outpatient department and solo/group physicians)
Tatelbaum et al. (1978)	Local comparison (hospital clinic)

NOTE: Excluded studies with populations only in elementary schools.

Community-Based Health Centers

Community-based health centers are a fundamental component of the safety-net primary care system. They offer a broad array of primary care services for populations that frequently lack access to traditional services or do not find such services acceptable for meeting their needs.

Several examples of community-based programs that serve more vulnerable adolescents are described in Chapter 4. The adolescents served by these programs often are difficult to engage in mainstream primary care centers for many reasons, such as a lack of insurance or a history of trauma and victimization. Community-based centers frequently emphasize outreach to difficult-to-reach or -serve populations (sometimes through the use of paraprofessionals or peer educators), case management and social support programs, and comprehensive medical and behavioral health services. They attract personnel who are trained in adolescent health and development, are skilled in establishing trust with more vulnerable adolescents, and are comfortable in discussing sensitive health issues with young people. While many community-based health centers have the capacity to offer reproductive health or behavioral health services, few have the resources to provide routine or specialized oral health services for adolescents.

These free-standing centers are frequently housed in locations that provide easy access to and opportunities for unscheduled encounters with adolescents in need. In some places, drop-in centers and mobile units have been used to deliver health services to particularly vulnerable populations, including those who are homeless, are from families that have recently immigrated, or live in rural settings (Diaz-Parez Mde, Farley, and Cabanis, 2004; C. A. Jones et al., 2005; Lee and O'Neal, 1994; Slesnick et al., 2008).

Populations	Findings
Children and adolescents under age 17	Only 17 percent of children and adolescents received high-quality care
Local community	High rates of center utilization for adolescent boys (63%) and girls (81%) in center
Children and adolescents with asthma	Higher visit rates for asthma compared with both; lower emergency department utilization compared with hospital; higher hospitalization rates compared with solo/group physicians
Adolescents, high proportion receiving Medicaid	Lower rates of anemia and pre-eclampsia in pregnant adolescents

Such centers often encourage interdisciplinary teams and integrated case management among their staff; in some situations, they assist adolescents in resolving housing, school, employment, legal, and family problems that contribute to their health conditions.

Community-based adolescent health centers frequently are vulnerable to the same limitations that characterize many other community-based programs: they serve a limited population of adolescents; they have a low-volume patient base; they are often poorly reimbursed for services associated with counseling, team interaction, and case management; they frequently rely on part-time health care providers and have difficulty attracting and retaining skilled personnel (because of limited funding, time demands, and difficulty securing malpractice insurance); and they often require supplemental funds from local or state health departments, the federal government, private donors, or other sources since fee-based services alone are not sufficient to support their programs (Institute of Medicine, 2000). Little is known about the effectiveness of different service models used by community-based health centers in reaching these particularly vulnerable adolescents for disease prevention, case management, and health promotion.

Hospital-Affiliated Primary Care Services

A number of hospital centers have established adolescent clinics that function as community health clinics and serve the primary care needs of adolescents; examples include Mount Sinai Hospital in New York City, Denver Health in Colorado, and the Arkansas Children's Hospital and

Adolescent Center in Little Rock (see Chapter 4). These adolescent clinics may be located within the hospital itself or organized as a satellite facility elsewhere within the community. Most offer basic primary care services and also emphasize reproductive health care; some have specialized expertise in the management of specific disorders, such as STIs, substance use, or mental health disorders (Fisher and Kaufman, 1996; Macfarlane and Blum, 2001).

One important feature of safety-net care associated with hospital-based settings is adolescents' high utilization of emergency care services at public hospitals for acute injuries and illnesses, as well as for routine primary care needs (a topic discussed later in this chapter). Surprisingly, few studies document trends in this area or identify strengths and gaps associated with the accessibility, acceptability, appropriateness, or effectiveness of health services for adolescents in emergency departments. A few specialized protocols for treatment and brief motivational interventions for adolescents (e.g., related to substance use) have been developed for use by emergency care providers (Burke, O'Sullivan, and Vaughan, 2005).

School-Based Health Centers

One important source of primary care for adolescents is schools, especially those with school-based health centers. Almost 30 years ago, New York State launched the first state-funded grant program to support school-based health centers (Brindis et al., 2003). By last count, the number of such centers nationwide had reached 1,709 in 45 states (Juszczak, Schlitt, and Moore, 2007). While school-based health centers serve students from kindergarten through high school, more than 50 percent serve mainly adolescents.

Since schools are where most school-aged adolescents spend a significant portion of their time, school-based health centers appear to be a logical means of improving access, efficiency, and economies of scale in adolescent health services. Significant debate has persisted, however, about the relative merits and disadvantages of a population-based versus a selective high-risk approach to offering primary care services in school-based health centers. As noted in the 1997 IOM report *Schools and Health: Our Nation's Investment* (Institute of Medicine, 1997), the population-based approach can have a large impact on the population as a whole, but the benefits for selected individuals may be small. Most adolescents in school already have access to and utilize mainstream primary care services. Yet many high-risk adolescents—a significant and growing segment of the population according to the 1997 IOM study—may be better served by providers in school-based health centers if they lack access to other community health personnel or do not find their local providers to be sensitive to their needs.

While no single model exists for school-based health centers, many share certain common characteristics. Centers are located inside the school building or on the school campus. Philip J. Porter, MD, an early architect of school-based health centers, once said, "Health services need to be where students can trip over them. Adolescents do not carry appointment books, and school is the only place where they are required to spend time" (The Center for Health and Health Care in Schools, 1993). In most instances, the centers are sponsored by mainstream health organizations. One study found that hospitals were the leading organizers of school-based health centers, sponsoring 32 percent of the total number. Health departments and federally funded community health centers each sponsored 17 percent, school districts 15 percent, and community-based nonprofit organizations 12 percent (Juszczak et al., 2003).

Students receive care in school-based health centers from a multidisciplinary team of professionals. Typically, a medical assistant supports a nurse practitioner or physician assistant. More than half of the centers provide mental health services, most frequently through a master's-level social worker, psychologist, or substance abuse counselor. A part-time pediatrician or family physician may also be part of the staff. A center may have access to part-time professionals as well, including nutritionists, health educators, social services case managers, dentists, dental hygienists, substance abuse counselors, and others, depending on the needs of the students and the resources available in the community (Juszczak, Schlitt, and Moore, 2007).

The fundamental reason school-based health centers have drawn support is their capacity to increase access to basic health care for low-income children and adolescents. Data on large numbers of such centers document their acceptability to students and families, as well as their capacity to address the critical needs of the adolescents they serve (Dryfoos, 1994, Institute of Medicine, 1997). And because the centers can be targeted to schools that enroll large numbers of underserved racial and ethnic minorities, they have the potential to foster equity in access to care and to improve in health outcomes among the most vulnerable populations.

Despite this evidence that school-based health centers have moved from the margin to the mainstream, however, two issues—funding and debate about the role and mission of the centers and their place in community health systems—represent a potential constraint on their growth.

Funding remains an issue because state governments subject to pay-as-they-go constraints are reluctant to create new programs that require annual infusions of large amounts of state funds. The tendency is to hope that programs can be funded through existing public revenues, most commonly Medicaid. The experience thus far has been that patient care revenues are

TABLE 3-3 Potential Strengths and Weaknesses of School-Based Health Centers

Type of Primary Care	Strengths	Weaknesses
First-contact care	Eliminates many barriers to access; reaches underserved, low-income, and high-risk populations; often is the sole source of care.	Tight budgets restrict hours and days of operation, resulting in access problems.
Continuous care	Can serve as "health care homes."	High turnover of personnel prevents long-term relationships between students and staff. Coverage must be arranged during summer, other vacations, evenings, and weekends.
Comprehensive care	A wide range of essential health services is usually provided to meet the physical, mental, and social needs of adolescents.	Little research has evaluated the adequacy and quality of the apparently wide range of services provided against the actual needs of the populations served. The scope of provided services is largely a function of funding. Provider availability may dictate the scope of services offered. Many centers are unable to provide a full range of reproductive health care services on site. Many are not able to employ full-time providers.

Coordinated care	Data management and outcome analysis systems are increasingly being used. Some programs have successfully coordinated services with managed care organizations.	Difficulties are faced in coordinating care with other community providers. Overall, little coordination with managed care organizations occurs.
Community-oriented care	Incorporating a community or population perspective can meet the needs of all children and adolescents, involve the community in planning and governance, and provide an impetus for community needs assessment and resource mapping.	Few are able to expand their services beyond the student population.
Family-centered care	Meets health care needs without disrupting everyday family functions. Limited data suggest popularity with parents and families. Efforts are made to respect both confidentiality and the right of the family to be informed. Creative ways of involving families are being developed.	Care is usually not provided to the entire family. This limits the gathering of family information and the development of client management strategies.
Culturally competent care	Provides care for culturally diverse populations.	Few data exist to allow assessment of cultural competence. A shortage of adequately trained bilingual or bicultural providers exists.

SOURCE: Institute of Medicine (1997), adapted, with permission, from Santelli et al. (1995) The Women's and Children's Health Policy Center, The Johns Hopkins Bloomberg School of Public Health, Copyright (1995).

insufficient to support school-based health centers, and additional core grants are required to sustain quality programs.

The other major challenge in developing primary care services for adolescents in school-based health centers lies in the relationship between the U.S. health system, which is predominantly private, and the U.S. education system, which is publicly financed through local and state funds. The low levels of financing for school-based health centers restrict their ability to attract the necessary providers, and conversely, local providers are frequently not aware of or well integrated into the centers' system of care. The fundamental mismatch and lack of engagement between the health and education systems remains a source of persistent concern. Table 3-3, drawn from the above-mentioned IOM report (Institute of Medicine, 1997) and a study by Santelli and colleagues (1995), highlights the strengths and shortcomings of school-based health centers.

Summary

Safety-net health centers play an important role in addressing the inequities and shortcomings of mainstream primary care services, especially for more vulnerable populations of uninsured or underinsured adolescents. Hospital-, community-, and school-based health centers provide valuable services for adolescents who have difficulty gaining access to mainstream primary care services or who require additional support in engaging with health care providers. While an extensive literature on the quality of school-based health services for adolescents is available, few studies have examined the quality of hospital- or community-based primary care services for adolescents. Safety-net centers constitute an important community resource within the broader public health and primary care system of each region. Safety-net centers depend largely on public funding rather than fee-for-service reimbursement.

Findings:

- *Evidence shows that safety-net health services for adolescents are:*
  - *accessible to many adolescents who are uninsured or do not find private office-based services acceptable for their needs.*
  - *frequently more acceptable to adolescents who are uncomfortable with private office-based primary care providers, especially when they can establish relationships with providers who are sensitive to their needs and promote open communication.*
  - *sometimes able to offer a more appropriate mix of skills and counseling services that address risky behaviors.*

- *able to provide effective disease prevention and health promotion services while also addressing issues related to risky behavior. However, such centers often can become unstable during times of fiscal uncertainty and may experience frequent personnel transitions. They also face unique challenges associated with financing of prevention and health promotion services that cannot be reimbursed.*
- *important mechanisms for resolving the disparities and inequities that exist within private office-based primary care.*

SPECIALITY CARE SERVICES

The preceding section reviewed knowledge of and experience with an array of programs and centers that offer primary care services for adolescents. This section focuses on specialty services in the areas of mental health, sexual and reproductive health, oral health, and substance use treatment and prevention. While some of these specialty services may be integrated into comprehensive primary care programs, they are more frequently located in separate sites and systems, which makes it difficult to blend them with primary care.

Mental Health

As noted in Chapter 2, mental disorders are common among adolescents and may impose a tremendous health burden for this population.[2] Emotional and behavioral symptoms often co-occur with other health problems seen in the health system and in the juvenile justice and foster care systems (see Chapter 2). Traditionally, the mental health sector has been responsible for treatment of adolescents with mental disorders. This sector comprises a diverse workforce of psychiatrists, psychologists, social workers, and other, lesser-trained individuals organized into loose networks of providers. The reimbursement system for mental health services has traditionally focused on the severely and persistently mentally ill, and has limited capacity to address emerging mental illness and adolescents who are functioning but not healthy. In case studies in four major cities, mental health providers reported that insurers rarely covered telephone calls to parents, teachers,

---

[2]Although an appreciation for the importance of mental disorders in adolescence has emerged over the past two decades, changes made to enhance mental health services for adolescents have been modest at best. For the purposes of this report and brevity, discussion of this subject—which can involve the use of various terms, including "mental health problems," "mental disorders," "emotional and behavioral disorders," "psychosocial problems," "emotionally disturbed," "mentally ill," and the like—is limited to mental disorders and related services.

and primary care providers; team conferences; or care coordination. In addition, these mental health providers reported that few insurers accepted diagnostic codes for psychosocial problems not yet considered diagnosable mental disorders (McManus, Shejavali, and Fox, 2003).

Treatment for adolescents with mental disorders generally involves the use of psychotropic medication and/or psychotherapy. Effective therapeutic interventions with fewer adverse effects have emerged in both areas over the last two decades. Unfortunately, despite the lack of effectiveness of usual clinical care, most routine community practices fail to incorporate evidence-based therapies for mental health problems into their delivery systems (Weisz, Hawley, and Doss, 2004; Weisz et al., 1995, 2005). In other words, community practices rarely incorporate effective care for mental disorders as assessed through randomized trials; therefore, the benefits of effective therapeutic interventions are not available to the majority of adolescents and families seeking care for mental health problems within their communities. In most communities, effective treatment is also hampered by severe shortages of trained professionals, limited coverage of useful care, and poor coordination among providers from different disciplines (Ben-Dror, 1994; McManus, Shejavali, and Fox, 2003). These factors have contributed to long waiting lists, low levels of satisfaction, and little evidence of effectiveness for routine community mental health services.

An analysis of 2003 data from the National Survey of Children's Health reveals that a significant percentage of adolescents need but fail to receive mental health or counseling services. On a national basis, 36 percent of adolescents aged 12–17 with current behavioral problems that require treatment or counseling do not receive mental health services; this percentage ranges from 63 percent in Texas to 10 percent in Wyoming (Child and Adolescent Health Measurement Initiative, 2008).

Sexual and Reproductive Health

The American Medical Association and the American College of Obstetricians and Gynecologists, among others, recommend that adolescents receive guidance and counseling on responsible sexual behavior, including abstinence, methods of birth control, and prevention of STIs and HIV infection (American Medical Association, 1997; Committee on Adolescent Health and American College of Obstetricians and Gynecologists, 2006). Current guidelines recommend that adolescents who have had sexual intercourse be screened for STIs.

According to data from the 2002 National Survey of Family Growth, approximately half (49 percent) of all adolescent girls aged 15–19 had visited a medical provider for reproductive health services[3] in the previous year (Suellentrop, 2006b). This proportion varies according to age and race or ethnicity. As young adolescents mature, their use of reproductive health services increases. Slightly more than one-third (38 percent) of adolescent females aged 15–17 reported receiving reproductive health services in the past year, increasing to 65 percent for those aged 18–19 (Chandra et al., 2005; Suellentrop, 2006b). Non-Hispanic black and non-Hispanic white adolescent females were more likely than Hispanic adolescent females to report the use of reproductive health services in the past year (57 percent, 49 percent, and 41 percent, respectively). Eight of ten sexually experienced adolescent females had visited a provider in the past year for reproductive health services (Suellentrop, 2006b). Female adolescents who had received reproductive health services in the past year reported that they had visited private doctors or managed care providers (55 percent) at around the same rate as clinics (53 percent). Older adolescents (aged 18–19), however, were significantly more likely than younger adolescents (aged 15–17) to report going to a private doctor or managed care organization as opposed to a clinic (Suellentrop, 2006b).

A Pap test and birth control were the most commonly reported reproductive health services. Almost three-quarters of adolescent females (71 percent) reported receiving a Pap test in the past year. Hispanic adolescent females were much less likely than non-Hispanic black adolescent females and non-Hispanic white adolescent females to have received a Pap test in the past year (55 percent, 80 percent, and 72 percent, respectively) (Suellentrop, 2006b). Approximately two-thirds of adolescent females who had used reproductive health services (64 percent) had received birth control or a prescription for birth control in the past year. Almost half reported receiving counseling or information about birth control (Suellentrop, 2006b).

Counseling on different methods of birth control is particularly important for adolescent girls and may be helpful in reducing the proportion of girls who discontinue using their method of contraception. In 2002, almost one third of sexually experienced adolescent girls indicated that they had ever stopped using a method of contraception, and more than half reported that they had stopped using a method because of side effects (53 percent). A majority of the adolescent girls who reported that they had stopped using a method of contraception were using the pill (Suellentrop, 2006c).

---

[3]Reproductive health services include family planning services and/or related medical services. Family planning services include such services as receipt of a birth control method or prescription, a test or checkup for a birth control method, or counseling or information about birth control from a medical provider. Medical services include, for example, a Pap smear, a pelvic exam, counseling, testing or treatment for STIs, or a pregnancy test.

Adolescent boys have particularly low rates of use of primary care—1.7 visits annually reported in 2000, compared with 2.2 visits annually for adolescent females (Ma, Wang, and Stafford, 2005). According to the National Survey of Family Growth, almost one-third of adolescent boys reported that they had received no health services in the past year. Among those who had visited a health care provider in the past year, approximately one-quarter had received counseling or advice from their provider about methods of birth control, STIs, or HIV/AIDS. Close to one in five adolescent boys reported that they had visited a family planning clinic for health services. Sexually experienced adolescent boys were more likely than inexperienced adolescent boys to report having visited a family planning clinic (Suellentrop, 2006a).

Studies evaluating the effectiveness of clinic services tailored specifically to adolescents have found that clinic interventions can increase adolescents' use of contraception, reduce rates of adolescent pregnancy, and increase adolescents' knowledge about sexual and other reproductive health issues (Burlew and Philliber, 2007). In 1995, approximately two-thirds of all family planning agencies (such as Planned Parenthood) are estimated to have provided one service specifically tailored to adolescents (Frost and Bolzan, 1997). Such tailoring usually involves offering longer appointment times, having specific counseling appointments, offering a variety of support services, or spreading a visit over two appointments (the first for counseling and the second for a pelvic exam). The convenience of a clinic in terms of location, hours of operation, types of services offered, and costs also affects its use by adolescents. Research suggests that adolescents are more inclined to rely on clinics when they offer a wide range of services in addition to family planning, when the services are provided at little or no cost, and when confidentiality is ensured. In a recent study, 59 percent of adolescent girls (under age 18) who were attending a Planned Parenthood clinic indicated that they would refuse family planning services and delay STI testing and treatment if their parents were notified that they were being prescribed oral contraceptives (Reddy, Fleming, and Swain, 2002). (See the section on confidentiality and privacy later in this chapter.)

Active outreach strategies are also important to draw adolescent clients to a clinic and ensure that the right services are being offered. Such strategies include forming partnerships with other organizations in the community, maintaining a presence at community events, and inviting adolescents to refer their peers to the clinic. Clinic personnel, especially those interested in and dedicated to working with adolescents, can also influence the clinic's success (Burlew and Philliber, 2007).

Oral Health

Dentistry has significantly different characteristics from medicine that directly influence the quantity, quality, accessibility, and affordability of dental services for adolescents. Service characteristics associated with oral health also result in environmental constraints that impede coordination of care with other basic medical and developmental health services; foster varying systems of professional education and training, financing, staffing, service delivery, accreditation, licensure, and professional governance; and contribute to differing involvement in government health programs and sometimes profound differences in professional culture, mores, and norms. As a result, observations and recommendations based on the medical professions typically cannot easily be extrapolated to dental services.

Dental services are used with approximately the same frequency as medical services among adolescents (see Table 3-4). Orthodontic and aesthetic concerns generate dental visits, and dental pathologies are both common and often symptomatic among adolescents. This frequent contact gives dentists both opportunities and responsibilities to engage their adolescent patients in promoting salutary health behaviors, to detect eating disorders and risky behaviors, and to identify health conditions that require referral. Despite the frequency with which adolescents visit dentists, however, the dental profession and its pediatric specialty have until recently focused relatively little on adolescence beyond orthodontic issues.

While 80 percent of adolescents' parents report that they obtained a dental visit in a year on the National Health and Nutrition Examination Survey (NHANES) in Table 3-4, overreporting of dental services is a well-recognized problem that is evidenced by discrepancies between federal surveys (Macek et al., 2002). This may result from the social expectation that all children should receive two preventive dental visits each year, an expectation that is not shared with medical care. Because of its more intensive surveillance approach, the Medical Expenditure Panel Survey (MEPS) is regarded as the most reliable national data source on adolescents' use of dental services. MEPS reports that 53 percent of adolescents ages 6 through 20 received at least one dental visit in the year 2004, virtually unchanged from 51 percent reported in 1996 (Manski and Brown, 2007). A variety of recognized barriers to dental care, including coverage inadequacies, workforce shortages, and adolescents' failure to use dental services (as occurs with medical services), combine to reduce utilization of dental care among adolescents. The percentages of adolescents who report dental care needs reflect compromised oral health status among the adolescent population: half of those aged 10–19 (53.5 percent) are reportedly in need of dental care (National Institute of Dental and Craniofacial Research, 1994, NHANES III data 1988–1994).

TABLE 3-4 Doctor and Dentist Visits by Children and Adolescents (aged 6–17) in Last 12 Months

	Doctor Visit (%)	Dentist Visit (%)
Age (years)		
6–10	87	82
11–14	85	83
15–17	83	80
Sex		
Male	85	81
Female	86	83
Race/Ethnicity		
White	89	86
Black	84	79
Hispanic	77	70
Other	82	81
Total	85	82

NOTE: Data from 2005 National Health Interview Survey child sample questionnaire.
SOURCE: Reprinted, with permission, from Schuchter and Fairbrother (2008). Copyright (2008) by Cincinnati Children's Hospital.

National surveys reveal higher levels of unmet need among racial and ethnic minorities relative to whites. For children aged 6–18, parents report rates of unmet need that are 1.6 times higher for blacks and 2.1 times higher for Mexican Americans than for whites (Vargas and Ronzio, 2002). Minority status may be confounded by other characteristics of social disadvantage, such as parental educational attainment. Two to three times more parents with only or less than a high school education (3.0 times and 2.3 times, respectively) than parents with more than a high school education report that their children aged 6–18 have unmet needs for dental care. Parents of children and adolescents with special health needs also report higher unmet dental needs (Schultz, Shenkin, and Horowitz, 2001). Data compiled by Schuchter and Fairbrother (2008) reveal increases in unmet need for dental care with advancing age, as well as variations by race or ethnicity and gender (see Table 3-5). Unmet need for preventive dental care among children and adolescents who have not seen a dentist in the past year increases steadily by age to one in five adolescents aged 12–17 (Maternal and Child Health Bureau, 2005).

Substance Use Treatment and Prevention

Studies of referral patterns for alcohol and drug treatment centers indicate that schools infrequently detect substance use disorders among

TABLE 3-5 Unmet Dental Needs, Last 12 Months

Characteristic	Percentage
Age (years)	
11–14	9
15–17	9
18–21	12
22–24	17
Sex	
Male	9
Female	12
Race/Ethnicity	
White	9
Black	11
Hispanic	14
Other	7

NOTE: Data from 2005 National Health Interview Survey.
SOURCE: Reprinted, with permission, from Schuchter and Fairbrother (2008). Copyright (2008) by Cincinnati Children's Hospital.

adolescents and make referrals for treatment. In 2004, only 11 percent of admissions to alcohol and drug treatment for adolescents aged 12–17 were due to school referrals (Substance Abuse and Mental Health Services Administration, 2006a). Schools may be more likely to handle drug use by punishing students than to refer them to or provide treatment (McAndrews, 2001).

Rates of substance use are particularly high among adolescents who are engaged with certain institutional sectors. For example, in one county in California, Aarons and colleagues (2001) found high proportions of adolescents (under age 18) with substance use disorders in the juvenile justice system (62 percent), the mental health system (41 percent), and the foster care system (19 percent). Prevalence rates for older youths aged 18–25 in institutional care are thought to be even higher. The criminal justice system is the major source of referrals for adolescent substance use treatment. In 2004, for example, the criminal justice system accounted for 52 percent of referrals for admission to treatment among adolescents aged 12–17, and the same percentage was reported for older adolescents aged 18–21 (Substance Abuse and Mental Health Services Administration, 2006a).

According to data from the National Survey on Drug Use and Health (2003–2004), 6.1 percent of adolescents aged 12–17 needed treatment for alcohol use, and 5.4 percent needed treatment for illicit drug use (Substance Abuse and Mental Health Services Administration, 2006b). Of those adolescents who needed treatment for alcohol use, however, only 7.2 percent had received specialty treatment (including inpatient hospitalization, treatment in a rehabilitation facility, or treatment in a mental health center) in the past year. The corresponding figure for treatment for illicit drug use was 9.1 percent.

Many adolescents, however, do not perceive a need for or seek treatment and may not volunteer information about their use of substances unless they have established a rapport with a health professional or counselor. In the National Survey on Drug Use and Health (2003–2004), among those who were classified as needing treatment but had received no specialty treatment in the past year, only 2.2 percent perceived a need for treatment for alcohol use problems and only 3.5 percent for drug use problems (Substance Abuse and Mental Health Services Administration, 2006b). Similar findings were reported in the Cannabis Youth Treatment Study: 80 percent of adolescents saw no need for treatment (Mensinger et al., 2006). Adolescents who experience more negative consequences from their substance use show more motivation to change (Battjes et al., 2003; Breda and Heflinger, 2004).

Several studies have identified certain characteristics associated with successful treatment outcomes for adolescents who use substances. These characteristics include severity and comorbidity (Dobkin et al., 1998; Grella and Joshi, 2003; Hser et al., 2001; Rounds-Bryant, Kristiansen, and Hubbard, 1999; Tomlinson, Brown, and Abrantes, 2004) and longer periods of time in treatment (Hser et al., 2001), especially for those with comorbid psychiatric disorders. Recent research suggests that substance use may affect neural systems that are important for reward and for self-regulation and inhibition. If adolescents suffer from these substance use–related changes in neural systems, sufficient duration of treatment may be important for addressing these problems (Kalivas and Volkow, 2005; Leshner, 1997; Volkow and Li, 2005). While duration is important, however, providers frequently have difficulty retaining adolescents in treatment programs. Retention in treatment is predicted by the presence of fewer deviant peers, the absence of emotional problems due to substance use, and a positive assessment of the counselor's skills on the part of the patient (Battjes et al., 2004). Treatment success is also associated with characteristics of the post-treatment environment, such as not being involved with others who engage in risky behavior (family substance use, peer networks), taking part in support groups (e.g., Alcoholics Anonymous or Narcotics Anonymous), and participating in substance-free leisure activities (Godley et al., 2005).

One problem with the delivery of substance use treatment may be a lack of professional training and certification in working with adolescents. As of 2002, for example, no U.S. state had adolescent-specific provider certification for such treatment. And as of 2004, the certification program of the National Association of Alcoholism and Drug Abuse Counselors had no adolescent-specific requirements (McLellen and Meyers, 2004). Another problem is that, despite their availability, appropriate screening instruments and treatment guidelines are not routinely incorporated into substance use treatment programs for adolescents (see the discussion of screening later in this chapter). One study of 144 "highly regarded programs" found that the average program score for these elements was 23.8 out of a possible 45 (Brannigan et al., 2004).

The low levels of availability, accessibility, and acceptability of effective treatment services for adolescents with substance use disorders are particularly disturbing in light of evidence demonstrating the effectiveness of such interventions (Brannigan et al., 2004). Positive treatment effects for significant reductions in marijuana use, heavy drinking, and other illicit drug use have been found for many different types of interventions, including multisystemic therapy, family therapy, contingency management, cognitive-behavioral therapy, 12-step programs, and motivational enhancement therapy (Williams, Chang, and the Addiction Centre Research Group, 2000). More time in treatment is associated with better outcomes (Hser et al., 2001).

Although a number of treatment approaches are promising (Deas and Thomas, 2001; Liddle and Dakof, 1995; Szapocznik et al., 2006; Waldron and Kaminer, 2004; Winters et al., 2000), studies of the relative effectiveness of a limited number of adolescent substance use treatment programs have been unable to demonstrate that one particular program or approach consistently works better than others (Godley et al., 2004; Morral et al., 2006; White, White, and Dennis, 2004). In the absence of evidence-based studies supporting the choice of any one treatment method, government and professional organizations have identified key principles of effective treatment that can serve as the basis for adolescent treatment strategies (Bukstein et al., 2005; Drug Strategies, 2003; National Institute on Drug Abuse, 1999). Examples of these principles include adapting treatment interventions to individual needs; continuing treatment for an adequate period of time; continuously monitoring for possible drug use; using developmentally appropriate programs; and attending to individuals' multiple needs, not just their drug use.

Positive outcomes for certain treatment strategies generally involve short-term effects, and relapse rates remain high (Winters, 1999). Some forms of relapse may be related to the above-noted structural changes in the brain that involve inhibition and reward centers (Kalivas and Volkow, 2005). Treatment regimens may therefore best be derived from a chronic disease management rather than an acute care model (National Institute on Drug Abuse, 2006; Volkow and Li, 2005). Important lessons for treatment and prevention services for adolescents can be drawn from treatments for diabetes and hypertension in older populations (which involve chronically relapsing and remitting disorders with major challenges of adherence to treatment regimens).

At present, aftercare for adolescents with substance use disorders remains inadequate, and comorbid mental health problems receive insufficient attention. One review of 53 studies found that fewer than half of adolescents discharged from treatment programs (38 percent) remained abstinent from substance use after 6 months, even when aftercare plans were in place (Williams, Chang, and the Addiction Centre Research Group, 2000). Data reported by Godley and colleagues (2007) for some aftercare models, such as "assertive" continuing care (in which the clinician rather than the patient has responsibility for linkage and retention), suggest that these models can improve linkage to aftercare for adolescents who have received residential drug treatment. However, while the authors found that substance use decreased as expected when these models were employed, the results were not significant (low statistical power, which limited conclusions). A recent (as yet untested) approach is for aftercare programs to implement "adaptive" interventions, which vary in focus and intensity in response to changes in individual needs (McKay, 2006).

Summary

Evidence-based therapies are available for adolescents in the specialty areas of mental health, sexual and reproductive health, oral health, and substance use treatment and prevention. Yet these interventions are commonly not integrated into routine health care practices, particularly for those who depend on public financing for their routine care. Many adolescents have difficulty gaining access to specialized services because of financial restrictions, shortages of skilled personnel, and the lack of appropriate or convenient settings that are suitable for their stage of development. Adolescents with comorbid conditions (such as mental health, sexual, and substance use conditions) are especially difficult to serve within the current fragmented array of health care services and settings.

Findings:

- *Evidence shows that specialty care services for the adolescent population are not accessible to most adolescents. Existing specialty services in the areas of mental health, sexual and reproductive health, oral health, and substance use treatment and prevention are generally insufficient to meet the needs of many adolescents. While evidence-based therapies are available in a number of these areas, they are not integrated into many practice settings.*

- *Even when specialty services are accessible, many adolescents do not find them acceptable because of concerns about disclosure of treatment in sensitive areas (such as substance use or sexual health).*
- *Many specialty providers lack appropriate training to address the needs of adolescent patients, and certification programs for treating adolescents are frequently unavailable in many specialty areas.*
- *The lack of appropriate specialty services that are suitable for adolescents means that effective treatment is often delayed, care is of limited duration, and services are poorly reimbursed.*
- *Limitations in the quality of or access to specialty services are especially prevalent among at-risk adolescents in whom problems in the above areas frequently co-occur, contributing to health care inequities and disparities.*

INPATIENT HOSPITAL SERVICES FOR ADOLESCENTS

Most hospitals in the United States do not have a sufficient volume of adolescent patients to justify the creation of specific inpatient services for this population. During the 1970s and 1980s, many youth advocates called for the creation of adolescent inpatient units. The Society for Adolescent Medicine estimated that there were 40–60 such units in the United States by the mid-1990s (Fisher and Kaufman, 1996; Macfarlane and Blum, 2001). In some cases, however, these units were simply sections within other wards. Although adolescent specialists have consistently advocated for separate adolescent inpatient units in both pediatric and general hospitals as an optimal approach to the delivery of developmentally appropriate health care for this population (Watson, 1998), it is unlikely that this ideal will be realized in response to current trends.

More commonly, hospitals rely on a multidisciplinary team approach involving health professionals with interest and expertise in adolescent health to meet the inpatient needs of adolescents. The Society for Adolescent Medicine has formulated guidelines for the care of adolescents in hospitals so that those with the greatest expertise in and awareness of developmental issues pertinent to adolescence can be involved with young people's care (Fisher and Kaufman, 1996).

Adolescents aged 13–17 account for 11 percent of all hospital stays by those aged 0–17. Adolescents are a distant second to neonates (less than 1 year of age), who account for 71 percent of hospital stays by children and adolescents (Owens et al., 2003).

Adolescent pregnancy is one of the most important reasons for hospitalizations before age 18, accounting for 3 percent of all pediatric hospitalizations. Adolescent girls (aged 10–17) have the highest rates of obstetrical trauma (e.g., perineal lacerations) during delivery among all females and are 35 percent more likely than older females to experience such trauma without instrument assistance (Owens et al., 2003).

Medicaid bears a larger burden of care for pregnant adolescents than private insurance—more than two-thirds of all adolescent admissions for pregnancy or childbirth are billed to state Medicaid programs, while one-fourth are billed to primary insurance—the converse of the distribution of pregnancy expenses for adult women (Owens et al., 2003). While adolescent deliveries are more likely to involve diagnoses of early or threatened labor, hypertension complicating pregnancy, and excess amniotic fluid, pregnant adolescents with no health insurance coverage are the least likely to deliver by Caesarian section, a fact that raises questions about the influence of insurance status on the choice of procedures (Owens et al., 2003).

Mental health disorders (primarily depression) are one of the ten main reasons for hospitalization among children. By age 13–17, affective disorders are the most common cause of hospitalization for conditions not related to pregnancy (Owens et al., 2003). Injuries, including leg injuries, medication poisonings, and head injuries, are also a primary reason for hospital stays among those aged 13–17 (Owens et al., 2003). Adolescents from low-income families are more likely to be admitted to the hospital through the emergency department than are adolescents from higher-income areas (Owens et al., 2003).

ADOLESCENTS' USE OF HEALTH SERVICES

Understanding the extent to which adolescents report access to and use of health services in various settings is useful in identifying differences between service capacity and utilization rates. Such information can also be helpful in understanding variations in unmet need and the quality of care available to young people.

Usual Sources of Medical Care

Most adolescents (aged 11–17) have a usual source of medical care—92 percent according to parental reports—while 75 percent of young people aged 18–21 report that they have a usual source of care (Schuchter and Fairbrother, 2008[4]) (see Figure 3-1). This is an important sign of access to health services and is a key indicator to monitor.

---

[4]Schuchter and Fairbrother (2008) use 2005 National Health Interview Survey (NHIS) data that are based on adolescents aged 18 and over reporting for themselves and parents reporting for those under age 18. This is the standard methodology for most national household surveys.

CURRENT ADOLESCENT HEALTH SERVICES 169

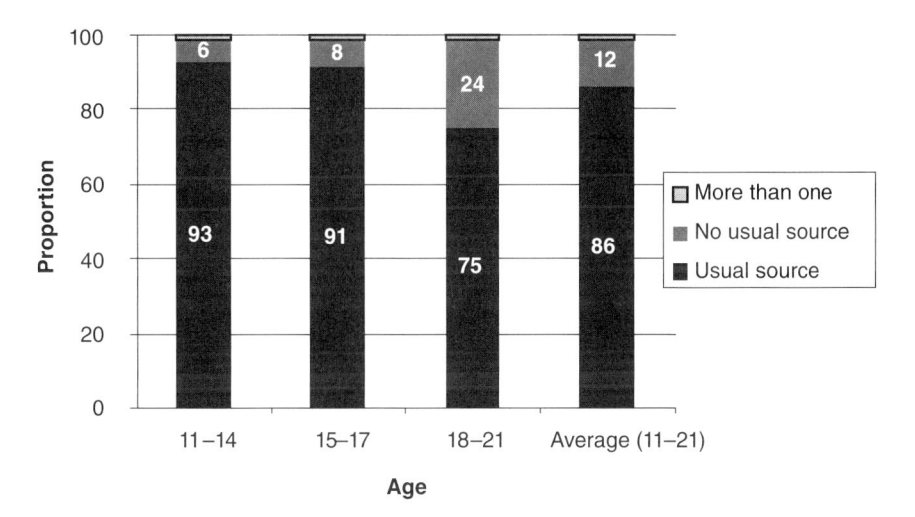

FIGURE 3-1 Percentage of adolescents with a usual source of care, 2005 National Health Interview Survey.
NOTE: Percents may not add to 100 because of rounding and small categories of less than 1 percent. Adolescents aged 18 and over answer for themselves; parents answer for those under 18.
SOURCE: Reprinted, with permission, from Schuchter and Fairbrother (2008). Copyright (2008) by Cincinnati Children's Hospital.

Adolescents who have a usual source of medical care rely predominantly on a doctor's office or managed care organization (approximately 77 percent) or a clinic or health center (a little over 20 percent). Privately insured adolescents aged 11–17 are more likely than publicly insured adolescents to report a doctor's office or managed care organization as their usual source of care (85 percent versus 66 percent) (see Table 3-6) (Schuchter and Fairbrother, 2008). These rates remain generally consistent as adolescents grow older, as indicated in Figure 3-2.

Publicly insured adolescents are more likely than their privately insured counterparts to name a clinic or health center as their usual source of medical care (30 percent versus 14 percent) (Schuchter and Fairbrother, 2008). Low reimbursement rates in public insurance programs (Medicaid and SCHIP) may cause many providers to limit the number of publicly insured patients they see, contributing to these disparities (Cunningham and Nichols, 2005; Tang, Yudkowsky, and Davis, 2003). A very small proportion of adolescents report nontraditional sites, such as school-based health centers, hospital emergency departments, or family planning centers, as their usual source of

TABLE 3-6 Usual Source of Care (%), by Age and Insurance Type, 2005 National Health Interview Survey

Insurance Type	Source of Care	Age (years) 11–14	15–17	18–21	Average (11–21)
Private					
	Doctor's office or HMO	85	85	80	83
	Clinic or health center	14	14	17	15
Public					
	Doctor's office or HMO	64	68	62	65
	Clinic or health center	32	28	32	31

NOTE: HMO = health maintenance organization.
SOURCE: Reprinted, with permission, from Schuchter and Fairbrother (2008). Copyright (2008) by Cincinnati Children's Hospital.

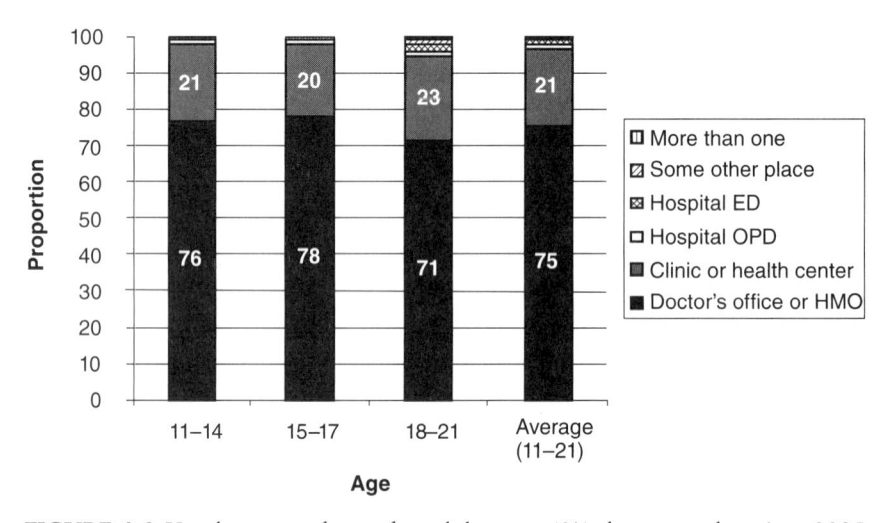

FIGURE 3-2 Usual source of care for adolescents (%), by age and setting, 2005 National Health Interview Survey.
NOTES: ED = Emergency Department, HMO = health maintenance organization, OPD = Outpatient Departments. Those aged 18 and over answer for themselves; parents answer for those under 18. Respondents are not asked about well-child checkups after age 17.
SOURCE: Reprinted, with permission, from Schuchter and Fairbrother (2008). Copyright (2008) by Cincinnati Children's Hospital.

medical care (about 1 percent in each category) (Schuchter and Fairbrother, 2008). Almost half of uninsured adolescents (aged 10–17) have at least one unmet health service need (MacKay and Duran, 2007).

Those with special health conditions, such as chronic illnesses or acute injuries, may have frequent encounters with health professionals. The usual source of care for these adolescents may not embody all aspects of a medical home; for example, a recent analysis from the Child and Adolescent Health Measurement Initiative 2005–2006 found that fewer than half of adolescents with special health needs experienced all facets of a medical home (Maternal and Child Health Bureau, 2008).

Visits with Health Care Providers

While the majority of adolescents visit a health care provider during the course of a year, the proportion decreases with age, especially in later adolescence as young people move into young adulthood. The sharpest decrease occurs at age 18, as adolescents age out of public insurance. Significant differences in utilization rates are also seen by gender.

In 2005, according to the NHIS, 83 percent of adolescents aged 10–19 reported having seen a doctor or other health care provider in the past year (MacKay and Duran, 2007). Males aged 18–19 were much less likely to have made a recent health visit than their younger counterparts; in contrast, health care utilization was much more consistent across the adolescent and young adult age spectrum for females. More than 34 percent of males aged 18–19 reported not having a health care visit in the past 12 months compared with 16 percent of females in the same age group (MacKay and Duran, 2007).

Especially noteworthy are adolescents' reported high rates of use of hospital emergency departments for routine as well as emergency care, rates that increase with age among both male and female adolescents. Adolescents frequently rely on emergency departments for both urgent and nonurgent health conditions, and their rates of utilization for routine, nonurgent health services in emergency settings are higher than those of any other age group (Nawar, Niska, and Xu, 2007).

Summary

Most adolescents have a usual source of medical care and see a health care provider annually. The types of settings where adolescents receive health services vary with their insurance plans: those with private insurance are more likely to receive health services in a private provider's or managed care office, while adolescents with public insurance are more likely to see providers in a local clinic or health center. A very small proportion of adolescents report nontraditional sites, such as school-based health centers, hospital emergency departments, or family planning centers, as their usual source of care (about 1 percent in each category).

As adolescent males grow older, their annual visits to health care providers decline significantly. The sharpest decrease occurs at age 18, a time when many adolescents age out of insurance, both public and private. Older adolescent females show much less of a decline in annual health care visits.

MISSED OPPORTUNITIES FOR PREVENTION AND HEALTH PROMOTION AMONG ADOLESCENTS

As reviewed in Chapter 2, more than 70 percent of all deaths among adolescents aged 10–19 can be attributed to three causes: unintentional injuries (including motor vehicle crashes), homicides, and suicide (National Center for Injury Prevention and Control, 2007). Furthermore, unhealthful habits and risky behaviors that are initiated in adolescence extend into adulthood and contribute directly to poor health conditions and significant morbidity and mortality in the short and long terms (Kolbe, Kann, and Collins, 1993). In one national survey, for example, 78 percent of adolescents had not eaten five or more servings of fruits and vegetables a day during the week preceding the survey, 33 percent had not participated in a sufficient amount of physical activity, and 14 percent were overweight. Moreover, 22 percent of high school students had smoked cigarettes in the month preceding the survey (Grunbaum et al., 2004). There is a need, then, for adolescent health services focused on prevention and health promotion.

Current Status of Prevention and Health Promotion Services for Adolescents

Standardized screening instruments, structured tools, and professional guidelines are available to address risky adolescent behaviors, as is discussed in more detail in Chapter 4. Despite the availability of these resources, studies have shown that practitioners fail to provide the recommended screening, counseling, and health education services. Health personnel frequently rely on adolescents or their parents to initiate discussions of health concerns that may involve the use of alcohol, tobacco, or other substances; risky sexual practices; or other problematic behaviors. The frequent practice in some domains, such as mental health, is simply to ask whether there are any general areas of concern during annual health maintenance visits or routine physical examinations or to use specific trigger questions around a particular topic (Olson et al., 2001). This lack of communication about high-risk issues may be especially problematic for adolescents who are marginalized or perceive themselves to be socially distant from health care providers, such as those who are LGBT. For example, there are clear differences in the identification and treatment of mental disorders among racial and ethnic groups, and rates of identification are lower for those who perceive greater social distance from their physicians (Cuffe et al., 1995; Strakowski et al., 1995).

In a review of preventive care for children and adolescents, Chung and colleagues (2006) found that in most studies, fewer than half of children had received developmental or psychosocial screening, and fewer than half of adolescents had been asked about various health risks or screened for chlamydia. Bethell and colleagues (2001) report that only 18 percent of adolescents aged 14–18 said they had received counseling on risky behavior (such as smoking, use of alcohol or street drugs, sexual/physical abuse, and violence); 23 percent had received preventive screening and counseling on emotional health and relationship issues; and 36 percent had received preventive screening and counseling on sexual activity and STIs. Furthermore, despite the national concern about obesity, only half of adolescents said they had received preventive screening regarding weight, diet, and exercise (Bethell, Klein, and Peck, 2001).

Adolescents generally do not receive routine preventive services for substance use, even though the guidelines of national professional organizations, such as the American Academy of Pediatrics, suggest that they should be screened for drug, alcohol, and cigarette use (Institute for Clinical Systems Improvement, 2007; Kulig and Committee on Substance Abuse, 2005). A 1995 survey of pediatricians showed that fewer than 50 percent screened adolescents for substance use (American Academy of Pediatrics and Division of Child Health Research, n.d.). Another survey from 1991–1996 showed that only a minority of physicians counseled adolescents about smoking (Thorndike et al., 1999).

While several studies have found that routine screening is uncommon for adolescents, providers do target counseling to the highest-risk adolescents, a finding that indicates a relationship between engagement of adolescents in risky behavior and receipt of counseling for that behavior (Bethell, Klein, and Peck, 2001; Fairbrother et al., 2005; Klein and Wilson, 2002). Many at-risk adolescents, however, do not receive counseling. A survey by Klein and Wilson (2002) found that 71 percent of adolescents engaged in one of eight behaviors with potential health risks. Among this at-risk group, 63 percent had not spoken to their doctor about any of these risks. Fairbrother and colleagues (2005) found that approximately one-third of low-income adolescents in New York City who reported having sexual intercourse had not been counseled about STIs. Even more striking, among adolescents reporting symptoms of depression, almost 70 percent had not been counseled about these feelings.

There are a number of reasons for the lack of preventive screening and counseling. First, routine screening requires the use of reliable screening instruments and standardized screening measures. Several such instruments are available for primary care settings (e.g., for substance use—Knight et al., 2002, 2003), yet they are absent or infrequently used in many practices that provide adolescent health care. Second, reimbursement for screening and counseling is inadequate (as discussed in Chapter 6). Third, studies demonstrate that some physicians may avoid screening because they regard it as too time-consuming or fear alienating patients. In the case of substance use, physicians may be unaware of positive treatment outcomes or lack information on treatment resources for adolescents (Kulig and Committee on Substance Abuse, 2005; Van Hook et al., 2007).

Another barrier to routine screening for risky and unhealthful behaviors in adolescents may be the lack of training in screening and counseling among health care providers. Research has demonstrated that educational interventions can improve providers' screening and counseling of adolescents. One project, for example, offered training and tools for providers to improve their screening and counseling regarding tobacco, alcohol, and drug use; sexual behavior; and safety. The study found significantly increased screening and counseling rates among providers who had received the intervention compared with those who continued to provide their usual standard of care. The average proportion of adolescents screened and counseled increased from 58 percent to 83 percent and from 52 percent to 78 percent, respectively, while no significant increases occurred in the comparison group during the same period. The authors report that the training appeared to account for most of this increase, with the tools sustaining the effects of the training (Ozer et al., 2005). Yet while significant increases in screening may occur as a result of such training programs, they are often difficult to sustain for the reasons outlined above.

In dealing with adolescents' risky behaviors, health care providers may need to interact with the education, legal, and/or social service sectors. Addressing another level of coordination, one project sought to improve adolescent screening and counseling through a broad community-level initiative involving partnerships among state Medicaid, managed care plans, and community leaders. Increases in screening and counseling for use of tobacco and other substances for Medicaid populations and improved HIV counseling for all populations were reported, although the gains were more modest than those seen with the training intervention described above (Klein et al., 2003).

Differences in the prevalence of unhealthful and risky behaviors among different populations of adolescents raise important questions about the extent to which all adolescents should be screened for use of selected substances or unhealthful practices. Given the specificity and sensitivity of many screening instruments, it is necessary to determine whether they are appropriate for use in a general or selected population. Some screening instruments may produce a high number of false positives or false negatives that would discount their value in many clinical settings. For example, the Centers for Disease Control and Prevention has provided new guidelines (Branson et al., 2006) for all health care providers in various primary care settings regarding routine screening for HIV in adolescents, especially those participating in risky behaviors leading to exposure to HIV. Moreover, some instruments may be more or less appropriate for diverse populations served in primary care settings. While several screening tools are available in many languages and in both audio and printed formats, others are more limited. Understanding the demographics of the primary care panel is critical to any screening process.

Summary

Health maintenance visits and health supervision are important components of primary care services for adolescents. As noted earlier in this chapter, most adolescents visit health care providers annually. Yet few providers screen adolescents for risk factors and unhealthful behaviors, and most providers fail to offer services or resources that could help adolescents improve their future health status as young adults.

Findings:

- *Routine screening for risk factors and unhealthful behaviors that emerge during adolescence is not available or accessible for most adolescents.*
- *Many health care providers who treat adolescents fail to adhere to recommended prevention guidelines, to screen for appropriate risk factors and unhealthful behaviors that emerge during adolescence, and to provide effective counseling that would reduce risks and foster health promotion.*

HEALTH DISPARITIES AND RACIAL AND ETHNIC BIASES

Research reported in both the adult and pediatric literature (Cooper and Powe, 2004; Flores and Ngui, 2006; Mayberry, Mili, and Ofili, 2000; West et al., 2006) has shown that disparities and biases in the delivery of health services are unwanted realties that deserve priority attention by both private organizations and federal agencies (Kaiser Family Foundation, 2007). The emphasis in this research has been on general access and service delivery; most of the work has focused on adults or the general pediatric population, with little specific attention to the needs of adolescents who are racial or ethnic minorities.

Existing Disparities in Adolescent Health Services

The 2001 U.S. Surgeon General's report emphasized adolescent health needs, with particular attention to violence and health care disparities. Other than this report, little attention has been directed toward strategies for reducing health service disparities among adolescents.

A review of racial and ethnic disparities and patient safety by Flores and Ngui (2006) focused on mental health among adolescents. The study found that white psychotherapists who were presented with identical case scenarios rated black less likely than white adolescents to display pathological behavior and that providers were less distressed by minority youths' reporting aggressive, deviant behavior or hating their mothers. This study reaffirmed earlier research indicating that black adolescents are underdiagnosed for depression and other mental health concerns (Adebimpe, 1981; Martin, 1993; Strakowski et al., 2003).

In a review of the literature on disparities in emergency department care, Heron, Stettner, and Haley (2006) found that Hispanic and black adolescents presenting with trauma had an increased rate of testing for drugs and alcohol compared with white adolescents (Marcin et al., 2003). The more frequent testing rates could not be clinically justified as there was no difference in the frequency of positive results. This same review documented disparities in the care for Hispanic adolescents who presented to the emergency department for brain injuries (O'Connor and Haley, 2003). The authors found health care disparities for all pediatric age groups in areas including asthma management (Heron, Stettner, and Haley, 2006).

Over the last 5 years, there has been an increase in studies examining disparities in health service delivery. In reviewing data from California and New York, Guagliardo and colleagues (2003) found racial and ethnic disparities in the rate of appendix rupture. Compared with white children and adolescents aged 4–18, Hispanic and Asian children and adolescents had higher odds (1.30 [1.14–1.48] and 1.21 [0.92–1.58], respectively) of a rupture in California; in New York, Asian and black adolescents had higher odds (2.09 [1.36–3.21] and 1.44 [1.07–1.95], respectively). The authors conclude that immigrant groups were more at risk for delayed emergency care in these communities as adjustments for other demographic factors did not fully explain the disparities.

Disparities have also been reported for a population of adolescents undergoing hemodialysis. A substantial proportion of minority adolescents (averaging age 12) had received inadequate hemodialysis (Leonard et al.,

2004). Similarly, these findings could not be explained by such factors as center size, age, or renal diagnosis.

In a review of 31 studies that spanned asthma services, mental health care, reproductive health services, and primary care, racial and ethnic disparities that could not be explained by socioeconomic status were found in all service areas (Elster et al., 2003). The authors offer four findings: (1) there is less utilization of health services among racial and ethnic minority adolescents, after controlling for insurance status and socioeconomic status; (2) despite the absence of differences in the prevalence of mental disorders among black, Hispanic, and white adolescents, there is less utilization of mental health services among minority adolescents; (3) minority youths receive more reproductive health services than white adolescents; and (4) socioeconomic status has a modest impact on health service delivery but does not completely account for the disparities seen.

Summary

Health disparities and biases are a persistent feature of the health care delivery system for racial and ethnic minority adolescents, although little research has been focused on this particular age group. Disparities have been reported in studies of mental health services and emergency department care, as well as in research on adolescents who receive hemodialysis and asthma treatment. While social and economic differences account for some of these disparities, researchers have found that these differences alone cannot explain significant variations in rates of utilization of health services and health outcomes.

Finding:

- *Disparities and biases affect the quality of health services for adolescents and deserve serious consideration in any efforts to improve access to appropriate services and reduce inequities in the health system.*

CONFIDENTIALITY OF HEALTH SERVICES

The extent to which visits with health care providers are kept confidential between adolescents and their providers can impact adolescents' utilization of health services. While some young people may be comfortable sharing their health care needs and information with their parents, others may find it embarrassing or fear disapproval or punishment, particularly for health services related to sexual activity, mental health, or substance use. Additionally, there is a body of overlapping and sometimes conflicting statutes, court decisions, and regulations that are relevant to adolescent health services. Various studies have examined the role of confidentiality generally in adolescents' willingness to seek health care and disclose information to health care professionals. This evidence demonstrates that ensuring access to care that is acceptable to adolescents is important in delivering quality health services.

Acceptability

Various studies have examined the role of confidentiality generally in adolescents' willingness to seek health care and disclose information to health care professionals. Ford and colleagues (1997) found through a randomized controlled trial that increased assurance of confidentiality produced an increase in adolescents' willingness to provide information about sexuality, mental health, and substance use (from 39 percent to 46.5 percent). Such candor with health care professionals who are taking a health history is critical to adolescents' receiving the most appropriate care. Other positive outcomes, such as willingness to make a return visit, were noted as well. These findings are consistent with those of an earlier statewide survey (Cheng et al., 1993) in which substantial numbers of adolescents in Massachusetts cited deep concern regarding confidentiality that affected how and when they sought care. Further, studies have examined the impact of limiting confidentiality on adolescents' use of specific health services, such as those addressing sexual and reproductive health, mental health, and substance use.

Sexual and Reproductive Health Services

Evidence suggests that adolescents' willingness to seek sexual and reproductive health services is negatively affected by a lack of confidentiality, and that a variety of health outcomes with potentially adverse consequences including STIs, pregnancy, and abortion are likely to increase if access to confidential care is restricted. In one national study of 1,526 female adolescents under age 18 using publicly funded clinics for reproductive health services, 60 percent of respondents reported that a parent knew of their access to these services. A majority said they would continue to use the clinic services even if parental notification were required, but 18 percent said they would go to a private physician under those circumstances. One in five said they would use no contraception at all or would rely on withdrawal, while only one out of a hundred said they would simply stop having sex in response (R. K. Jones et al., 2005; note that some respondents gave multiple responses).

These findings are broadly consistent with those of similar statewide surveys. For instance, Reddy and colleagues (2002) surveyed adolescents using family planning clinics in Wisconsin and found that 47 percent would stop using all clinic services if parental notification were mandatory for prescription contraceptives; an additional 12 percent said they would delay testing or treatment for HIV or STIs or discontinue use of specific health services. An urban subset was asked about alternative practices; 29 percent indicated these would include unprotected sex and withdrawal. Of interest, parental notification in one area appears to affect how adolescents view a wider range of reproductive health services: many adolescents said they would alter their use of other health services—STI and HIV testing and treatment or pregnancy testing—even if parental notification were required only for birth control. A commentary on this work underscores the dangers to adolescent health indicated by these findings and cites smaller-scale studies that reinforce this concern (Ford and English, 2002).

Mental Health Services

Most of the studies cited above and in the literature as a whole pertain to sexual and reproductive health, but recent studies suggest that the situation is similar with respect to mental health. One regional study of 878 adolescents who reported receiving needed mental health treatment in the past found that 57 percent had foregone treatment at least once. Of these, 36 percent identified confidentiality concerns as a barrier to seeking treatment. Notably, girls and adolescents living with two parents were more likely than others to forego treatment (Samargia, Saewyc, and Elliott, 2006). Wissow and colleagues (2002) discuss the importance of confidentiality for mental health more broadly and review the earlier literature, finding broad consensus that confidentiality is crucial in getting adolescents to seek treatment.

Substance Use Services

One barrier to adolescent engagement with services to prevent substance use is the lack of opportunity for a private visit with a health professional. Research by Klein and colleagues (1999), for example, indicates that a third of adolescents failed to seek care that they felt they needed because they wanted to hide the visit from their parents. Similar work by Bethell and colleagues (2001) reveals that only half of adolescents had an opportunity for a private visit.

Accessibility

In addition to the importance of confidentiality to adolescents' willingness to seek health services and disclose information to health care providers, it is necessary to ensure access to these confidential services.

Consent

The protection of confidentiality cannot be considered outside of the legal framework for consent, as it is in the law governing consent to care that difficulty arises in protecting the secrets of adolescents. As the twentieth century progressed, it became clear that there was some role for children in medical decision making, especially for adolescents approaching adulthood. Scholars increasingly argued that medical care decisions were infused with value considerations and that adolescents had strong feelings about these values. Scholars also pointed out the overlapping interests of child, parent, physician, and the state in how these decisions are made (Bennet, 1976).

By common law, at least one parent had to consent to medical care for a child under age 18 except in an emergency, when no parent might be available and when it was assumed that the parent would consent if available. In addition to this emergency exception, a doctrine known as the mature minor doctrine was developed by statute and in the courts and became an accepted part of the law in many states (Johnson, 1998–1999). According to this doctrine, an older adolescent may give consent to care when it is exclusively for his or her benefit; it is in the mainstream of medical practice; and the minor has been informed of the risks and benefits, is capable of giving informed consent, and has not been coerced into agreement.

By statute, every state has established a right for minors to consent to their own care in a variety of circumstances. The circumstances vary from state to state, but each state has at least some laws that allow minors to consent on the basis of one or more categories of status (mature, emancipated, living apart from parents, over a certain age, married, or parenting) and one or more categories of services being sought (general health care, contraception, pregnancy-related care, STI/HIV care, drug and alcohol care, or outpatient mental health services). Although not every state recognizes each of these categories, every state recognizes some. The most commonly recognized and those supported by the American Medical Association are diagnosis and treatment for STIs, contraceptive services, pregnancy-related care (excluding abortion), and counseling or treatment for drug and alcohol problems (American Medical Association, 1997).

By constitutional precedent, the right of privacy protects minors' choices regarding contraception and abortion. With respect to contraception, the U.S. Supreme Court has decided that access to contraception is protected.

With respect to abortion, minors must be allowed, at a minimum, to give their own consent for abortion without first involving their parents. The majority of states have enacted statutes requiring parental consent or notification, but creating a judicial bypass procedure that allows minors to make their own decision if they are mature and to receive an abortion with court approval and without parental involvement if it would be in their best interest.

Thus, through a combination of common-law decisions, statutory enactments, and constitutional precedents, the legal framework for health care consent developed over the past half-century has authorized adolescents who are minors to give their own consent for health care in a wide variety of circumstances. This framework not only is consistent with ethical principles applicable to consent for medical care, but also is the foundation for confidentiality protections in adolescent health services (English, 1999).

Confidentiality

Legal protections of confidentiality in adolescent health services derive from numerous sources in federal and state law, including evidentiary privileges, funding statutes, medical privacy and medical records laws, minor consent laws, and the constitutional right of privacy. It is also important to recognize that a host of nongovernmental institutions, especially universities, have their own regulations that may involve parental notification, especially with respect to substance use and mental health. Universities responding to lawsuits increasingly notify parents or even expel students facing such problems (Bombardieri, 2006; Kinzie, 2006).

Federal-level provisions At the federal level, there are (1) specific programs that fund health services incorporating confidentiality provisions that protect adolescents, and (2) general privacy regulations that affect adolescents. The major federal funding programs at issue are Medicaid and the Title X clinics funded under the Public Health Service Act, both of which provide for minors' receipt of confidential family planning services ("without regard to age" in the case of Title X, 42 Code of Federal Regulations § 59.5). Other programs, such as SCHIP, either defer largely to states or, like the Maternal and Child Health Block Grant, simply are less explicit in their requirements for confidentiality protection for adolescents (Dailard and Turner Richardson, 2005; English and Morreale, 2001; Jones and Boonstra, 2004).

Also at the federal level, the Privacy Rule of the Health Insurance Portability and Accountability Act includes general regulatory requirements governing the disclosure of private health information, including information pertaining to minors. The rule generally provides a "floor" of privacy protection, which states may choose to exceed. On the question of parents' access to the private information of minors, however, the rule defers to "state or other applicable law." Although the rule does create some new rights for adolescents to control the release of personal information, it is deferential to other authorities on the question of parental access to information. Thus, if state or other law prohibits disclosure of information to parents without the permission of the adolescent minor, the information may not be disclosed; if state or other law requires disclosure, the information must be disclosed; and if state or other law permits disclosure or is silent on the issue, the health care provider has the discretion to disclose or not (English and Ford, 2004). The situation is similar with respect to substance use treatment: the federal government has not established its own consent and confidentiality guidelines in that domain, but has added its regulatory weight to existing state frameworks (English and Kenney, 2003).

State-level provisions At the state level, there is broad variation with respect to the degree of confidentiality protection accorded adolescents, as recently reviewed by Fox and Limb (2008). Often, confidentiality protections track the circumstances in which minors are authorized to consent to their own care, granting them a correlative right to control disclosure of the information. Sometimes, however, states are silent on the question of confidentiality or explicitly permit, without requiring, health professionals to disclose information to parents; often when they do so, states articulate criteria related to the minor's health for how that discretion should be exercised. Except with respect to abortion, it is rare for states to mandate disclosure to parents, especially when the minor has the right to consent. When physicians or other health professionals are granted discretion to disclose, the exercise of that discretion should be guided by sound ethical principles and the overriding importance of the adolescent's health and safety.

Some of the laws and regulations concerning adolescents' access to confidential care have been intensely contested at both the federal and state levels, in both legislatures and courts (for specific examples, see Arons, 2000; English and Morreale, 2001; Jones and Boonstra, 2004). Proposed legislative changes are often aimed at requiring parental consent and/or notification for such services as abortion, contraception, treatment for substance use, or even diagnosis and treatment for STIs, but sometimes they are aimed at requiring notification of sexual activity by minors in general (Rudoren, 2006). Numerous national organizations advocate for increased parental involvement and restrictions on confidential access.

In summary, as others have pointed out, the body of overlapping and sometimes conflicting statutes, court decisions, and regulations that are relevant to adolescent health services is extremely heterogeneous and is subject to ongoing change (U.S. Congress and Office of Technology Assessment, 1991). Nevertheless, the overall trend, with the exception of abortion, has been to protect the confidentiality of adolescents' health information when they are legally allowed to consent to their own care. When exceptions are made, such as to grant health professionals discretion to disclose information to parents even when the minor has consented to the care and objects to disclosure, they are usually grounded in the importance of protecting the health of adolescents or others.

Findings:

- *Evidence shows that health services that are confidential increase the acceptability of services and the willingness of adolescents to seek them, especially for issues related to sexual behavior, reproductive health, mental health, and substance use.*
- *Existing state and federal policies generally protect the confidentiality of adolescents' health information when they are legally allowed to consent to their own care.*

SUMMARY

This chapter has presented a review of current health services for adolescents and the settings where those services are typically received, with a focus on both the array of mainstream and safety-net primary care services and specialty services. It has also proposed the five objectives of accessibility, acceptability, appropriateness, effectiveness, and equity as a valuable framework for assessing health services and health care models that serve adolescents. Available evidence shows that health services for all adolescents, including those who are particularly vulnerable because of their demographic characteristics or other circumstances, do not reliably and consistently meet these objectives. Evidence also shows the lack of a system that provides coordinated health promotion, disease prevention, and behavioral health services for adolescents—all important elements for appropriately and effectively addressing the adolescent health needs discussed in Chapter 2.

REFERENCES

Aarons, G., Brown, S., Hough, G., Garland, A., and Wood, P. (2001). Prevalence of adolescent substance use disorders across five sectors of care. *Journal of American Academy of Child and Adolescent Psychiatry, 40,* 419–426.

Adebimpe, V. R. (1981). Overview: White norms and psychiatric diagnosis of black patients. *American Journal of Psychiatry, 138,* 279–285.

American Academy of Pediatrics and Division of Child Health Research. (n.d.). *Periodic Survey of Fellows* (No. 31). Available: www.aap.org/research/periodicsurvey/ps31a.htm [January 22, 2008].

American Medical Association. (1997). *Guidelines for Adolescent Preventive Services (GAPS), Recommendations Monograph*. Chicago, IL: American Medical Association.

Anderson, M. E., Freas, M. R., Wallace, A. S., Kempe, A., Gelfand, E. W., and Liu, A. H. (2004). Successful school-based intervention for inner-city children with persistent asthma. *Journal of Asthma, 41*, 445–453.

Armbruster, P., and Lichtman, J. (1999). Are school based mental health services effective? Evidence from 36 inner city schools. *Community Mental Health Journal, 35*, 493–504.

Arons, J. R. (2000). Misconceived laws: The irrationality of parental involvement requirements for contraception. *William and Mary Law Review, 41*, 1093–1131.

Barnet, B., Duggan, A. K., and Devoe, M. (2003). Reduced low birth weight for teenagers receiving prenatal care at a school-based health center: Effect of access and comprehensive care. *Journal of Adolescent Health, 33*, 349–358.

Battjes, R. J., Gordon, M. S., O'Grady, K. E., Kinlock, T. W., and Carswell, M. A. (2003). Factors that predict adolescent motivation for substance abuse treatment. *Journal of Substance Abuse Treatment, 24*, 221–232.

Battjes, R. J., Gordon, M. S., O'Grady, K. E., and Kinlock, T. W. (2004). Predicting retention of adolescents in substance abuse treatment. *Addictive Behaviors, 29*, 1021–1027.

Ben-Dror, R. (1994). Employee turnover in community mental health organization: A developmental stages study. *Community Mental Health Journal, 30*, 243–257.

Bennet, R. (1976). Allocation of child medical care decision-making authority: A suggested interest analysis. *Virginia Law Review, 62*, 285–330.

Bethell, C., Klein, J., and Peck, C. (2001). Assessing health system provision of adolescent preventive services: The Young Adult Health Care Survey. *Medical Care, 39*, 478–490.

Bombardieri, M. (2006). Parents strike settlement with MIT in death of daughter. *The Boston Globe*, April 4. Available: http://www.boston.com/news/local/articles/2006/04/04/parents_strike_settlement_with_mit_in_death_of_daughter [July 22, 2006].

Brabin, L. (2002). *Adolescent Friendly Health Services: An Impact Model to Evaluate Their Effectiveness and Cost*. Geneva: World Health Organization.

Brannigan, R., Schackman, B. R., Falco, M., and Millman, R. B. (2004). The quality of highly regarded adolescent substance abuse treatment programs: Results of an in-depth national survey. *Archives of Pediatrics and Adolescent Medicine, 158*, 904–909.

Branson, B. M., Handsfield, H. H., Lampe, M. A., Janssen, R. S., Taylor, A. W., Lyss, S. B., and Clark, J. E. (2006). Revised recommendations for HIV testing of adults, adolescents, and pregnant women in health-care settings. *Morbidity and Mortality Weekly Reviews: Recommendations and Reports, 55*(RR14), 1–17.

Breda, C., and Heflinger, C. (2004). Predicting incentives to change among adolescents with substance abuse disorder. *American Journal of Drug and Alcohol Abuse, 30*, 251–267.

Brindis, C. D., Klein, J., Schlitt, J., Santelli, J., Juszczak, L., and Nystrom, R. J. (2003). School-based health centers: Accessibility and accountability. *Journal of Adolescent Health, 32*, 98–107.

Britto, M. T., Klostermann, B. K., Bonny, A. E., Altum, S. A., and Hornung, R. W. (2001). Impact of a school-based intervention on access to health care for underserved youth. *Journal of Adolescent Health, 29*, 116–124.

Bukstein, O., Bernet, W., Arnold, V., Breitchman, J., Shaw, J., Benson, S., Kinlan, J., McCellan, J., Stock, S., Ptakowski, K., and the Work Group of Quality Issues. (2005). AACAP official action. Practice parameters for the assessment and treatment of children and adolescents with substance use disorders. *Journal of the American Academy of Child and Adolescent Psychiatry, 44*, 609–621.

Burke, P. J., O'Sullivan, J., and Vaughan, B. L. (2005). Adolescent substance use: Brief interventions by emergency care providers. *Pediatric Emergency Care, 21*, 770–776.

Burlew, R., and Philliber, S. (2007). *What Helps in Providing Contraceptive Services for Teens.* Washington, DC: The National Campaign.

The Center for Health and Health Care in Schools. (1993). *The Answer Is at School: Bringing Health Care to Our Students.* Washington, DC: The George Washington University.

Center for Reproductive Health Research Policy. (n.d.). *Adolescent Sexuality and Reproductive Health.* Available: http://reprohealth.ucsf.edu/research/researchareas/as_and_rh.html#IIID [October 10, 2007].

Chandra, A., Martinez, G. M., Mosher, W. D., Abma, J. C., and Jones, J. (2005). Fertility, family planning, and reproductive health of U.S. women: Data from the 2002 National Survey of Family Growth. National Center for Health Statistics. *Vital Health and Statistics, 23*(25).

Chatterji, P., Caffray, C. M., Crowe, M., Freeman, L., and Jensen, P. (2004). Cost assessment of a school-based mental health screening and treatment program in New York City. *Mental Health Services Research, 6*, 155–166.

Cheng, T. L., Savageau, J. A., Sattler, A. L., and DeWitt, T. G. (1993). Confidentiality in health care: A survey of knowledge, perceptions, and attitudes among high school students. *Journal of the American Medical Association, 269*, 1404–1407.

Child and Adolescent Health Measurement Initiative. (2008). *2003 National Survey of Children's Health: Health Care Access and Utilization Indicator 4.5.* Available: http://www.nschdata.org/ [May 1, 2008].

Chung, P. J., Lee, T. C., Morrison, J. L., and Schuster, M. A. (2006). Preventive care for children in the United States: Quality and barriers. *Annual Review of Public Health, 27*, 491–515.

Committee on Adolescent Health and American College of Obstetricians and Gynecologists. (2006). ACOG Committee Opinion No. 335. The initial reproductive health visit. *Obstetrics and Gynecology, 107*, 1215–1219.

Cooper, L. A., and Powe, N. R. (2004). *Disparities in Patient Experiences, Health Care Processes, and Outcomes: The Role of Patient-Provider Racial, Ethnic, and Language Concordance.* New York: The Commonwealth Fund.

Crespo, R. D., and Shaler, G. A. (2000). Assessment of school-based health centers in a rural state: The West Virginia experience. *Journal of Adolescent Health, 26*, 187–193.

Cuffe, S. P., Waller, J. L., Cuccaro, M. L., Pumariega, A. J., and Garrison, C. Z. (1995). Race and gender differences in the treatment of psychiatric disorders in young adolescents. *Journal of the American Academy of Child and Adolescent Psychiatry, 34*, 1536–1543.

Culligan, V. (2002). *Connecticut Association of School Based Health Centers. Patient Satisfaction Survey Summary.* North Haven: Connecticut Association of School-Based Health Centers.

Cunningham, P. J., and Nichols, L. M. (2005). The effects of Medicaid reimbursement on the access to care of Medicaid enrollees: A community perspective. *Medical Care Research and Review, 62*, 676–696.

Dailard, C., and Turner Richardson, C. (2005). Teenagers' access to confidential reproductive health services. *Guttmacher Report on Public Policy, 8*, 6–11.

Deas, D., and Thomas, S. E. (2001). An overview of controlled studies of adolescent substance abuse treatment. *American Journal of Addiction, 10*, 178–189.

Diaz-Perez Mde, J., Farley, T., and Cabanis, C. M. (2004). A program to improve access to health care among Mexican immigrants in rural Colorado. *Journal of Rural Health, 20*, 258–264.

Dobkin, P. L., Chabot, L., Maliantovitch, K., and Craig, W. (1998). Predictors of outcome in drug treatment of adolescent inpatients. *Psychological Reports, 83*, 175–186.

Donovan, C., Mellanby, A., Jacobson, L., Taylor, B., and Tripp, J. (1997). Teenagers' views on the general practice consultation and provision of contraception. *British Journal of General Practice, 47,* 715–718.

Dougherty, D. (2007). *Adolescent Research: Effectiveness, Quality and Costs of Community- and School-based Health Programs/Settings.* Presentation at the Research Workshop on Adolescent Health Care Services and Systems, January 22, Washington, DC.

Drug Strategies. (2003). *Treating Teens: A Guide to Adolescent Drug Programs.* Washington, DC: Drug Strategies.

Dryfoos, J. (1994). Medical clinics in junior high school: Changing the model to meet demands. *Journal of Adolescent Health, 15,* 549–557.

Ellen, J. M., Franzgrote, M., Irwin, C. E., Jr., and Millstein, S. G. (1998). Primary care physicians' screening of adolescent patients: A survey of California physicians. *Journal of Adolescent Health, 22,* 433–438.

Elster, A., Jarosik, J., VanGeest, J., and Fleming, M. (2003). Racial and ethnic disparities in health care for adolescents: A systematic review of the literature. *Archives of Pediatric and Adolescent Medicine, 157,* 867–874.

English, A. (1999). Health care for the adolescent alone: A legal landscape. In J. Blustein, C. Levine, and N. N. Dubler (Eds.), *The Adolescent Alone: Decision Making in Health Care in the United States* (pp. 78–99). Cambridge, UK: Cambridge University Press.

English, A., and Ford, C. A. (2004). The HIPAA privacy rule and adolescents: Legal questions and clinical challenges. *Perspectives on Sexual and Reproductive Health, 36,* 80–86.

English, A., and Kenny, K. (2003). *State Minor Consent Laws: A Summary* (2nd Ed.). Chapel Hill, NC: Center for Adolescent Health and the Law.

English, A., and Morreale, M. (2001). A legal and policy framework for adolescent health care: Past, present, and future. *Houston Journal of Health Law and Policy, 1,* 63–108.

Fairbrother, G., Scheinmann, R., Osthimer, B. J. D., Dutton, M. J., Newell, K. A., Fuld, J., and Klein, J. D. (2005). Factors that influence adolescent reports of counseling by physicians on risky behavior. *Journal of Adolescent Health, 37,* 467–476.

Fisher, M., and Kaufman, M. (1996). Adolescent inpatient units: A position statement of the Society for Adolescent Medicine. *Journal of Adolescent Health, 18,* 307–308.

Flores, G., and Ngui, E. (2006). Racial/ethnic disparities and patient safety. *Pediatric Clinics of North America, 53,* 1197–1215.

Ford, C. A., and English, A. (2002). Limiting confidentiality of adolescent health services: What are the risks? *Journal of the American Medical Association, 288,* 752–753.

Ford, C., Millstein, S., Halpern-Felsher, B., and Irwin, C. E. (1997). Influence of physician confidentiality assurances on adolescents' willingness to disclose information and seek future health care: A randomized control trial. *Journal of the American Medical Association, 278,* 1029–1034.

Fox, H. B., and Limb, S. J. (2008). *State Policies Affecting the Assurance of Confidential Care for Adolescents* (Fact Sheet No. 5). Washington, DC: Incenter Strategies.

Fox, H. B., McManus, M. A., and Reichman, M. B. (2003). Private health insurance for adolescents: Is it adequate? *Journal of Adolescent Health, 32*(6), 12–24.

Fox, H. B., Limb, S. J., and McManus, M. A. (2007). *Preliminary Thoughts on Restructuring Medicaid to Promote Adolescent Health* (Issue Brief No. 1). Washington, DC: Incenter Strategies.

Frost, J., and Bolzan, M. (1997). The provision of public-sector services by family planning agencies in 1995. *Family Planning Perspectives, 29,* 6–14.

Gance-Cleveland, B., Costin, D. K., and Degenstein, J. A. K. (2003). School-based health centers. Statewide quality improvement program. *Journal of Nursing Care Quality, 18,* 288–294.

Ginsburg, K., Slap, G., Avital, C., Forke, C., Balsley, C., and Rouselle, D. (1995). Adolescents' perceptions of factors affecting their decisions to seek health care. *Journal of the American Medical Association, 273,* 1913–1918.

Godley, S. H., Jones, N., Funk, R., Ives, M., and Passetti, L. L. (2004). Comparing outcomes of best-practice and research-based outpatient treatment protocols for adolescents. *Journal of Psychoactive Drugs, 36,* 35–48.

Godley, M. D., Kahn, J. H., Dennis, M. L., Godley, S. H., and Funk, R. R. (2005). The stability and impact of environmental factors on substance use and problems after adolescent outpatient treatment for cannabis abuse or dependence. *Psychology of Addictive Behaviors, 19,* 62–70.

Godley, M. D., Godley, S. H., Dennis, M. L., Funk, R. R., and Passetti, L. L. (2007). The effect of assertive continuing care on continuing care linkage, adherence, and abstinence following residential treatment for adolescents with substance use disorders. *Addiction, 102,* 81–93.

Grella, C. E., and Joshi, V. (2003). Treatment processes and outcomes among adolescents with a history of abuse who are in drug treatment. *Child Maltreatment, 8,* 7–18.

Grunbaum, J. A., Kann, L., Kinchen, S., Ross, J., Hawkins, J., Lowry, R., Harris, W. A., McManus, T., Chyen, D., and Collins, J. (2004). Youth risk behavior surveillance—United States, 2003. *Morbidity and Mortality Weekly Report. Surveillance Summaries, 53,* 1–96.

Guagliardo, M. F., Teach, S. J., Huang, Z. J., Chamberlain, J. M., and Joseph, J. G. (2003). Racial and ethnic disparities in pediatric appendicitis rupture rate. *Academy of Emergency Medicine, 10,* 1218–1227.

Guo, J. J., Jang, R., Keller, K. N., McCracken, A. L., Pan, W., and Cluxton, R. J. (2005). Impact of school-based health centers on children with asthma. *Journal of Adolescent Health, 37,* 266–274.

Halpern-Felsher, B. L., Ozer, E. M., Millstein, S. G., Wibbelsman, C. J., Fuster, C. D., Elster, A. B., and Irwin, C. E., Jr. (2000). Preventive services in a health maintenance organization: How well do pediatricians screen and educate adolescent patients? *Archives of Pediatric and Adolescent Medicine, 154,* 173–179.

Heron, S. L., Stettner, E., and Haley, L. L. (2006). Racial and ethnic disparities in the emergency department: A public health perspective. *Emergency Medicine Clinics of North America, 24,* 905–923.

Hoffman, J. (2007). Treating the awkward years. *The New York Times,* p. F1, April 24.

Hser, Y. I., Grella, C. E., Hubbard, R. L., Hseieh, S. C., Fletcher, B. W., Brown, B. S., and Anglin, M. D. (2001). An evaluation of drug treatments for adolescents in 4 US cities. *Archives of General Psychiatry, 58,* 689–695.

Institute for Clinical Systems Improvement. (2007). *Health Care Guideline: Preventive Services for Children and Adolescents.* Bloomington, MN: Institute for Clinical Systems Improvement.

Institute of Medicine. (1997). *Schools and Health: Our Nation's Investment.* Washington, DC: National Academy Press.

Institute of Medicine. (2000). *America's Health Care Safety Net: Intact but Endangered.* Washington, DC: National Academy Press.

Institute of Medicine. (2001). *Crossing the Quality Chasm: A New Health System for the 21st Century.* Washington, DC: National Academy Press.

Institute of Medicine. (2003). *The Future of the Public's Health in the 21st Century.* Washington, DC: The National Academies Press.

Johnson, P. (1998–1999). Refusal of treatment by children and the mature minor doctrine. *Quality of Care Newsletter, 74*(Fall–Winter). Available: http://www.cqcapd.state.ny.us/newsletter/74cclong.htm [May 29, 2008].

Jones, C. A., Clement, L. T., Hanley-Lopez, J., Morphew, T., Kwong, K. Y., Lifson, F., Opas, L., and Guterman, J. J. (2005). The Breathmobile Program: Structure, implementation, and evolution of a large-scale, urban, pediatric asthma disease management program. *Disease Management, 8,* 205–222.

Jones, R. K., and Boonstra, H. (2004). Confidential reproductive health services for minors: The potential impact of mandated parental involvement for contraception. *Perspectives on Sexual and Reproductive Health, 36,* 182–191.

Jones, R. K., Purcell, A., Singh, S., and Finer, L. B. (2005). Adolescents' reports of parental knowledge of adolescents' use of sexual health services and their reactions to mandated parental notification for prescription contraception. *Journal of the American Medical Association, 293,* 340–348.

Juszczak, L., Schlitt, J., Odium, M., Baragon, C., and Washington, D. (2003). *School-Based Health Centers National Census School Year 2001–2002.* Washington, DC: National Assembly on School-Based Health Care. Available: http://www.nasbhc.org/atf/cf/{CD9949F2-2761-42FB-BC7A-CEE165C701D9}/EQ_2001census.pdf [January 9, 2008].

Juszczak, L., Schlitt, J., and Moore, A. (2007). *School-Based Health Centers. National Census School Year 2004–2005.* Washington, DC: National Assembly on School-Based Health Care. Available: http://www.nasbhc.org/atf/cf/%7BCD9949F2-2761-42FB-BC7A-CEE165C701D9%7D/Census2005.pdf [October 11, 2007].

Kaiser Family Foundation. (2007). *Key Facts: Race, Ethnicity, and Medical Care.* Menlo Park, CA: Kaiser Family Foundation.

Kalafat, J., and Illback, R. J. (1998). A qualitative evaluation of school-based family resource and youth service centers. *American Journal of Community Psychology, 26,* 573–604.

Kalivas, P. W., and Volkow, N. D. (2005). The neural basis of addiction: A pathology of motivation and choice. *American Journal of Psychiatry, 162,* 1403–1413.

Kang, M., Bernard, D., Booth, M., Quine, S., Alperstein, G., Usherwood, T., and Bennett, D. (2003). Access to primary health care for Australian young people: Service provider perspectives. *British Journal of General Practice, 53,* 947–952.

Key, J. D., Washington, E. C., and Hulsey, T. C. (2002). Reduced emergency department utilization associated with school-based clinic enrollment. *Journal of Adolescent Health, 30,* 273–278.

Kinzie, S. (2006). GWU suit prompts questions of liability. *The Washington Post,* p. A01, March 10.

Kisker, E. E., and Brown, R. S. (1996). Do school-based health centers improve adolescents' access to health care, health status, and risk-taking behavior? *Journal of Adolescent Health, 18,* 335–343.

Klein, J. D., and Wilson, K. M. (2002). Delivering quality care: Adolescents' discussion of health risks with their providers. *Journal of Adolescent Health, 30,* 190–195.

Klein, J. D., Wilson, K. M., McNulty, M., Kapphahn, C., and Collins, K. S. (1999). Access to medical care for adolescents: Results from the 1997 Commonwealth Fund Survey of the Health of Adolescent Girls. *Journal of Adolescent Health, 25,* 120–130.

Klein, J. D., Sesselberg, T. S., Gawronski, B., Handwerker, L., Gesten, F., and Schettine, A. (2003). Improving adolescent preventive services through state, managed care, and community partnerships. *Journal of Adolescent Health, 32,* 91–97.

Knight, J. R., Sherritt, L., Shrier, L. A., Harris, S. K., and Chang, G. (2002). Validity of the CRAFFT substance abuse screening test among adolescent clinic patients. *Archives of Pediatrics and Adolescent Medicine, 156,* 607–714.

Knight, J. R., Sherritt, L., Harris, S. K., Gates, E., and Chang, G. (2003). Validity of brief alcohol screening tests among adolescents: A comparison of the AUDIT, POSIT, CAGE, and CRAFFT. *Alcoholism: Clinical and Experimental Research, 27,* 67–73.

Kolbe, L. J., Kann, L., and Collins, J. L. (1993). Overview of the Youth Risk Behavior Surveillance System. *Public Health Reports*, 108(Suppl. 1), 2–10.

Kulig, J. W., and Committee on Substance Abuse. (2005). Tobacco, alcohol, and other drugs: The role of the pediatrician in prevention, identification, and management of substance abuse. *Pediatrics*, 115, 816–821.

Lee, E. J., and O'Neal, S. (1994). A mobile clinic experience: Nurse practitioners providing care to a rural population. *Journal of Pediatric Health Care*, 8, 12–17.

Leonard, M. B., Stablein, D. M., Ho, M., Jabs, K., and Feldman, H. I. (2004). Racial and center differences in hemodialysis adequacy in children treated at pediatric centers: A North American Pediatric Renal Transplant Cooperative Study (NAPRTCS) Report. *Journal of the American Society of Nephrology*, 15, 2923–2932.

Leshner, A. I. (1997). Addiction is a brain disease and it matters. *Science*, 278, 45–47.

Liddle, H. A., and Dakof, G. A. (1995). Family-based treatment for adolescent drug use: State of the science. *NIDA Research Monographs*, 156, 218–254.

Lieberman, H. M. (1974). Evaluating the quality of ambulatory pediatric care at a neighborhood health center. *Clinical Pediatrics (Philadelphia)*, 13, 52–55.

Ma, J., Wang, Y., and Stafford, R. S. (2005). U.S. adolescents receive suboptimal preventive counseling during ambulatory care. *Journal of Adolescent Health*, 36, 441.e1–441.e7.

Macek, M. D., Manski, R. J., Vargas, C. M., and Moeller, J. F. (2002). Comparing oral health care utilization estimates in the United States across three nationally representative surveys. *Health Services Research*, 37, 499–521.

Macfarlane, A., and Blum, R. (2001). Do we need specialist adolescent units in hospitals? *British Medical Journal*, 322, 941–942.

MacKay, A. P., and Duran, C. (2007). *Adolescent Health in the United States, 2007*. Hyattsville, MD: National Center for Health Statistics.

Mangione-Smith, R., DeCristofaro, A. H., Setodji, C. M., Keesey, J., Klein, D. J., Adams, J. L., Schuster, M. A., and McGlynn, E. A. (2007). The quality of ambulatory care delivered to children in the United States. *New England Journal of Medicine*, 357, 1515–1523.

Manski, R. J., and Brown, E. (2007). *Dental Use, Expenses, Private Dental Coverage, and Changes, 1996 and 2004*. MEPS Chartbook No. 17. Rockville, MD: Agency for Healthcare Research and Quality.

Marcin, J. P., Pretzlaff, R. K., Whittaker, H. L., and Kon, A. A. (2003). Evaluation of race and ethnicity on alcohol and drug testing of adolescents admitted with trauma. *Academy of Emergency Medicine*, 10, 1253–1259.

Martin, T. W. (1993). White therapists' differing perceptions of black and white adolescents. *Adolescence*, 28, 281–289.

Maternal and Child Health Bureau. (2005). *The Oral Health of Children: A Portrait of States and the Nation, 2005*. Rockville, MD: U.S. Department of Health and Human Services, Health Resources and Services Administration.

Maternal and Child Health Bureau. (2008). *The National Survey of Children with Special Health Care Needs Chartbook 2005–2006*. Rockville, MD: U.S. Department of Health and Human Services.

Mayberry, R. M., Mili, F., and Ofili, E. (2000). Racial and ethnic differences in access to medical care. *Medical Care Research and Review*, 57(Suppl.), 108–145.

McAndrews, T. (2001). Zero tolerance policies (ERIC Documentation Reproduction Service No. ED451579). *ERIC Digest*, 146, 1–7.

McKay, J. (2006). Continuing care in the treatment of addictive disorders. *Current Psychiatry Reports*, 8, 355–362.

McLellan, A. T., and Meyers, K. (2004). Contemporary addiction treatment: A review of systems problems for adults and adolescents. *Biological Psychiatry*, 56, 764–770.

McManus, M. A., Shejavali, K. I., and Fox, H. B. (2003). *Is the Health Care System Working for Adolescents? Perspectives from Providers in Boston, Denver, Houston, and San Francisco.* Washington, DC: Maternal and Child Health Policy Research Center.

Mensinger, J. L., Diamond, G. S., Kaminer, Y., and Wintersteen, M. B. (2006). Adolescent and therapist perception of barriers to outpatient substance abuse treatment. *American Journal on Addictions, 15*(Suppl. 1), 16–25.

Millstein, S. G., and Marcell, A. V. (2003). Screening and counseling for adolescent alcohol use among primary care physicians in the United States. *Pediatrics, 111,* 114–122.

Millstein, S. G., Igra, V., and Gans, J. (1996). Delivery of STD/HIV preventive services to adolescents by primary care physicians, *Journal of Adolescent Health, 19,* 249–257.

Morral, A. R., McCaffrey, D. F., Ridgeway, G., Mukherji, A., and Beighley, C. (2006). *The Relative Effectiveness of 10 Adolescent Substance Abuse Treatment Programs in the United States* (RAND Technical Report No. 346). Santa Monica, CA: RAND Corporation.

National Center for Injury Prevention and Control. (2007). *Leading Causes of Death and Fatal Injury Reports* (2004 data). Available: http://www.cdc.gov/ncipc/wisqars/ [July 30, 2007].

National Institute of Dental and Craniofacial Research. (1994). *NIDCR CDC Oral Health Data Query System.* Available: http://apps.nccd.cdc.gov/dohdrc/dqs/entry.html [June 6, 2007].

National Institute on Drug Abuse. (1999). *Principles of Drug Addiction Treatment: A Research-Based Guide* (NIH Publication No. 00-4180). Bethesda, MD: National Institutes of Health.

National Institute on Drug Abuse. (2006). *Principles of Drug Abuse Treatment for Criminal Justice Populations: A Research-Based Guide* (NIH Publication No. 06-5316). Bethesda, MD: National Institutes of Health.

National Research Council. (1999). *Risks and Opportunities: Synthesis of Studies of Adolescence.* M. D. Kipke (Ed.). Washington, DC: National Academy Press.

National Research Council and Institute of Medicine. (2002). *Community Programs to Promote Youth Development.* J. Eccles and J. A. Gootman (Eds.). Washington, DC: National Academy Press.

Nawar, E. W., Niska, R. W., and Xu, J. (2007). National Hospital Ambulatory Medical Care Survey: 2005 emergency department summary. *Advance Data from Vital and Health Statistics, 386*(June 29).

O'Connor, K. G., Johnson, J., and Brown, R. T. (2000). *Barriers to Providing Health Care for Adolescents: The Pediatrician's View.* Presented at the Association for Health Services Research Annual Meeting, June, Los Angeles, CA. Available: http://www.aap.org/research/periodicsurvey/ps42ahsr.htm [March 8, 2008].

O'Connor, R. E., and Haley, L. (2003). Disparities in emergency department health care: Systems and administration. *Academy of Emergency Care, 10,* 1193–1198.

Olson, A. L., Kelleher, K. J., Kemper, K. J., Zuckerman, B. S., Hammond, C. S., and Dietrich, A. J. (2001). Primary care pediatrician's roles and perceived responsibilities in the identification and management of depression in children and adolescents. *Ambulatory Pediatrics, 1,* 91–98.

Orso, C. L. (1979). Delivering ambulatory health care: The successful experience of an urban neighborhood health center. *Medical Care, 17,* 111–126.

Owens, P. L., Thompson, J., Elixhauser A., and Ryan, K. (2003). *Care of Children and Adolescents in U.S. Hospitals.* HCUP Fact Book No. 4; AHRQ Publication No. 04-0004. Rockville, MD: Agency for Healthcare Research and Quality.

Ozer, E. M., Adams, S. H., Lustig, J. L., Gee, S., Garber, A. K., Gardner, L. R., Rehbein, M., Addison, L., and Irwin, C. E., Jr. (2005). Increasing the screening and counseling of adolescents for risky health behaviors: A primary care intervention. *Pediatrics, 115,* 960–968.

Rand, C. M., Shone, L. P., Albertin, C., Auinger, P., Klein, J. D., and Szilagyi, P. G. (2007). National health care visit patterns of adolescents. Implications for delivery of new adolescent vaccines. *Archives of Pediatrics and Adolescent Medicine*, 161, 252–259.

Reddy, D. M., Fleming, R., and Swain, C. (2002). Effect of mandatory parental notification on adolescent girls' use of sexual health care services. *Journal of the American Medical Association*, 288, 710–714.

Rounds-Bryant, J. L., Kristiansen, P. L., and Hubbard, R. L. (1999). Drug abuse treatment outcome study of adolescents: A comparison of client characteristics and pretreatment behaviors in three treatment modalities. *American Journal of Drug and Alcohol Abuse*, 25, 573–591.

Rudoren, J. (2006). Judge blocks law to report sex under 16. *The New York Times*, April 19. Available: http://www.nytimes.com/2006/04/19/us/19kline.html [July 19, 2006].

Samargia, L., Saewyc, E., and Elliott, B. (2006). Foregone mental health care and self-reported access barriers among adolescents. *Journal of School Nursing*, 22, 17–24.

Santelli, J., Morreale, M., Wigton, A., and Grason, H. (1995). *Improving Access to Primary Care for Adolescents: School Health Centers as a Service Delivery Strategy* (MCH Policy Research Brief). Baltimore, MD: The Johns Hopkins University School of Hygiene and Public Health.

Schuchter, J., and Fairbrother, G. (2008). *Health Services Utilization among Adolescents from the 2005 NHIS*. An analysis of 2005 National Health Interview Survey data. Report to the Institute of Medicine Committee on Adolescent Health Care Services and Models of Care for Treatment, Prevention, and Health Development. Available: http://www.cincinnatichildrens.org/assets/0/78/1067/1395/1833/1835/1849/1853/960a6652-5045-4946-ba64-191c919cefb7.pdf [March 19, 2008].

Schultz, S. T., Shenkin, J. D., and Horowitz, A. M. (2001). Parental perceptions of unmet dental need and cost barriers to care for developmentally disabled children. *Pediatric Dentistry*, 23, 321–325.

Shields, A. E., Finkelstein, J. A., Comstock, C., and Weiss, K. B. (2002). Process of care for Medicaid-enrolled children with asthma: Served by community health centers and other providers. *Medical Care*, 40, 303–314.

Slade, E. P. (2002). Effects of school-based mental health programs on mental health service use by adolescents at school and in the community. *Mental Health Services Research*, 4, 151–166.

Slesnick, N., Kang, M. J., Bonomi, A. E., and Prestopnik, J. L. (2008). Six- and twelve-month outcomes among homeless youth accessing therapy and case management services through an urban drop-in center. *Health Services Research*, 43, 211–229.

Strakowski, S. M., Lonczak, H. S., Sax, K. W., West, S. A., Crist, A., Mehta, R., and Thienhaus, O. J. (1995). The effects of race on diagnosis and disposition from a psychiatric emergency service. *Journal of Clinical Psychiatry*, 56, 101–107.

Strakowski, S. M., Keck, P. E., Jr., Arnold, L. M., Collins, J., Wilson, R. M., Fleck, D. E., Corey, K. B., Amicone, J., and Adebimpe, V. R. (2003). Ethnicity and diagnosis in patients with affective disorders. *Journal of Clinical Psychiatry*, 64, 747–754.

Substance Abuse and Mental Health Services Administration. (2006a). Characteristics of young adults (aged 18–25) and youth (aged 12–17) admissions: 2004. *The DASIS Report*, 21.

Substance Abuse and Mental Health Services Administration. (2006b). Substance use treatment need among adolescents: 2003–2004. *The NSDUH Report*, 24.

Suellentrop, K. (2006a). Adolescent boys' use of health services. *Science Says*, 26. Washington, DC: National Campaign to Prevent Teen Pregnancy.

Suellentrop, K. (2006b). Adolescent girls' use of health services. *Science Says*, 28. Washington, DC: National Campaign to Prevent Teen Pregnancy.

Suellentrop, K. (2006c). Teen contraceptive use. *Science Says, 29*. Washington, DC: National Campaign to Prevent Teen Pregnancy.

Szapocznik, J., Lopez, B., Prado, G., Schwartz, S. J., and Pantin, H. (2006). Outpatient drug abuse treatment for Hispanic adolescents. *Drug and Alcohol Dependence, 84*, S54–S63.

Tang, S. S., Yudkowsky, B. K., and Davis, J. C. (2003). Medicaid participation by private and safety net pediatricians, 1993 and 2000. *Pediatrics, 112*, 368–372.

Tatelbaum, R., Adams, B., Kash, C., McAnarney, E., Roghmann, K., Coulter, M., Charney, E., and Plume, M. (1978). Management of teenage pregnancies in three different health care settings. *Adolescence, 13*, 713–728.

Thorndike, A. N., Ferris, T. G., Stafford, R. S., and Rigotti, N. A. (1999). Rates of U.S. physicians counseling adolescents about smoking. *Journal of the National Cancer Institute, 91*, 1857–1862.

Todd, K. H., Deaton, C., D'Adamo, A. P., and Goe, L. (2000). Ethnicity and analgesic practice. *Annals of Emergency Medicine, 35*(1), 11–16.

Tomlinson, K. L., Brown, S. A., and Abrantes, A. (2004). Psychiatric comorbidity and substance use treatment outcomes of adolescents. *Psychology of Addictive Behaviors, 18*, 160–169.

Tylee, A., Haller, D. M., Graham, T., Churchill, R., and Sanci, L. A. (2007). Youth-friendly primary-care services: How are we doing and what more needs to be done? *Lancet, 369*, 1565–1573.

U.S. Congress and Office of Technology Assessment. (1991). *Adolescent Health* (OTA-H-466, 467, and 468). Washington, DC: U.S. Government Printing Office.

U.S. Department of Health and Human Services. (2000). *Healthy People 2010* (2nd Ed.). Washington, DC: U.S. Government Printing Office.

U.S. Department of Health and Human Services. (2007). *21 Critical Health Objectives for Adolescents and Young Adults*. Centers for Disease Control and Prevention. Available: http://www.cdc.gov/HealthyYouth/AdolescentHealth/NationalInitiative/pdf/21objectives.pdf [October 17, 2007].

U.S. Preventive Task Force and Agency for Healthcare Research and Quality. (2004). *Screening for Family and Intimate Partner Violence*. Available: http://www.ahrq.gov/clinic/uspstf/uspsfamv.htm [March 11, 2008].

U.S. Surgeon General. (2001). *Youth Violence: A Report of the Surgeon General*. Washington, DC: U.S. Department of Health and Human Services.

Van Hook, S., Harris, S. K., Brooks, T., Carey, P., Kossack, R., Kulig, J., Knight, J. R., and New England Partnership for Substance Abuse Research. (2007). The "Six T's": Barriers to screening adolescents for substance abuse in primary care. *Journal of Adolescent Health, 40*, 456–461.

Vargas, C. M., and Ronzio, C. R. (2002). Relationship between children's dental needs and dental care utilization: United States, 1988–1994. *American Journal of Public Health, 92*, 1816–1821.

Veit, F. C., Sanci, L. A., Coffey, C. M., Young, D. Y., and Bowes, G. (1996). Barriers to effective primary health care for adolescents. *The Medical Journal of Australia, 165*, 131–133.

Volkow, N. D., and Li, T. K. (2005). Drugs and alcohol: Treating and preventing abuse, addiction, and their medical consequences. *Pharmacological Therapy, 108*, 3–17.

Waldron, H. B., and Kaminer, Y. (2004). On the learning curve: The emerging evidence supporting cognitive-behavioral therapies for adolescent substance abuse. *Addiction, 99*(Suppl. 2), 93–105.

Watson, S. (1998). A ward of their own. *Nursing Standard, 12*, 12–13.

Weisz, J. R., Donenberg, G. R., Han, S. S., and Kauneckis, D. (1995). Child and adolescent psychotherapy outcomes in experiments versus clinics: Why the disparity? *Journal of Abnormal Child Psychology, 23,* 83–106.

Weisz, J. R., Hawley, K. M., and Doss, A. J. (2004). Empirically tested psychotherapies for youth internalizing and externalizing problems and disorders. *Child and Adolescent Psychiatric Clinics of North America, 13,* 729–815.

Weisz, J. R., Sandler, I. N., Durlak, J. A., and Anton, B. S. (2005). Promoting and protecting youth mental health through evidence-based prevention and treatment. *The American Psychologist, 60,* 628–648.

West, J. C., Herbeck, D. M., Bell, C. C., Colquitt, W. L., Duffy, F. F., Fitek, D. J., Rae, D., Stipec, M. R., Snowden, L., Zarin, D. A., and Narrow, W. E. (2006). Race/ethnicity among psychiatric patients: Variations in diagnostic and clinical characteristics reported by practicing clinicians. *Focus, 4,* 48–56.

White, M., White, W. L., and Dennis, M. L. (2004). Emerging models of effective adolescent substance abuse treatment. *Counselor, The Magazine for Addiction Professionals, 5,* 24–28.

Williams, R. J., Chang, S. Y., and the Addiction Centre Research Group. (2000). A comprehensive and comparative review of adolescent substance abuse treatment outcome. *Clinical Psychology: Science and Practice, 7,* 138–166.

Winters, K. C. (1999). Treating adolescents with substance use disorders: An overview of practice issues and treatment outcome. *Substance Abuse, 20,* 203–225.

Winters, K. C., Stinchfield, R. D., Opland, E., Weller, C., and Latimer, W. W. (2000). The effectiveness of the Minnesota Model approach in the treatment of adolescent drug abusers. *Addiction, 95,* 601–612.

Wissow, L., Fothergill, K., and Forman, J. (2002). Confidentiality for mental health concerns in adolescent primary care. *Bioethics Forum, 18,* 43–54.

World Health Organization. (1999). *Programming for Adolescent Health and Development: Report of a WHO/UNFPA/UNICEP Study Group on Programming for Adolescent Health* (WHO Technical Report Series 886). Geneva: World Health Organization.

World Health Organization. (2001). *Global Consultation on Adolescent Health Services. A Consensus Statement.* Geneva: Department of Child and Adolescent Health and Development, World Health Organization.

4

Improving Systems of Adolescent Health Services

SUMMARY

Developing improved health systems for adolescents will require attention to several fundamental goals:

- Emphasize the capacity of primary health care services to provide high-quality screening, assessment, health management, referral, and care management of specialty services, especially for behaviorally based health problems.
- Coordinate behavioral, reproductive, mental health, and dental services in practice and community settings.
- Incorporate health promotion, disease prevention, and youth development throughout the health system and within the community.
- Focus attention on the health and health service needs of those adolescents who are most vulnerable to risky behavior and poor health.
- Ensure consent and confidentiality for adolescents seeking care.

Chapter 3 described the current array of primary and specialty care health services for adolescents, with a particular emphasis on reviewing the evidence on the gaps and shortcomings in the accessibility, acceptability, appropriateness, effectiveness, and equity of these services. The evidence presented underscores the importance of adolescent health services that meet these quality objectives; the scarcity of current services that consistently do so; and the lack of systems that provide coordinated health promotion, disease prevention, and behavioral health services for adolescents. Whereas Chapter 3 focused primarily on findings with respect to problems with adolescent health services, this chapter focuses on ways to address these problems and achieve improved adolescent health systems that embody the above quality objectives. The strategies recommended are informed by three of the behavioral and contextual characteristics presented in Chapter 1. First, *participation matters*: effective health services for young people invite engagement with clinicians by adolescents and their families. Second, *family matters*: at the same time that adolescents are growing in their autonomy, families continue to affect their health and overall well-being and to influence what health services they use; young people without adequate family support are particularly vulnerable to risky behavior and poor health and thus require additional support in health service settings. Third, *community matters*: good health services for adolescents include population-focused as well as individual and family services since the environment that adolescents live in as well as the supports provided in the community are important.

Efforts to improve the availability of health services for adolescents and the accessibility of those services are insufficient by themselves to meet the health needs of today's adolescents. Those needs increasingly involve health problems resulting from behaviors that can best be addressed before the onset of obvious morbidity or during the early stages of experimentation in such areas as diet and exercise, substance use (including tobacco and alcohol), driving, and sexual behavior. Therefore, adolescent health services need to do a better job of incorporating prevention and health promotion, while also being more tailored to the developmental stage of adolescents.

Evidence is insufficient to suggest that one particular setting or practice structure for adolescents can achieve significantly better outcomes than other approaches. While a small number of comprehensive clinics and facilities focused on adolescents do exist, these service approaches are not easily applied to larger populations or most communities because of a lack of professionals specializing in adolescent health. However, the five criteria of accessibility, acceptability, appropriateness, effectiveness, and equity provided the committee with a framework for assessing the use, adequacy, and quality of adolescent health services, and comparing and contrasting the extent to which different services, settings, and providers meet the health needs of adolescents in the United States.

To meet these needs, improved systems of adolescent health services will be necessary. These systems must encompass (1) evidence-based and standardized screening tools and management and referral processes in adolescent-friendly primary care settings, including primary care provider offices, community-based health centers, hospital-affiliated primary care services, and school-based health centers; (2) facilitated linkages between providers of primary and specialty care services, especially for specific subpopulations of more vulnerable adolescents; and (3) expanded connections between primary care settings and community agencies providing health promotion, disease prevention, behavioral health, and youth development services that are delivered by health professionals with appropriate training in adolescent medicine. In short, it will be necessary to modify the structure and design of primary care (including safety-net services), specialty care (including mental health, sexual and reproductive health, oral health, and substance abuse treatment and prevention services), organizational arrangements, workforce development, and financial systems so that adolescent health services can place greater emphasis on health promotion, disease prevention, and youth development. The latter three emphases are particularly lacking for the most underserved and high-risk groups of adolescents, such as those who are poor; are members of a racial or ethnic minority; are in the foster care system; are homeless; are in families that have recently immigrated to the United States; are lesbian, gay, bisexual, or transgender; or are in the juvenile justice system.

This chapter describes elements of adolescent health services that can best meet the needs of all adolescents. It emphasizes the importance of integrating efforts to identify and address risky behavior with interventions aimed at health promotion, disease prevention, and youth development in settings that serve adolescents. The first section identifies selected features of health services (including screening, assessment, health management, referral, and care management of specialty services) that, when incorporated into primary care services, may enable those services to better address unhealthful habits and risky behaviors of adolescents. Next is a discussion of strategies that can be used for enhanced coordination of primary care services with more specialized behavioral, nutritional, oral, and sexual and reproductive health services. The third section examines strategies for fostering health promotion, disease prevention, and youth development, with the goal of improving the health of all adolescents. This section also considers how public health objectives for adolescents (the 21 critical objectives within the broader set of Healthy People 2010 goals and the Healthy People 2010 adolescent oral health objectives) can be linked to the health system for adolescents through a population-based approach (U.S. Department of Health and Human Services, 2000, 2007). The ultimate goal is to identify strategies that can foster service integration and coordination across public and private health systems so the two sectors can complement each other in addressing the health needs of today's adolescents, strengthen adolescents' capacity to become healthy and productive adults, and ultimately achieve the objectives for adolescents of Healthy People 2010. The fourth section reviews the roles and responsibilities of various stakeholders in ensuring adolescents' access to confidential health services. This is followed by a discussion of innovations in adolescent health services, including the increasing use of health information technology, as well as some examples of current efforts to deliver health services to this population through a variety of approaches.

IDENTIFYING AND ADDRESSING UNHEALTHFUL HABITS AND RISKY BEHAVIORS AMONG ADOLESCENTS

As reviewed in Chapter 2, unhealthful habits and risky behaviors that are initiated during adolescence extend into adulthood and contribute directly to poor health conditions and significant morbidity and mortality in the short and long terms (Kolbe, Kann, and Collins, 1993). Health systems can play a critical role in the early identification, management, and monitoring of adolescents who are already experimenting with unhealthful habits and risky behaviors or associating with peers who do so. Systematic efforts to identify and respond appropriately to these behaviors can delay their onset or reduce their severity and duration, as well as prevent the initiation of other, co-occurring behaviors, such as use of alcohol, drugs, and tobacco products; unprotected sex; violence; and hazardous driving. Designing interventions to address unhealthful habits and risky behaviors requires attention to several key components of primary care: screening, assessment, health management, referral, and care management of specialty services. Each of these components is discussed below, with a focus on selected research findings that may influence the development of more effective health services for adolescents.

Screening

As discussed in Chapter 3, screening and counseling are critical for adolescents, since unhealthful and risky behaviors are the leading cause of morbidity and mortality among individuals in this age group and also affect their future health status as adults. A general physician inquiry, the screening method most frequently relied upon by health care practitioners, frequently falls short in screening for unhealthful habits and risky behaviors. An alternative to a general physician inquiry is the use of standardized screening tools. Such tools, however, are used infrequently in primary care settings for adolescents (Gardner et al., 2003). Those that are used often focus on only a single risky behavior, such as sexual practices or substance use (McPherson and Hersch, 2000), so that clinicians must administer several screens to have a comprehensive battery. Internal factors, such as physician attitudes or inadequate training of personnel who must administer the screens, and external factors, such as cost, time, inadequate referral resources, and a lack of guidance on the use of the tools, may be an additional barrier to their use (Horwitz et al., 2007; Ozer et al., 2005).

Several national organizations, including the American Medical Association (AMA) and the American Academy of Pediatrics (AAP), recommend that, at a minimum, all adolescents receive routine structured screening for a variety of behavioral and health risks as part of the annual health maintenance visit (Elster and Kuznets, 1994; Green and Palfrey, 2002). Not only do such tools increase the identification of targeted behaviors or symptoms, but they also may minimize disparities in care by increasing standardization of practice (Miranda et al., 2003). Numerous regulatory and advisory bodies are in general agreement on criteria for the use of standardized screening tools (Calonge, 2001; Feightner and Lawrence, 2001). These criteria include the availability of practical, sensitive, and specific instruments; a high prevalence of morbidity or mortality associated with the target condition(s); access to effective intervention(s) for the condition(s); and positive benefits from the early initiation of intervention.

Despite their infrequent use, a number of routine screening instruments for unhealthful habits and risky behaviors are available for use in primary care settings. Common instruments for alcohol and drug use include the Problem Oriented Screening Instrument for Teenagers (POSIT) (Rahdert, 1991), the Alcohol Use Disorders Identification Test (AUDIT) (Babor et al., 2001), and the RAFFT (Relax, Alone, Friends, Family, and Trouble) (Riggs and Alario, 1989) and CRAFFT (Car, Relax, Alone, Forget, Family, Trouble) tests for adolescent substance use (Knight et al., 1999). Similar instruments are available for depression and suicidality. Routine urine tests for sexually transmitted infections (STIs), such as chlamydia, are recommended for all sexually active adolescents (American Medical Association, 1997). HEADSS (Home, Education, Activities, Drug use and abuse, Sexual behavior, Suicidality and depression; or Home, Education, Alcohol, Drugs, Smoking, Sex) has also been used for many years as a provider-driven questionnaire for assessing unhealthful habits and risky behaviors in adolescents (Cohen, Mackenzie, and Yates, 1991; Van Amstel, Lafleur, and Blake, 2004). Instruments for assessing nutrition and exercise for adolescents in primary care have not been extensively studied.

An alternative to surveys or questionnaires completed by patients and families is semistructured questionnaires for clinicians to administer to patients. An example, issued by the AMA, is *Bright Futures: Guidelines for Health Supervision of Infants, Children and Adolescents* (GAPS), which consolidates national guidelines of multiple professional organizations (e.g., AMA, AAP) for preventive screening, counseling, and health education services for both adolescents and children into one set of recommendations endorsed by all these organizations (American Medical Association, 1997).

Recommendations for adolescents are organized into four types of services that address 14 separate topics or health conditions (see Box 4-1).

These guidelines offer physicians recommendations for identifying adolescents at risk and helping them change or prevent unhealthful behaviors. They suggest specific questions providers can ask their young patients as gateways for addressing concerns in such areas as physical, social, and emotional development; oral health habits; and sexual practices. These guidelines emphasize periodic health care visits for health education and preventive screening to provide opportunities for counseling, anticipatory guidance, early identification, and referral for medical, behavioral, and emotional risks. According to the GAPS, health care providers should ask all adolescents about risky behaviors every year, including their use of tobacco products, alcohol, and other substances; behaviors or emotions that indicate recurrent or severe depression or risk of suicide; and any sexual behavior that may result in unintended pregnancy or STIs. The guidelines further specify that at-risk adolescents should be counseled about how to reduce their risks.

It should be noted that the GAPS are based on consensus among experts and are not required to be evidence based. In contrast, the U.S. Preventive Services Task Force (USPSTF) also issues recommendations for clinical preventive services, but does so only if evidence for the effectiveness of the counseling or screening is available, and only after using study results to weigh the benefits against possible harm. Because research-based evidence is often not available, the recommendations of the USPSTF are less extensive than the GAPS. For example, the USPSTF has not issued a recommendation with respect to preventing obesity because an evidence base to support the effectiveness of such counseling does not exist. On the other hand, the USPSTF does recommend both chlamydia screening and counseling on family violence (U.S. Preventive Task Force and Agency for Healthcare Research and Quality, 2004, 2007).[1]

As discussed previously, the unhealthful habits and risky behaviors targeted for screening in primary care are highly prevalent among adolescents and are associated with significant morbidity and mortality both during and after adolescence. Moreover, many of these behaviors could be mitigated by early treatment. Less clear, however, is whether adolescents who screen positive for these behaviors will have the insurance benefits, transportation access, or cultural predisposition to take advantage of such treatment.

It is clear that most criteria for the implementation of screening for unhealthful habits and risky behaviors as part of adolescent primary care, especially those related to depression, substance use, and violence, are not met in most settings that treat large numbers of adolescents, but should

---

[1] See www.ahrq.gov/clinic/prevenix.htm.

> **BOX 4-1**
> **Guidelines for Adolescent Preventive Services (GAPS)**
>
> GAPS recommendations are organized into **four types of services** that address 14 separate topics or health conditions:
>
> - Three recommendations pertain to the delivery of health care services.
> - Seven recommendations pertain to the use of health guidance to promote the health and well-being of adolescents and their parents or guardians.
> - Thirteen recommendations describe the need to screen for specific conditions that are relatively common among adolescents and that cause significant suffering either during adolescence or later in life.
> - One recommendation pertains to the use of immunizations for the primary prevention of selected infectious diseases.
>
> The **14 topics or health conditions** addressed by GAPS are divided into those aimed at health promotion and those aimed at disease prevention:
>
> **Promotion**
> - Parents' ability to respond to the health needs of their adolescents
> - Adjustment to puberty and adolescence
> - Safety and injury prevention
> - Physical fitness
> - Healthy dietary habits and prevention of eating disorders and obesity
> - Healthy psychosexual adjustment and prevention of the negative health consequences of sexual behaviors
>
> **Prevention**
> - Hypertension
> - Hyperlipidemia
> - The use of tobacco products
> - The use and abuse of alcohol and other drugs
> - Severe or recurrent depression and suicide
> - Physical, sexual, and emotional abuse
> - Learning problems
> - Infectious diseases
>
> SOURCE: American Medical Association (1997).

be a priority. Primary care systems must assess their capacity to process screening results, the prevalence of various problems in their community, and the capacity of local treatment services to respond before deciding whether to initiate screening in each risk area. With regard to expanding the capacity of local treatment services to respond, primary care providers for adolescents may have a role to play, including direct management in the primary care setting. Changes in screening practices and treatment capacity are likely to benefit marginalized and more vulnerable adolescents the most since carefully worded instruments and standardized services would eliminate some barriers to inquiry about unhealthful and risky behaviors that are especially salient for these individuals.

Such changes are unlikely to come about quickly or at all without major external impetus. Significant financing changes currently under way are especially likely to move screening to the forefront. Specifically, the increased willingness of payors to reimburse primary care clinicians for screening and assessment activity and the rapid expansion of pay-for-performance contracting that rewards early detection, as well as the greater availability of automated screening tools and brief paper tools, are all likely to encourage clinicians to consider universal screening during adolescent visits.

Assessment

Research has identified a developmental sequence in the emergence of unhealthful habits and risky behaviors such as substance use. Yet the use of one drug does not inevitably lead to the use of more potent drugs (Golub and Johnson, 1994), nor does it mean that current use will extend indefinitely (Chen and Kandel, 1995). Uncertainty about the strength of the pathway hypothesis creates challenges for assessment of the meaning and implications of positive results of screening for unhealthful habits and risky behaviors, especially those involving substance use. The substantial heterogeneity of the adolescent population and the absence of predictive models make it difficult to distinguish adolescents who are at substantial risk of chronic or problematic substance use or dependency from those who engage in one-time or short-term experimentation with hazardous substances or behaviors as part of normal adolescent development and peer interaction.

Positive results of a screen for substance use or other unhealthful habits or risky behaviors must therefore be carefully assessed to determine the characteristics, severity, and duration of the problem and to identify an appropriate course of treatment and follow-up. Many health care providers feel ill equipped to provide detailed assessments of positive screens or suspicions of behavioral, reproductive, or developmental concerns for their adolescent patients (Horwitz et al., 2007). As a result, they tend to refer their patients to specialty practices that may focus on only one dimension of unhealthful habits and risky behaviors that frequently co-occur (treatment for alcohol use, for example, in the presence of smoking and unprotected sex). Substantial delays may occur between initial screening and assessment, during which other risk factors or behaviors may emerge that complicate the determination of a best course of action. Alternatively, new protective factors (such as family reunification, positive peer interactions, athletic success, or improved school achievement) may emerge that could mitigate the results of the initial screen and alter the preferred course of action.

Concerns about privacy and confidentiality (discussed in detail later in this chapter) are particularly significant during screening and assessment, when sensitivity to stigma and bias may affect the adolescent patient's willingness to trust and communicate with health professionals or return for follow-up care. Low-income and minority adolescents are at particular risk of being labeled with certain risk factors prior to an in-depth assessment of their overall health status and history. For example, African American youths are more likely to be diagnosed with conduct disorder and less likely to be diagnosed with depression than comparable white youths (Cuffe et al., 1995). High-risk populations also are especially likely to lack access to effective care management and treatment services, as discussed in later chapters.

Health Management

Health management of unhealthful habits and risky behaviors in primary care settings has a limited research base except for some studies of specific domains or risks. For example, there has been considerable research on the prescription of psychotropic drugs for the management of depression and attention-deficit hyperactivity disorder (ADHD) in primary care settings (Harpaz-Rotem and Rosenheck, 2006; Hoagwood et al., 2000; Murray et al., 2005; Rushton, Clark, and Freed, 2000; Zito et al., 1999). Primary care clinicians are the most common prescribers of psychotropic drugs to adolescents, in part because of the large number of younger adolescents receiving stimulants for ADHD. Rapid growth was also seen in the prescribing of antidepressants for adolescents until the U.S. Food and Drug Administration issued recent warnings about possible associations with suicidal ideation (U.S. Food and Drug Administration, 2007). The provision of effective services for adolescents with mental health and substance use disorders will continue to require that primary care clinicians manage psychiatric medications for large numbers of adolescent patients because there will never be a sufficient number of child psychiatrists to do so. To accomplish medication management effectively, primary care clinicians need specific training in the use of these medications and better processes for monitoring side effects and adherence, attendance at follow-up visits, and changes in symptoms and functioning. Such activities are almost impossible to conduct within a small primary care practice without additional staff. Multiple practices employing common records, in partnership with pharmacy benefit programs, disease management organizations, or health plans, likely must coordinate such efforts through guild organizations or managed care plans.

Since counseling takes time, new organizational structures and physician-extender professionals may be needed to permit a shift from treatment to prevention. Physicians and other health workers dealing with adolescents may need to acquire new skills in such promising techniques as solution-focused interviewing, the medication interest model, and motivational interviewing (Cheng, 2007). The latter technique has been shown in college students to reduce risky behavior related to alcohol (LaBrie et al., 2007b), increase condom use (LaBrie et al., 2007a), potentially improve patient involvement in dental care and smoking cessation counseling by dentists (Koerber, Crawford, and O'Connell, 2003), and potentially enable patients to control diabetes (Dale et al., 2007). Although many physicians feel comfortable interviewing patients and families, formal physician training in these manual-based techniques, including role play, has been shown to improve satisfaction and outcomes for patients (Wissow et al., 2008).

While primary care management of mental health disorders such as ADHD and depression is fairly well documented, much less evidence exists on the primary care management of high-risk sexual activity, substance use disorders, adolescent obesity, or other nutritional problems. In part, this is attributable to the lack of pharmaceutical interventions for these problems, from which clear data for research on ADHD and depression management are generated. It is also true, however, that ideal services for primary care interventions for these other problems have not been well described. For example, few successful interventions for adolescent obesity have been documented in any settings (Hawley, Beckman, and Bishop, 2006; O'Brien, Holubkov, and Reis, 2004; Quintos and Castells, 2006). Similarly, primary care management strategies for adolescent substance use are largely unstudied.

Because these problems are so understudied, many researchers have focused on the importance of the clinician–patient relationship in adolescent primary care. Relationships between adolescents and parents, families, peers (especially best friends), and extrafamilial individuals play a significant role in adolescent development (Collins and Laursen, 2000). Although research in this area has not explicitly addressed relationships between adolescents and their health care providers, it offers intriguing opportunities to study the attributes and processes that attract (or repel) adolescents to certain providers and care environments.

The presence or absence of supportive relationships provides a context for socialization and the inculcation of social norms, as well as models for future relationships, including the capacity to relate effectively to others (Hartup, 1986; Maccoby, 1984). The affective quality of the relationship between a health care provider and an adolescent can therefore be as important as the content or quality of the service provided, especially if it reinforces the adolescent's positive experience with a parent–child relationship or addresses dimensions that lie beyond the sphere of parent–child communications. Through their relationships with health care providers, adolescents can be encouraged to disclose health conditions and behaviors of concern and to become attentive to risks and protective factors that influence their current and future health status. Significant attention is therefore warranted to understand how supportive relationships can be cultivated and sustained in the provision of health services in ways that lead to positive health outcomes for adolescents, especially those in vulnerable circumstances. Of course, such relationships and their benefits are greatly enhanced by longitudinal care provided over many years to adolescents and their families. When care is less continuous and youths are seen only once every few years, the potential benefits are much more difficult.

In addition to the establishment of close ties with adolescents, primary care management will increasingly require monitoring strategies. Adolescents are particularly vulnerable to low rates of attendance at follow-up appointments, failure to adhere to medication instructions, and inadequate communication with health care providers. Numerous strategies for improving communication and monitoring have shown promise. These range from better communication links, such as automated calls and messages through cell phones and the Internet (described later in this chapter), to contact that involves problem solving and motivational interviewing between visits. As with other components of high-quality primary care for adolescents, regional coordination across multiple practices and settings can diminish the cost of such interventions for individual practices.

Referral

Once an adolescent patient has been screened and assessed, the provider must determine what course of action is most appropriate. In some cases, the patient may need to be referred to another care setting for treatment.

In many situations, the primary care provider may not be familiar with community resources that are appropriate to address the behavior in question. This is the case especially for patients who have difficulty navigating traditional health service settings or those whose insurance panel providers may not include the resource considered most appropriate. Indeed, primary care clinicians cite a lack of referral sources as a major barrier to their identifying and meeting the mental health needs of adolescents and their families (Horwitz et al., 2007). Strategies that may support providers in finding and engaging with community partners are described below. For purposes of efficiency, these strategies may be pursued by groups of clinicians or practices in partnership.

Specialists in pediatrics, oral health, mental health, and substance abuse can help primary care clinicians with diagnosis and/or therapy. Ideally, the primary care clinician will develop or have access to a community specialty or mental health resource guide, cross-referenced by the type of third-party payment each provider accepts and the types of evidence-based therapies offered. Such directories have been a central focus of early intervention programs nationwide and have been important in increasing referrals for young children with developmental disabilities (Dunst and Trivette, 2004). For mental health, specific evidence-based psychotherapies are documented online by the Substance Abuse and Mental Health Services Administration[2] and the American Psychological Association,[3] along with their supporting evidence.

Directories that can provide a starting point for clinicians seeking mental health and/or substance abuse resources may be available from the local health department, community mental health or substance abuse agency, emergency department, or 211/311 resource line, or from family and consumer advocacy groups (such as the National Alliance on Mental Illness, Mental Health America, the Federation of Families for Children's Mental Health, or Children and Adults with Attention Deficit/Hyperactivity Disorder). Initially, information can be collected through a mailed questionnaire, but having a mental health professional speak personally with mental health agency representatives or individual mental health or substance abuse clinicians is invaluable in clarifying qualifications and services. A community can seek funding for this process from nonprofit or governmental sources; frequently, the public mental health agency will fund and staff its continuation.

In some regions, family support networks—organizations aimed at linking families to resources for adolescents with special health needs—are available to clinicians. There may be a state, regional, or local office that maintains a directory of resources and/or provides live referrals and strategies for negotiating the system. While community networks and directories may have been available for many years, in some domains, such as behavioral health and domestic violence, primary care clinician referrals are low, and clinicians report being unfamiliar with such resources.

In many areas of the country, managed care "carve outs"—separate insurance plans for the delivery of specialty oral health, mental health, and substance abuse benefits—provide their insured customers with a limited panel of professionals who may or may not have expertise in working with adolescents and may or may not provide evidence-based interventions. Furthermore, the primary care clinician may have no access to the list of

---

[2] See http://www.nrepp.samhsa.gov/.
[3] See http://www.apa.org/practice/ebpreport.pdf.

professionals on an insurance plan's mental health panel. Typically, families must access these services directly, often through a 1-800 number or other "gatekeeper" arrangement. In these situations, primary care clinicians must focus advocacy efforts on regional directors of these ambulatory managed care plans and on insured families and their employers to make them more knowledgeable about adolescent needs.

It is important to include school contacts in community mental health resource directories. Schools are the largest de facto provider of mental health services (Burns et al., 1995), although most school-based mental health personnel (guidance counselors, social workers, psychologists) typically focus on attendance, testing, course selection, and college preparation rather than on mental health needs unless they are part of more comprehensive systems.

Care Management of Specialty Services

One of the most challenging aspects of the decentralized U.S. health system is the absence of resources devoted to managing specialty care services and easing transitions across multiple settings for the treatment of chronic, complex, or comorbid health conditions. While these challenges exist for all populations, they are especially problematic for adolescents and their families who lack experience in navigating transitions between primary and specialized care settings. Appropriate care management practices can help avoid unnecessary or duplicative tests and assessments and align services and treatments so they complement and reinforce each other, instead of producing adverse effects or confusing outcomes.

Care management duties can be time-consuming and often are uncompensated by most current U.S. payors. They involve such tasks as identifying appropriate providers, scheduling appointments, requesting information on the results of laboratory and other diagnostic tests, reviewing the relative merits of alternative treatment regimens, responding to adverse effects or uncertain treatment outcomes, and assessing medications and therapies to identify potentially harmful interactions. While many office personnel are capable of scheduling appointments, other care management tasks (such as identification of the interactions of multiple medications and periodic assessments of health status) require greater expertise.

The responsible performance of care management duties can make the adolescent patient more willing to comply with recommended treatments and specialty care. In the absence of such support and assistance, the adolescent or family members may bear sole responsibility for care management. Experience with delays, unexpected complications, repetitive or duplicative tests and assessments, and financial burdens can lead to frustration and ultimately to refusal to comply with referrals that require the navigation of complex procedures or health systems.

Recent studies of medical errors, patient safety, and patient-centered care have called attention to the importance of smoothing transitions across multiple providers and care settings (Institute of Medicine, 2000, 2001, 2004, 2007b). While information technology may help resolve some of these problems, adolescents require additional support in care management, particularly when their parents or other adults are not available to assist them in making decisions or to help them navigate fragmented health services.

Summary

Health settings can play a critical role in the early identification, management, and monitoring of adolescents who are experimenting with unhealthful habits and risky behaviors. Fulfilling this role, however, requires an intentional and systematic process of screening, assessment, health management, referral, and care management of specialty services. When incorporated into routine primary care services, these elements can contribute to more effective health services for adolescents.

LINKAGES BETWEEN PRIMARY AND SPECIALTY CARE SERVICES

To meet the health needs of adolescents, it is critical for general health settings and especially primary care sites to improve their ability to identify, assess, and manage risky behaviors and emerging behavioral, nutritional, oral, and sexual and reproductive health issues. Yet a critical deficiency of current adolescent primary care is the linkage with specialty health services in these important areas. Adolescents referred for specialty services frequently fail to connect effectively to these services. For some types of services, such as mental health, the vast majority of adolescents referred for care fail to complete a minimum number of sessions (Gardner et al., 2004; Rushton, Bruckman, and Kelleher, 2002). Establishing strong linkages to the various specialty services, as well as mechanisms for monitoring successful transitions between primary and specialty care, would improve the accessibility, acceptability, and appropriateness of health services for adolescents, particularly those who are more vulnerable. Mechanisms for improving linkages between primary care settings and various specialty services generally fall into three categories: specific referral practices, referral management, and specialty consultation (see Federal Expert Work Group on Pediatric Subspecialty Capacity et al., 2006).

Referral practices can be improved through referral guidelines—specific algorithms for clinical management that clarify particular assessment plans in primary care and specialty settings, criteria for referral, and planned follow-up. Referral practices can also be improved through preappointment management of referrals by specialists. In such cases, specialists briefly review prior records and results to determine the extent of specialty and primary care coordination and management required. Preappointment management reduces specialty waiting lists, improves communication, and enhances coordination.

Referral management is the term used for comprehensive case management of referral processes employing support services that are specific to individual patient and family needs, including transportation assistance, structured telephone reminders, encouragement to attend, babysitting for a parent's other children, and related services. Such services have been used for high-risk populations in urban, low-income settings to increase service use and for homeless families or adolescents with substance use disorders.

Finally, specialty consultation approaches can be used to strengthen the interface between primary care and specialty services for adolescents. For the past several decades, child psychiatrists have provided consultation and liaison psychiatry services primarily to adolescents in academic medical centers. New models have been developed, however, for organizing and financing such services in community primary care settings for both rural (Campo et al., 2005) and urban (Williams, Shore, and Foy, 2006) adolescents. Even more promising, telephone support services provided by regional child psychiatrists for primary care clinicians seeing adolescents with psychiatric medication needs have expanded greatly in the past 5 years, with some early success (Connor et al., 2006; Young and Ireson, 2003).

The historical dichotomy between the delivery of dental and medical care requires special attention to linkages between these two care systems. The dental care delivery system functions separately from the medical care system; lacks a discrete adolescent focus; is rarely collocated with medical services for adolescents; and is overwhelmingly private, with only a small safety-net component that is readily accessible to the socially and medically disadvantaged. Physicians typically do not screen for dental caries and periodontal disease, the two most common oral health problems in adolescence. They are therefore less likely to consider targeted referrals for resolution of these as compared with other conditions. Conceptually, a closer linkage between dental and medical care is inherently worth promoting because dental and medical conditions share common risk factors, and because systemic and oral diseases often have complementary presentations and consequences. As described in Chapter 2, drug, tobacco, and alcohol use, as well as driving, firearm use, sports, and sexual activity, all can manifest as oral trauma and pathology, and poor eating patterns and food choices are directly associated with dental caries. Because many adolescents come in frequent contact with dental professionals through routine preventive dental visits and orthodontic treatment, there are also opportunities for dentists to screen adolescents and refer them to primary medical care.

All of these linkages between primary care clinicians and specialists caring for high-risk adolescents will benefit to the extent that expectations and responsibilities for each are clearly articulated. The use of service agreements between primary care and specialty providers, besides specifying the types of services offered at each site, can clarify and expedite the transfer of information and referrals between sites and facilitate processes for handoffs of care to and from specialty settings. Specification of waiting times and facilitated appointments may be part of such agreements. Comanagement or multidisciplinary approaches are often reserved for the few adolescents with multiple disorders or conditions requiring complex services with high costs. In such cases, team communication is the essential element. Collocation of specialty, dental, and primary care services is beneficial in some settings, especially for adolescents with transportation and confidentiality concerns.

The shortages and inequitable distribution of mental health, oral health, sexual and reproductive health, nutritional, and other specialty services necessary for adolescents are long-standing problems. Several decades of calls for change and modest policy initiatives to alter both the volume and location of such services have met with very limited success (Kim and The American Academy of Child and Adolescent Psychiatry Task Force on Workforce Needs, 2003). In response to similar concerns in other fields, comprehensive regional plans have been developed. Thus, fields as diverse as neonatology, burn care, trauma, craniofacial surgery, pediatric oncology, and cystic fibrosis have developed and implemented regional coordinated services in pediatric and adult medical settings (American Academy of Pediatrics, American College of Critical Care Medicine, and Society of Critical Care Medicine, 2000; David, 1977; Klitzner and Chang, 2003; McCormick, Shapiro, and Starfield, 1985; Praiss, Feller, and James, 1980). Such services provide stepped care processes that aim to prevent problems, identify those that are in the early stages, manage early processes in local settings, and transfer complex cases to regional facilities as soon as possible. This stepped care model is usually coordinated at the regional level. Similar plans will be essential if there is to be any hope of maximizing the services provided by the scarce specialists with adolescent experience currently available.

In summary, the establishment of strong links between primary care and community prevention services, dental care, and various medical specialty services would contribute to making health services more accessible, acceptable, and appropriate for adolescents. Establishing mechanisms for monitoring successful transitions between primary care and community, specialty, and dental care could also improve services and health systems in the future.

HEALTH PROMOTION, DISEASE PREVENTION, AND YOUTH DEVELOPMENT

Some adolescents lack regular access to primary care services (Newacheck et al., 1999). This gap is frequently associated with poor insurance status, financial limitations, insurance coverage restrictions, and limited access to trained providers, as discussed in Chapters 5 and 6. But even for those adolescents who have routine access to primary care, their providers and the settings in which they receive health services are rarely equipped to provide guidance or resources that encourage them to adopt healthy behaviors in such basic areas as nutrition, physical activity, injury prevention, substance use (including drugs, alcohol, and tobacco), peer interactions, and sexual relationships. Various health settings or programs may provide opportunities to strengthen health promotion and disease prevention. As well, the area of youth development offers another approach to promoting health among adolescents.

Health Promotion

A population-based health care delivery system focuses not just on risk reduction, but also on the creation of environments and behaviors that promote healthy outcomes for adolescents. As with disease prevention (discussed below), health promotion for adolescents needs to involve multiple individuals, including the adolescent him- or herself, the primary care provider, the family, and the community. Dentists have a particular opportunity to promote not just oral but also systemic health given that, as noted Chapter 3, they are likely to have frequent and often lengthy visits with many adolescents, especially those undergoing orthodontic treatment. Tobacco use—including not only smoking, but also use of spit tobacco—is an example of a behavior with both oral and systemic health consequences that dentists can address with their patients.

The Society for Adolescent Medicine (SAM) has developed educational materials to help adolescents assume responsibility for their health and to guide them in seeking advice from health professionals. *Health Guide for America's Teens*, for example, is a brochure that includes explicit health guidance, as well as a list of more than a dozen resource centers that are equipped to address such problems as adolescent violence, child abuse, sexual assault, and teen pregnancy (Society for Adolescent Medicine, 2003).

Other adolescent-focused websites in the SAM brochure that offer health promotion guidance include http://www.teenwire.com (produced by the

Planned Parenthood Federation of America) and http://www.iwannaknow.org (produced by the American Social Health Association). Both websites focus predominantly on sexual and reproductive health issues. The website http://www.kidshealth.org/teen (produced by the Nemours Foundation) offers a broader network of educational materials, answers and advice, and adolescent profiles that cover such topics as food and fitness, drugs and alcohol, body and mind, school and jobs, and living with parents.

Despite the availability of these sources, little is known at present about the extent to which individual clinicians or health practices are aware of the existence of print and electronic health promotion materials or how these materials are used in providers' encounters with young patients. As a result, the impact of such advisories and educational materials on health outcomes for adolescents or adolescent engagement with health services remains uncertain. Through their national organizations and state chapters, providers should endeavor to present messages consistent with those of other groups and to encourage healthy behaviors through available educational materials.

Disease Prevention

As noted earlier in this chapter, unhealthful habits and risky behaviors directly related to leading causes of premature death and disease in adulthood are usually initiated in adolescence, but have consequences that extend into adulthood. These behaviors are interrelated and preventable, a fact that argues for a major shift from treatment to prevention in primary care for adolescents.

Interventions

Improved screening is the first step in disease prevention, and as discussed earlier, evidence suggests that this can be accomplished. The next step is to improve interventions, especially those focused on enhanced communication. Such improvement needs to occur at multiple levels, including the primary care provider, the family, and the community.

Personalized messages tailored to the needs of the adolescent are an important part of successful disease prevention programs. For example, physician-delivered personalized messages regarding weight management succeeded in producing weight loss in low-income obese African American women in one trial, and show great promise for adolescent care (Davis et al., 2006). To communicate such messages, practices will need to employ technologies used by adolescents, such as text messaging (Franklin et al., 2006), web-based feedback (Doumas and Hannah, 2007), and telephone messages (Burleson and Kaminer, 2007; Dale et al., 2007) (see also the discussion of health information technology later in this chapter).

Most successful prevention programs seek not only to respond to and reduce negative influences on the adolescent, but also to strengthen positive, protective factors. These protective factors operate within multiple domains—the individual, the family, the school, the peer group, the neighborhood, and the larger community.

Intervention with the family is an important component of most successful disease prevention programs. Brief family interventions have been found to be successful in preventing adolescent substance abuse (Spoth, Redmond, and Shin, 2001). Combining a school-based life skills training program with a program to strengthen parent–child bonds was much more successful in preventing alcohol initiation than was a life skills training program alone (Spoth et al., 2002).

Community-level interventions are also important. A great deal of research over the last two to three decades has shown that interventions in the community can be effective in preventing some high-risk behaviors and health problems in adolescents. Some of these interventions focus on selected local settings (the family, the school, the neighborhood, and the community); others emphasize changes that potentially affect all adolescents in the nation (such as tax increases on alcohol and tobacco or changes in labeling practices for foods and beverages). Primary care physicians can be powerful voices in these policy changes.

The most effective strategies for preventing smoking among adolescents are increases in the tax on cigarettes and media campaigns against smoking (Institute of Medicine, 2007a). Such approaches have been effective, can save thousands of lives (Rivara et al., 2004), and end up generating net revenue (Fishman et al., 2005). Community-based interventions to decrease underage adolescents' access to alcohol can reduce high alcohol consumption and decrease injuries and fatalities due to alcohol-related motor vehicle crashes (Holder et al., 2000; National Research Council and Institute of Medicine, 2004). Increasing taxes on alcohol and limiting advertising aimed at adolescents can be effective community-level interventions as well (Hollingworth et al., 2006).

Comprehensive communitywide interventions, such as the Communities That Care program, provide selected jurisdictions with the capacity to organize service delivery in ways that utilize disease prevention science. That program assesses community strengths and risks and matches the community's priorities to tested effective programs (Hawkins, Catalano, and Arthur, 2002).

Immunization

Immunization is a special case of disease prevention. Immunization care for adolescents is inextricably related to primary care and preventive health strategies. Unfortunately, as discussed in Chapter 3, the proportion of adolescents making any sort of a visit to a health care provider decreases as adolescents mature, as does the proportion making a health maintenance visit in particular (Schuchter and Fairbrother, 2008). Lessened contact with primary care settings impedes high immunization coverage levels. Immunization visits may be the draw for parents to bring their infants and young children to a physician. The fact that visits, particularly health maintenance visits, decline in adolescence is a barrier that needs to be overcome. Perhaps immunization requirements for adolescents can act as a draw for this group to come to primary care as well.

Impediments to achieving the goal of universal immunization of adolescents revolve around reimbursement and education. The National Vaccine Advisory Committee has recommended "substantial, but incremental changes to the current system," including expanded funding of the existing immunization grant program, expansion of the Vaccines for Children program, promotion of "first dollar" insurance coverage for immunizations, and assurance to the provider of adequate reimbursement for the administration of vaccines (Hinman, 2005). Other strategies for ensuring good vaccination coverage for adolescents involve education on the need for the vaccines and on the appropriate visit schedule (Middleman et al., 2006).

Although an annual health maintenance visit for adolescents has been recommended by multiple agencies and professional groups, there has in the past been no need for recommended immunizations and other services that would bring patients in this age group into care. The new recommended immunizations, such as those for the human papillomavirus (HPV) (Markowitz et al., 2007), necessitate standard visit platforms with recommendations that target age groups within the adolescent years.

SAM has endorsed a set of recommendations for improving immunization coverage of the adolescent population, including the following (Middleman et al., 2006):

- The use of all vaccines and vaccination schedules promulgated by the Advisory Committee on Immunization Practice for the adolescent age group.
- The development of three distinct vaccination visit platforms for adolescents (an 11- to 12-year visit, a 14- to 15-year visit, and a 17- to 18-year visit) to integrate and emphasize the role of vaccination in already recommended comprehensive health maintenance visits.

- The use of immunization standing orders, immunization screening tools, immunization registries, and immunization reminder and recall systems.
- The simultaneous administration of multiple vaccines to increase vaccination rates.
- The use of "noncomprehensive" visits (e.g., minor illness visits, camp/sports physical visits, precollege visits) and qualified "alternative" vaccination sites (e.g., pharmacies, schools) to administer vaccines.
- The continued and increased education of health care providers, parents, and adolescents regarding the disease prevention benefits of immunization.

While vaccinations are available for many pediatric and adolescent infectious diseases that were once far more common, a clinically effective immunization for dental caries has yet to be developed, despite a biological basis for its development (Taubman, and Nash, 2006). At this time, the most effective preventive interventions for caries are dental sealants and topical use of fluorides (Adair et al., 2001; National Institutes of Health Consensus Development Conference Statement, 2001). Widespread availability of these two preventive interventions holds strong promise for reducing caries among adolescents.

Youth Development

The 2002 report *Community Programs to Promote Youth Development* (National Research Council and Institute of Medicine, 2002) identifies a set of personal and social assets that facilitate youth development (see Box 4-2). These assets address four domains of development: physical, intellectual, psychological/emotional, and social. They are drawn from an extensive research base that highlights the importance of and relationships among these personal assets in contributing to an adolescent's capacity to navigate transitions from childhood to a productive adult life (Compas et al., 1986; Entwisle, 1990; Wentzel, 1991). The report also identifies positive features of youth settings that support the development of these assets (see Table 4-1). The key features are physical and psychological safety; appropriate structure; supportive relationships; opportunities to belong; positive social norms; support for efficacy and mattering; opportunities for skill building; and integration of family, school, and community efforts. The presence of these features has been demonstrated to foster the personal assets described in Box 4-2 and to contribute to the formation of settings that are helpful to adolescents (see National Research Council and Institute of Medicine, 2002, for a detailed review). Table 4-1 describes how these

BOX 4-2
Personal and Social Assets That Facilitate Positive Youth Development

Physical Development
- Good health habits
- Good health risk management skills

Intellectual Development
- Knowledge of essential life skills
- Knowledge of essential vocational skills
- School success
- Rational habits of mind—critical thinking and reasoning skills
- In-depth knowledge of more than one culture
- Good decision-making skills
- Knowledge of skills needed to navigate through multiple cultural contexts

Psychological and Emotional Development
- Good mental health, including positive self-regard
- Good emotional self-regulation skills
- Good coping skills
- Good conflict resolution skills
- Mastery motivation and positive achievement motivation
- Confidence in one's personal efficacy
- "Planfulness"—planning for the future and future life events
- Sense of personal autonomy/responsibility for self
- Optimism coupled with realism
- Coherent and positive personal and social identity
- Prosocial and culturally sensitive values
- Spirituality or a sense of a "larger" purpose in life
- Strong moral character
- A commitment to good use of time

Social Development
- Connectedness—perceived good relationships and trust with parents, peers, and some other adults
- Sense of social place/integration—being connected and valued by larger social networks
- Attachment to prosocial/conventional institutions, such as school, church, and nonschool youth programs
- Ability to navigate in multiple cultural contexts
- Commitment to civic engagement

SOURCE: Reproduced from National Research Council and Institute of Medicine (2002).

TABLE 4-1 Features of Positive Developmental Settings

	Descriptors	Opposite Poles
Physical and psychological safety	Safe and health-promoting facilities; practice that increases safe peer-group interaction and decreases unsafe or confrontational peer interactions.	Physical and health dangers, fear, feeling of insecurity, sexual and physical harassment, verbal abuse.
Appropriate structure	Limit setting, clear and consistent rules and expectations, firm-enough control, continuity and predictability, clear boundaries, and age-appropriate monitoring.	Chaotic, disorganized, laissez-faire, rigid, overcontrolled, autocratic.
Supportive relationships	Warmth, closeness, connectedness, good communication, caring, support, guidance, secure attachment, responsiveness.	Cold, distant, overcontrolling, ambiguous support, untrustworthy, focused on winning, inattentive, unresponsive, rejecting.
Opportunities to belong	Opportunities for meaningful inclusion, regardless of one's gender, ethnicity, sexual orientation, or disabilities; social inclusion, social engagement and integration; opportunities for sociocultural identity formation; support for cultural and bicultural competence.	Exclusion, marginalization, intergroup conflict.
Positive social norms	Rules of behavior, expectations, injunctions, ways of doing things, values and morals, obligations for service.	Normlessness, anomie, laissez-faire practices, antisocial and amoral norms, norms that encourage violence, reckless behavior, consumerism, poor health practices, conformity.

Support for efficacy and mastering	Youth-based empowerment practices that support autonomy, making a real difference in one's community, and being taken seriously. Practice that includes enabling, responsibility granting, meaningful challenge. Practices that focus on improvement rather than on relative current performance levels.	Unchallenging, overcontrolling, disempowering, disabling. Practices that undermine motivation and desire to learn, such as excessive focus on current relative performance level rather than improvement.
Opportunities for skill building	Opportunities to learn physical, intellectual, psychological, emotional, and social skills; exposure to intentional learning experiences; opportunities to learn cultural literacies, media literacy, communication skills, and good habits of mind; preparation for adult employment; opportunities to develop social and cultural capital.	Practice that promotes bad physical habits and habits of mind; practice that undermines school and learning.
Integration of family, school and community efforts	Concordance, coordination, and synergy among family, school, and community.	Discordance, lack of communication, conflict.

SOURCE: Reproduced from National Research Council and Institute of Medicine (2002).

features are made operational and also lists the characteristics associated with their absence.

Recent decades have seen the emergence of several organizations that offer technical assistance to community-based efforts to foster youth development. These efforts are seen as a complement to, and sometimes a substitute for, problem-based disease prevention and treatment programs, especially in such areas as substance abuse, juvenile delinquency, and risky sexual activity. The Center for Youth Development and Policy Research within the Academy of Educational Development,[4] for example, offers an extensive array of research publications and other resources that support the undertaking of such efforts in different communities.

Other groups have sought to translate the youth development framework to the particular circumstances of health settings. For example, the Mount Sinai Adolescent Health Center in New York City has prepared *A Guide for Positive Youth Development* (ACT for Youth Downstate Center for Excellence and ACT for Youth Upstate Center of Excellence, 2003) that is now used by the Los Angeles County Public Health Department to assist adolescents in positive growth. Los Angeles County health officials are drawing on the framework articulated in the Mount Sinai guide to shift their programs from a problem and deficit orientation toward one that highlights an adolescent's strengths, cultivates skill development, and promotes healthy relationships (Harding, 2007). The program is built around six principles of youth development (ACT for Youth Downstate Center for Excellence and ACT for Youth Upstate Center of Excellence, 2003):

- Strengths: Focus on the strengths rather than the deficits of adolescents.
- Youth engagement: View adolescents not just as recipients of services, but also as resources, contributors, and leaders in the program.
- Youth/adult relationships: Recognize that the interactions and relationships between adolescents and program staff are as important as the services provided.
- Youth voice: Provide an opportunity for adolescents to participate in the organization from which they are receiving services.
- Community involvement: Encourage the community, not just the family and professionals, to contribute to the health and well-being of adolescents.
- Long-term involvement: Recognize that commitment to a youth development approach requires long-term involvement and cannot be viewed as an isolated or time-limited event.

---

[4]See http://cydpr.aed.org.

In another locale, the City of Detroit's Department of Health and Wellness Promotion has created a Youth Development Institute (YDI) aimed at preventing the onset of or experimentation with drug use among adolescents, primarily those aged 12–18 (Anthony, 2007). The program is built on a framework similar to that of the Los Angeles program. Lessons learned from the Detroit YDI experience highlight the importance of providing transportation, especially for adolescents from families who depend on public transportation. Also important are having mentorship and counseling available during after-school hours and on weekends and fostering collaborations across diverse sectors.

ENSURING ACCESS TO CONFIDENTIAL SERVICES

As reviewed in Chapter 3, health care services that are confidential increase the acceptability of services and the willingness of adolescents to seek care, especially for sensitive issues such as sexual behavior, reproductive health, mental health, and substance use. Not only may the confidentiality of health services for patients increase utilization of health care, but it also may be morally appropriate. Providers argue that their ability to protect conversations and records is one of the pillars of the trusting relationship that is a precondition for patients' comfort in communicating their history, feelings, and symptoms. In support of the moral perspective on this issue, many argue that the personal history and secrets of a patient are the patient's to hold and to share only when he or she has made the decision to do so.

Confidentiality for the adolescent exists within this conversation but is complicated by tensions that do not exist in the adult realm (Friedland, 1994). Society generally accepts that an adult has a right to confidentiality that ends only at possible harm to self or others. Reflecting the latter restrictions, every jurisdiction has mandatory reporting laws that cover matters as disparate as gunshot and knife wounds, STIs, and communicable diseases. Most of these laws, even those that relate to violence, have a public health rationale and can be justified under the police power of the state. In addition, there is the complexity of child abuse reporting laws and, in a few jurisdictions, elder abuse reporting laws; these laws aim to protect, under the *parens patriae* power of the state, those who cannot secure their own welfare and protect their own well-being.

But adolescents fall under none of these analytic schemes. They are aging out of the parent–child relationship, and their claims to the confidentiality enjoyed by adults are evolving rather than already established. Clearly there is no absolute protection for the confidentiality of a small child. Yet even here some have argued that it is in the interest of the development of the child as a moral person that a confidence shared be guarded with the promise of protection (Murray, 1996). Obviously, keeping a secret that would have a negative impact in the present or the future cannot be ethically supported. But as the child ages and the consequences of keeping confidences have more to do with lifestyle and life choices and less to do with predictable, definable, immediate, or long-term harms, the more claim the adolescent has on the provider's maintaining confidentiality.

As described in Chapter 3, current state and federal policies generally protect the confidentiality of adolescents' health information when they are legally allowed to consent for their own care. Without these polices in place, adolescents could feel compelled to forego needed health services—particularly in such sensitive areas as sexual behavior, reproductive health, mental health, and substance use.

In addition to existing state and federal policies, studies have focused on the specific roles of providers, parents, health care professional organizations, and health care payors in dealing with confidentiality issues. Physicians and other health practitioners who care for adolescents understand that, as in medicine generally, the assurance of confidentiality in adolescent medicine is not an absolute. Given that the stakes are high for adolescents and their health and that the persons to whom confidences would be revealed are most often parents, health care professionals treating adolescents must constantly walk a fine line in determining how best to secure the trust of their adolescent patients and in deciding what to disclose and when.

Role of the Health Care Provider

As previously discussed, results of one study suggest that strategies for explaining conditional confidentiality in a way adolescents understand and feel comfortable with can be developed and used in positive ways to foster trust (Ford et al., 1997). This study looked at whether adolescents' concerns about privacy in clinical settings decreased their willingness to seek health care for sensitive problems and may have inhibited their communication with physicians. The authors of the study conclude that adolescents are more willing to communicate with and seek health care from physicians who assure them of confidentiality. They suggest that further investigation is needed to identify a confidentiality assurance statement that would explain the legal and ethical limitations of confidentiality without decreasing the likelihood that adolescents will seek future health services for routine and nonreportable sensitive health concerns.

Another study found that most physicians do not consistently discuss confidentiality with their adolescent patients. Those who do so assure adolescents of unconditional confidentiality, which is inconsistent with either professional guidelines or legal limitations (Ford and Millstein, 1997).

Role of the Parent

While professional guidelines for the practice of adolescent medicine stress the importance of privacy and confidentiality in interactions with adolescent patients, parents frequently receive information about their children's health services. In particular, although adolescents may have an opportunity to confer privately with their health care providers, the bills for their expenses are usually sent to the insured parent or guardian. These bills may disclose the types of services provided or the condition that prompted the visit.

Parents are deeply involved in their adolescent children's health care decisions, and medical professionals recognize both the fact and the importance of that involvement. The data cited earlier make this clear: even for intimate forms of care such as reproductive health services and even at public clinics, the great majority of parents are involved (Jones et al., 2005), and most organizations of health care professionals encourage communication between parents and adolescents about important health concerns and health services (Morreale, Stinnett, and Dowling, 2005).

Empirical evidence suggests that parents generally think parental notification laws make sense, although the majority holding this belief is not as large as some imagine. In one multistate investigation, Eisenberg and colleagues (2005) found that 55 percent of parents favored parental notification for access to contraception. However, a large majority also favored exceptions. Reinforcing the point made earlier that the health of adolescents is one very important value parents consider, but not the only one, most parents had realistic beliefs about the consequences of parental notification. Hardly any (3 percent) thought adolescents would respond by ceasing to have sex, and the parents understood that notification would lead to an increase in STIs and other adverse outcomes (although it is unclear what they believed the magnitude of those outcomes to be). Yet some parents still supported notification laws.

Results of another study suggest that parents' attitudes can be influenced by education. Hutchinson and Stafford (2005) demonstrated that the percentage of parents who initially disagreed with various forms of adolescent privacy dropped by roughly half after exposure to basic facts about the importance of privacy for adolescent health. Unfortunately, the interpretation of "adolescent privacy" in this study was not the same as that in the previous study (the focus was on allowing adolescents to speak with a doctor alone and "the general importance of teen privacy," not parental notification specifically). Also, the authors do not describe the facts that were presented to the parents to educate them, making it difficult to compare the two studies.

Although the evidence is not uniform, the findings of research completed over several decades have consistently supported several key points: (1) most adolescents share information with their parents and seek even sensitive services such as contraception with their parents' knowledge; (2) privacy concerns influence adolescents' willingness to seek services at all, their choice of provider, their candor in giving a health history, their willingness to accept specific services, and other important aspects of access to care; (3) few adolescents plan to stop risky behaviors if confidential care is unavailable; (4) some parents support the idea of parental notification; and (5) parents often understand the importance of privacy and confidentiality and their potential effect on health and access to health services.

Role of Health Care Professional Organizations

The confidentiality policies and ethical guidelines of health care professional organizations tend to acknowledge the important role played by parents in caring for adolescents while favoring confidential access to health care (for an exhaustive treatment, see Morreale, Stinnett, and Dowling, 2005). For example, SAM's position paper on confidential care for adolescents states that "health care professionals should support effective communication between adolescents and their parents or other caretakers. Participation of parents in the health care of their adolescents should usually be encouraged but should not be mandated," and "confidentiality protection is an essential component of health care for adolescents because it is consistent with their development of maturity and autonomy and without it, some adolescents will forgo care." The statement goes on to assert, "Laws that allow minors to give their own consent for all or some types of health care and that protect the confidentiality of adolescents' health care information are fundamentally necessary" (Ford, English, and Sigman, 2004, p. 1). Similarly, an American Academy of Pediatrics position statement says that "the issue of confidentiality has been identified, by both providers and young people themselves, as a significant barrier to access to health care." The statement goes on to urge providers to communicate with parents while saying that minors should "have an opportunity for examination and counseling apart from parents, and the same confidentiality will be preserved between the adolescent patient and the provider as between the parent/adult and the provider" (American Academy of Pediatrics, 1989, p. 9). A large number of similar position statements from professional medical organizations emphasize the importance of confidentiality for adolescent health (Morreale, Stinnett, and Dowling, 2005).

Role of the Health Care Payor

Even if adolescents are able to consent to care, this does not necessarily guarantee confidentiality. In the last 30 years, a number of factors have combined to limit the scope of protections that providers and patients have assumed to exist (Siegler, 1982). Private insurance third-party payors, Medicare and Medicaid, and managed care organizations all require that records be shared so that standards can be set, maintained, and enforced. In addition, the development of electronic medical records, while providing ease of access to patient records and helping to establish the basis for quality review and improvement, also allows for the possibility of electronic breach. Although many electronic systems boast more security than typical paper records, the potential for distribution after an electronic breach remains a concern.

Private and public insurance administrative and billing practices often counteract confidentiality protections. As reviewed by Fox and Limb (2008), commercial and public insurers have different explanation of benefits (EOB) policies, which vary by state, payor, and program. The EOB statements, which generally list the recipient's name, services provided, and other service-related information, may be mailed home directly to the adolescent, may be directed to the parent or head of the household, or not mailed at all. These policies may be in direct violation of state and federal laws that afford adolescents the right to consent for certain services.

INNOVATIONS IN ADOLESCENT HEALTH SERVICES

A greater focus on community resources, linkages to specialty care, and increased standardization of adolescent health services will not happen in a vacuum. Advances in health information technology for adolescents hold promise for facilitating the integration and coordination of adolescent health services across geographic areas. This section describes these innovations, and provides a brief discussion of the emerging field of personalized medicine. It also reviews a number of existing examples of health services and systems that have been shown to make services accessible, acceptable, appropriate, effective, and equitable for adolescents.

Health Information Technology

Changing the settings and system features associated with the delivery of adolescent health services can help create environments that promote key health objectives for adolescents, especially in the context of changes in health services that are occurring more broadly. This environmental approach requires careful attention to selected components that are ripe for change, so that health care providers can convey guidance and information that are consistent with the health objectives for adolescents and young adults of Healthy People 2010 (U.S. Department of Health and Human Services, 2007).

Most adolescents already have a sizable array of information and communication technologies at their disposal. Their comfort level with electronic communications and activity far exceeds that of their parents and other older family members, and for many, e-mail, the Internet, social networking sites, mobile phones, and text messaging are an integral form of communication. Health institutions, however, have not kept pace with their young patients in this regard, especially in considering how such technologies can improve health service delivery and reduce unhealthful habits and risky behaviors.

Interactive technologies such as instant messaging and text messaging have been redefining the social networks of today's adolescents. In 2005, 65 percent of American adolescents overall and 75 percent of those who were online used instant messaging (Lenhart, Madden, and Hitlin, 2005). Adolescents report that they use text messaging for keeping in touch and making plans with friends, playing games, and even asking someone out or ending a relationship (Bryant, Sanders-Jackson, and Smallwood, 2006).

The SexInfo program in San Francisco has capitalized on this trend by using text messaging to share health information with adolescents, particularly about STIs, HIV, birth control, and sexual health services. In response to rising rates of chlamydia and gonorrhea among African American adolescents in the city, a public–private partnership launched SexInfo, an information and referral program that helps adolescents learn about sexual health and obtain answers to common questions about STIs and pregnancy. A similar program in the United Kingdom was the model for this program (SexInfo, 2006).

Sweet Talk, a pilot text messaging program developed in the United Kingdom for diabetic patients (not aimed at adolescents in particular) delivers individually targeted text messages and general diabetes information to patients. The program offers a system of contact and support between clinic visits and aims to increase adherence to intensive insulin regimens and improve clinical outcomes (Franklin et al., 2003).

In Ireland, Headsup is a text service that provides adolescents access to a range of helplines and support services. Users simply text the word "Headsup" to a free 24-hour text service, through which adolescents can receive, direct to their mobile phones, up-to-date and accurate contact numbers for organizations that will provide advice on their problems (Rehab, 2007).

In addition to text messaging, online mental health services have been provided in some sites with results comparable to those of face-to-face services for some patients. Some rural sites have used real-time video links to deliver mental health services to adolescents. Such techniques are especially promising for areas of professional shortages or for patients who are unable to attend routine specialty care (Brick, Brick, and D'Alessandri, 2004; Sulzbacher, Vallin, and Waetzig, 2006).

Health information technology will play an increasing role in the health care system, providing real-time decision support for patients and clinicians, educating adolescents and families, encouraging the diffusion of health services from the office to the community, and assisting in the tracking and coordination of care across regions and providers.

Personalized Health Services

The new tools described above are part of an increasing array of techniques for individualized electronic assessment and intervention. The capacity to collect and analyze large amounts of data about individuals, including prior use of health services, previous diagnoses, behavioral issues, and even genomic or proteomic profiles, may make it possible to personalize therapeutic or preventive interventions for specific conditions. The use of such information is largely limited to research purposes at this time, although applications for adolescents may be emerging. However, the ethical, insurance, prognostic, and financial implications of these new initiatives are not well understood for any group of patients, let alone adolescents in particular.

Examples of Innovative Adolescent Health Services

A number of efforts are being undertaken across the United States to deliver health services to adolescents in innovative ways. These services are being provided in various settings, with diverse foci, and by a range of providers. These efforts demonstrate both the potential and the drawbacks of highly focused adolescent specialty sites. Almost all of them provide the types of services needed by adolescents—from reproductive services to counseling and mental health—in a more comprehensive way than do traditional primary care settings. In addition, these special sites and programs that cater to adolescents are able to offer numerous nonmedical services, such as vocational or safety classes and instruction. At least as important, all have created an environment that is accessible and acceptable to adolescents by reducing barriers related to confidentiality, transportation, and availability. At the same time, these efforts demonstrate the limitations of such highly specialized adolescent models. They rely on staff with adolescent expertise, a group in short supply. Moreover, they usually are not well connected with traditional medical services or with services for other members of adolescents' families. And they often rely on grants and governmental support to make ends meet.

These complexities, together with the limited evaluation of such innovations and the lack of a standard against which to study them, make it impossible to identify any one model for innovative service delivery for adolescents. Nonetheless, some descriptive, anecdotal reports offer insights into innovative primary care models that work for adolescents. The committee conducted site visits to understand the range of services, settings, and providers involved in these efforts. The sites visited serve as useful examples of adolescent-specific health services delivered in various settings and illustrate what might qualify as lead or coordinating centers in the provision of regional services for adolescents. This section describes the sites visited by the committee, as well as one site documented by Sandmaier and colleagues (2007).

Denver Health

Denver Health and Hospital Authority is a comprehensive, integrated health system that serves the city and county residents of Denver, Colorado. This system includes a public hospital (with a Level I trauma center), a public health department, and community health services (8 community health centers and 12 school-based centers located throughout the city). It also includes centers for poison, drug, and alcohol treatment; occupational health; behavioral health; and correctional care. A telephone advice line is provided as well. Generally, Denver Health provides the following services throughout the system: medical, dental, psychiatric, psychological, obstetric and gynecological, dermatological, and educational. Denver Health is funded by many sources, including federal (330 grants), state, and city funding and patient revenues; the school-based health centers also receive support from a variety of foundations and other partners. Denver Health manages all policies, procedures, protocols, registration, billing, quality assurance, staff development, strategic planning, grant management, utilization review, and outcome monitoring internally. The system also works with other community partners, including the local mental health authority, a substance abuse organization, two other local hospitals, Denver public schools, and other community services (Special Supplemental Nutrition Program for Women, Infants, and Children; immunization; early periodic screening, diagnosis, and treatment; and services for children with special health needs).

Adolescents utilize primarily Denver Health's 12 school-based health centers (39 percent of total visits to the Denver Health system), obstetrics and gynecology clinics (13 percent), pediatric/adolescent clinics (10 percent/18 percent), and family practice offices (14 percent) located in the community health service network. The community health centers serve mainly low-income neighborhoods. The most common services provided to adolescents in the school-based and community health centers are immunizations; health maintenance visits; asthma treatment; gynecological and reproductive health services (family planning, pregnancy testing); STI screening and treatment; behavioral services (e.g., for ADHD); tuberculosis screening; and treatment for depression, headaches, acne, and upper respiratory infections.

The school-based health centers provide clinical preventive services, acute injury and illness treatment, management of stable chronic conditions, mental health counseling, substance abuse intervention, health education, basic laboratory services, and basic prescriptions. They do not provide hospitalization, x-rays, nonroutine laboratory tests, dental services, vision care, or abortion counseling, nor do they prescribe contraceptives; patients are referred to other parts of the Denver Health system if these services are needed. Fully 77 percent of patients using the school-based health centers are Hispanic, and 53 percent have no insurance.

Howard Brown's Broadway Youth Center

Howard Brown is a regional, federally qualified health organization in Chicago that provides an expansive network of health programs and services to the Chicago community. It has a diverse and qualified staff of licensed doctors, nurses, mental and other health practitioners, renowned research professionals, and prominent community leaders. The Broadway Youth Center is one of a number of programs offered by Howard Brown. It offers comprehensive services to people aged 12–24, including:

- Drop-in services that offer a place to hang out and connect while providing computer and telephone access, a daily snack, hygiene supplies, showers, and materials on safe sex.
- Daily health and education workshops.
- Case managers available to help with everything from meeting basic needs to obtaining resources and skills to help with housing, job placement, and education.
- Free drop-in, anonymous HIV testing and confidential STI screening for chlamydia and gonorrhea, available daily, as well as medical treatment for those with symptoms of an STI.
- Free drop-in medical services and health education for common health issues, including acute illness, family planning, and STI treatment. Referrals to primary care services are also made for those in need of ongoing care.
- Free individual and group drop-in counseling to assist with such is-

sues as coming out, dating violence, substance use, and HIV status. Those seeking ongoing counseling can receive an initial assessment followed by an appropriate referral.
- Social and support groups focused on various subpopulations (e.g., those who are transgender, college-aged, or HIV-positive) and relevant activities (e.g., creative expression, activism, legal rights).
- Peer education and adult mentoring.
- Research activities that explore various health issues and treatments.

Arkansas Children's Hospital's Adolescent and Sports Medicine Center

The Adolescent and Sports Medicine Center is part of the Arkansas Children's Hospital system, which serves local residents of Little Rock as well as state residents. It is the only center in the region that provides health services focused on adolescents. The following services are offered by a multidisciplinary team: medical and wellness services, gynecology, sports medicine, athletic training, sports physical therapy, mental health services, nutrition counseling, diabetes treatment, substance abuse services, and treatment for eating disorders. The center also provides financial consulting, an in-house limited pharmacy, and laboratory services. Diagnosis and treatment of eating disorders are delivered offsite in a specialty clinic. Adolescents needing subspecialty services are referred to other parts of the Arkansas Children's Hospital system. The center is funded mainly through a clinical contract with the University of Arkansas for Medical Sciences; additional funding is received from other partners that support the Arkansas Children's Hospital and the center.

The Adolescent and Sports Medicine Center has 12 outreach sites for its Sports Medicine PLUS program in local senior high and middle schools that serve as entry points for the full range of adolescent health services. The center operates a weekly consultation clinic in northwest Arkansas, as well as at two Job Corps facilities. It also works with other community partners, including a Community Health Coalition with a local high school, the local school board, Planned Parenthood, and the University of Arkansas for Medical Services.

The center provides health services to those aged 12–21—65 percent female, 70 percent African American. It serves primarily low-income adolescents who are enrolled in the State Children's Health Insurance Program (SCHIP), but also provides services for those within the Arkansas Children's Hospital system, members of the local community, and those referred for consults and emergency room follow-up.

The center offers unique features, including an electronic sign-in service to ease registration and remind all staff of the patients waiting to be seen and a 24-hour Kids Care telephone resource staffed by registered nurses for all-hours advice on medical needs. The provision of sports medicine and physical therapy is well suited to an adolescent-specific health center. The offsite adolescent eating disorders clinic uses an interdisciplinary approach for diagnosis and treatment, and is the only adolescent-specific eating disorders clinic in the state of Arkansas. Partnership with the school district provides payment for the sports medicine program, while other services are covered by SCHIP. The center's medical staff make up the Adolescent Division of the Department of Pediatrics and enjoy considerable autonomy in the center's management and planning. The center's policies, procedures, strategic planning, and monitoring are largely within the purview of the Arkansas Children's Hospital administration, with consultation from the medical staff of the Adolescent Division. The hospital submits all outpatient billing and returns collections on physician and other professional charges to the Department of Pediatrics through a contractual agreement.

Jetson Center for Youth

Through a contract with the Louisiana State Office of Youth Development, the Louisiana State University (LSU) Health Sciences Center's Juvenile Justice Program provides multidisciplinary health services for youths in the state's long-term secure juvenile facilities. The Jetson Center for Youth is one of these long-term secure juvenile sites. It serves primarily the southern portion of the state of Louisiana, including New Orleans and Baton Rouge, and provides medical, dental, psychiatric, and psychological services, as well as other specialty services, including neurology, orthopedics, gastroenterology, audiology, radiology, and ophthalmology. The center also provides educational and vocational services. Many of the center's services are available onsite; however, youths have access to all LSU health services offsite as well. The services are fully funded by the state. All policies, procedures, protocols, billing, quality assurance, staff development, strategic planning, grant management, and utilization review and outcome monitoring are managed through the Office of Youth Development in partnership with LSU.

The Jetson Center for Youth provides health services to 150 to 200 males aged 12–21, 80 percent of whom are African American and most of whom come from low-income rural communities. The most common health issues for adolescents served by the center are mental disorders (40 percent of these adolescents have a serious mental health problem), STIs, behavioral problems, and bruises and broken bones and teeth due to physical encounters. A multidisciplinary health care team delivers the center's onsite health services. The team includes registered, licensed practical, and administrative nurses; psychologists; psychiatrists; social workers; pediatricians; an ophthalmologist; a dentist; a dental hygienist; and pediatric, physician assistant, and administrative personnel essential to the coordination of services. In addition to the onsite staff, there is access to other specialists, most notably an additional psychiatrist, who works offsite through telemedicine. This health team, employed by LSU and with several members available onsite at all times (24-hour nursing and on-call psychiatric/psychological staff), is eager to move from a correctional to a therapeutic model, particularly in dealing with serious mental illness, through ongoing planning, training, and evaluation with Office of Youth Development leadership.

Mount Sinai Medical Center

An adolescent health clinic associated with Mount Sinai Medical Center, established in 1968, is one of the largest and oldest examples of a freestanding health center that provides integrated, multidisciplinary services and also strives to help adolescents take responsibility for their own health. The center annually serves more than 10,000 youths (aged 12–22) in several sites, including one in East Harlem and two school-based health centers in other Manhattan neighborhoods (Sandmaier et al., 2007). About one-third of clients have public or private insurance, and the center helps young people enroll in such public insurance programs as Medicaid or SCHIP; even so, care is available to all patients without restriction. The center's diverse and multiethnic staff operates as a collaborative team focusing on coordinated, comprehensive, and highly individualized care. It includes 6 adolescent medicine specialists; 20 clinical social workers; 3 health educators; specialists in obstetrics/gynecology, mental and behavioral health, and nutrition; and nurse practitioners, physician assistants, and ambulatory care technicians (Sandmaier et al., 2007).

The Mount Sinai adolescent health clinic is especially noteworthy for its emphasis on youth empowerment through intentional engagement with adolescents and partners in understanding and ownership of their health. The Youth Advisory Board, a peer education program called SPEEK (Sinai Peers Encouraging Empowerment through Knowledge), and skill-building components in both primary and specialty care programs all reflect the center's focus on helping adolescents make healthy decisions and supporting their overall growth through mentoring, tutoring, legal advocacy, and preparation for taking such key tests as the General Educational Development, a high school equivalency degree (Sandmaier et al., 2007).

Erie Teen Health Center

The mission of the Erie Teen Health Center in Chicago is "both simple and challenging: to provide comprehensive, integrated, teen-sensitive care, focusing on helping adolescents to develop the strengths and skills that will allow them to become effective stewards of their own health" (Sandmaier et al., 2007, p. 12). The center serves approximately 2,200 adolescent patients per year, along with more than 500 babies and young children of patients. More than three-quarters of its clients are aged 18–21, and approximately 70 percent are Hispanic. The center has developed a nationally recognized group model of prenatal care—the Centering Pregnancy Program—that includes physician examinations, consultation with a nurse midwife, group discussion sessions, self-assessment instruments, and community support within the group. Assessments of program effectiveness are based on patient satisfaction surveys, as well as data on the center's reproductive health services. Those data show that 93 percent of the center's adolescent patients used birth control over the past 12 months without becoming pregnant, and that 86 percent of clients with STIs had been reached and treated by the center within 14 days of testing, a rate that exceeds the state goal of 73 percent (Sandmaier et al., 2007).

SUMMARY

Developing an improved health system for adolescents will require attention to several fundamental goals:

- Placing a greater emphasis on and enhancing the capacity of primary care providers to offer high-quality screening, assessment, health management, referral, and care management of specialty services for this population, especially for behaviorally based health problems.
- Coordinating behavioral, reproductive, mental health, and dental services in practice and community settings.
- Incorporating health promotion, disease prevention, and youth development throughout the health system, in coordination with such services in the community.
- Ensuring consent and confidentiality for adolescents seeking care.

Strengthening these features of the settings in which health services for adolescents are provided will require explicit attention to the ways in which service environments are structured and the training and clinical experiences of health care providers. It will also require comprehensive integration of electronic health records and electronic tools for communicating with adolescents, and the development of sustained partnerships with sectors such as education, the media, and the entertainment industry that are important parts of the adolescent culture. It will be necessary to introduce new incentives and assessment efforts, derived from population health research, aimed at realigning the health environment, provider services, and information resources, probably in regional centers with varying levels of expertise, to achieve a more explicit focus on accomplishing the national health objectives for adolescents outlined in Healthy People 2010 (as described in detail in Chapter 2). At the very least, primary care providers who care for large numbers of adolescents will need to organize support for comprehensive screening and monitoring initiatives that are likely to require electronic databases and trained staff. These initiatives should build upon the strengths of the existing diversity of health service settings while also attempting to move those settings toward greater coordination and a set of common objectives and screening and assessment methods that can enrich the quality of adolescent health services and ultimately lead to better health outcomes. These initiatives should also focus on the context of health services by building upon lessons learned from the delivery of services to marginalized and special subpopulations of adolescents with respect to those operational features and processes that foster adolescents' engagement with providers. Emphasis should be placed on improving the skills and capacity of all health personnel in primary care settings—not solely physicians—to serve the needs of all adolescents.

This chapter has proposed several approaches to improving health systems for adolescents to make services accessible, acceptable, appropriate, effective, and equitable. Such improvements are particularly important to support healthy development for those adolescents who are more vulnerable to poor health or unhealthful habits and risky behavior because of their demographic characteristics or other circumstances. Limited evidence is available on health outcomes associated with alternative service strategies. Therefore, the committee has attempted to highlight areas in which research could yield knowledge that would support quality improvements in the organization and delivery of health services for adolescents. For example, the evidentiary base currently does not support the formulation of performance standards and operational criteria that would make it possible to compare the strengths and limitations of different service delivery models in meeting the needs of all adolescents, as well as specific subpopulations. In particular, few evaluations provide insight into the validity and reliability of screening tools and counseling techniques for the most vulnerable groups of adolescents. Efforts to improve the knowledge base on the provision of services to these adolescents should therefore be a major priority in efforts to improve health services and the quality of care for adolescents.

REFERENCES

ACT for Youth Downstate Center for Excellence and ACT for Youth Upstate Center of Excellence. (2003). *A Guide to Positive Youth Development*. New York: Mount Sinai Adolescent Health Center.

Adair, S. M., Bowen, W. H., Burt, B. A., Kumar, J. V., Levy, S. M., Pendrys, D. G., Rozier, R. G., Selwitz, R. H., Stamm, J. W., Stookey, G. K., and Whitford, G. M. (2001). Recommendations for using fluoride to prevent and control dental caries in the United States. *Recommendations and Reports: Morbidity and Mortality Weekly Report, 50*(RR14), 1–42.

American Academy of Pediatrics. (1989). Confidentiality in adolescent health care. *AAP News, 5,* 9.

American Academy of Pediatrics, American College of Critical Care Medicine, and Society of Critical Care Medicine. (2000). Consensus report for regionalization of services for critically ill or injured children. *Pediatrics, 105,* 152–155.

American Medical Association. (1997). *Guidelines for Adolescent Preventive Services (GAPS), Recommendations Monograph*. Chicago, IL: American Medical Association.

Anthony, Y. E. (2007). The Youth Development Institute of the Detroit Department of Health and Wellness Promotion. *City Lights, 15*(1), Spring.

Babor, T. F., Higgins-Biddle, J. C., Saunders, J. B., and Montiero, M. G. (2001). *The Alcohol Use Disorders Identification Test: Guidelines for Use in Primary Care* (2nd Ed., WHO/MSD/MSB/01.6a). Geneva: World Health Organization.

Brick, J. E., Brick, J. E., and D'Alessandri, R. (2004). Mountaineer doctor television in West Virginia. *West Virginia Medical Journal, 100,* 92–93.

Bryant, J. A., Sanders-Jackson, A., and Smallwood, A. M. K. (2006). IMing, text messaging, and adolescent social networks. *Journal of Computer-Mediated Communication, 11*(2), article 10.

Burleson, J. A., and Kaminer, Y. (2007). Aftercare for adolescent alcohol use disorder: Feasibility and acceptability of a phone intervention. *American Journal of Addiction, 16,* 202–205.

Burns, B. J., Costello, E. J., Angold, A., Tweed, D., Stangl, D., Farmer, E. M. Z., and Erkanli, A. (1995). Children's mental health service use across service sectors. *Health Affairs, 14,* 147–159.

Calonge, N. (2001). New USPSTF guidelines: Integrating into clinical practice. *American Journal of Preventive Medicine, 20,* 7–9.

Campo, J. V., Shafer, S., Strohm, J., Lucas, A., Cassesse, C. G., Shaeffer, D., and Altman, H. (2005). Pediatric behavioral health in primary care: A collaborative approach. *Journal of the American Psychiatric Nurses Association, 11,* 276–282.

Chen, K., and Kandel, D. B. (1995). The natural history of drug use from adolescence to the mid-thirties in a general population sample. *American Journal of Public Health, 85,* 41–47.

Cheng, M. K. B. (2007). New approaches for creating the therapeutic alliance: Solution-focused interviewing, motivational interviewing, and the medication interest model. *Psychiatric Clinics of North America, 30,* 157–166.

Cohen, E., Mackenzie, R. G., and Yates, G. L. (1991). HEADSS, a psychosocial risk assessment instrument: Implications for designing effective intervention programs for runaway youth. *Journal of Adolescent Health, 12,* 539–544.

Collins, W. A., and Laursen, B. (2000). Adolescent relationships: The art of fugue. In C. Hendrick and S. Hendrick (Eds.), *Close Relationships: A Sourcebook* (pp. 59–70). Thousand Oaks, CA: Sage.

Compas, B. E., Wagner, B. M., Slavin, L. A., and Vannatta, K. (1986). A prospective study of life events, social support, and psychological symptomatology during the transition from high school to college. *American Journal of Community Psychology, 14,* 241–257.

Connor, D. F., McLaughlin, T. J., Jeffers-Terry, M., O'Brien, W. H., Stille, C. J., Young, L. M., and Antonelli, R. C. (2006). Targeted child psychiatric services: A new model of pediatric primary clinician—Child psychiatry collaborative care. *Clinical Pediatrics, 45,* 423–434.

Cuffe, S. P., Waller, J. L., Cuccaro, M. L., and Pumariega, A. J., and Garrison, C. Z. (1995). Race and gender differences in the treatment of psychiatric disorders in young adolescents. *Journal of the American Academy of Child and Adolescent Psychiatry, 34,* 1536–1543.

Dale, J., Caramlau, I., Docherty, A., Sturt, J., and Hearnshaw, H. (2007). Telecare motivational interviewing for diabetes patient education and support: A randomised controlled trial based in primary care comparing nurse and peer supporter delivery. *Trials, 8,* 18.

David, D. J. (1977). Craniofacial surgery: The team approach. *ANZ Journal of Surgery, 47,* 193–198.

Davis, M. P., Rhode, P. C., Dutton, G. R., Redmann, S. M., Ryan, D. H., and Brantley, P. J. (2006). A primary care weight management intervention for low-income African-American women. *Obesity, 14,* 1412–1420.

Doumas, D. M., and Hannah, E. (2007). Preventing high-risk drinking in youth in the workplace: A web-based normative feedback program. *Journal of Substance Abuse Treatment,* June 27, epub.

Dunst, C. J., and Trivette, C. M. (2004). Toward a categorization scheme of child find, referral, early identification, and eligibility determination practices. *Tracelines, 1*(2), 1–18.

Eisenberg, M. E., Swain, C., Sieving, R., Bearinger, L. H., Sieving, R. E., and Resnick, M. D. (2005). Parental notification laws for minors' access to contraception—What do parents say? *Archives of Pediatrics and Adolescent Medicine, 159,* 120–125.

Elster, A., and Kuznets, N. (Eds.). (1994). *AMA Guidelines for Adolescent Preventive Services (GAPS).* Baltimore, MD: Williams and Wilkins.

Entwisle, D. R. (1990). Schooling and the adolescent. In S. S. Feldman and G. R. Elliott (Eds.), *At the Threshold: The Developing Adolescent* (pp. 197–224). Cambridge, MA: Harvard University Press.

Federal Expert Work Group on Pediatric Subspecialty Capacity, McManus, P., Fox, H., Limb, S., and Carpinelli, A. (2006). *Promising Approaches for Strengthening the Interface between Primary and Specialty Pediatric Care.* Washington, DC: Maternal and Child Health Policy Research Center.

Feightner, J. W., and Lawrence, R. S. (2001). Evidence-based prevention and international collaboration. *American Journal of Preventive Medicine, 20*(3 Suppl.), 5–6.

Fishman, P. A., Ebel, B. E., Garrison, M. M., Christakis, D. A., Wiehe, S. E., and Rivara, F. P. (2005). Cigarette tax increase and media campaign: Cost of reducing smoking-related deaths. *American Journal of Preventive Medicine, 29,* 19–26.

Ford, C. A., and Millstein, S. G. (1997). Delivery of confidentiality assurances to adolescents by primary care physicians. *Archives of Pediatrics and Adolescent Medicine, 151,* 505–509.

Ford, C., Millstein, S., Halpern-Felsher, B., and Irwin, C. E. (1997). Influence of physician confidentiality assurances on adolescents' willingness to disclose information and seek future health care: A randomized controlled trial. *Journal of the American Medical Association, 278,* 1029–1034.

Ford, C., English, A., and Sigman, G. (2004). SAM position statement: Confidential health care for adolescents. *Journal of Adolescent Health, 35,* 1–8.

Fox, H. B., and Limb, S. J. (2008). *State Policies Affecting the Assurance of Confidential Care for Adolescents*. Fact Sheet No. 5. Washington, DC: Incenter Strategies, the National Alliance to Advance Adolescent Health.

Franklin, V., Waller, A., Pagliari, C., and Greene, S. (2003). "Sweet talk": Text messaging support for intensive insulin therapy for young people with diabetes. *Diabetes Technology and Therapy, 5*, 991–996.

Franklin, V. L., Waller, A., Pagliari, C., and Greene, S. A. (2006). A randomized controlled trial of Sweet Talk, a text-messaging system to support young people with diabetes. *Diabetes Medicine, 23*, 1332–1338.

Friedland, B. (1994). Physician-patient confidentiality. Time to re-examine a venerable concept in light of contemporary society and advances in medicine. *The Journal of Legal Medicine, 15*, 249–277.

Gardner, W., Kelleher, K. J., Pajer, K. A., and Campo, J. V. (2003). Primary care clinicians' use of standardized tools to assess child psychosocial problems. *Ambulatory Pediatrics, 3*, 191–195.

Gardner, W., Kelleher, K. J., Pajer, K., and Campo, J. V. (2004). Follow-up care of children identified with ADHD by primary care clinicians: A prospective cohort study. *The Journal of Pediatrics, 145*, 767–771.

Golub, A., and Johnson, B. D. (1994). The shifting importance of alcohol and marijuana as gateway substances among serious drug abusers. *Journal of Studies of Alcohol, 55*, 607–614.

Green, M., and Palfrey, J. (Eds.). (2002). *Bright Futures: Guidelines for Health Supervision of Infants, Children, and Adolescents* (2nd Ed.). Washington, DC: National Center for Education in Maternal and Child Health, Georgetown University.

Harding, C. (2007). Youth development—A perspective from Los Angeles. *City Lights, 15*(4), Spring.

Harpaz-Rotem, I., and Rosenheck, R. A. (2006). Prescribing practices of psychiatrists and primary care physicians caring for children with mental illness. *Child Care, Health, and Development, 32*, 225–237.

Hartup, W. W. (1986). On relationships and development. In W. W. Hartup and Z. Rubin (Eds.), *Relationships and Development* (pp. 1–26). Mahwah, NJ: Erlbaum.

Hawkins, J. D., Catalano, R. F., and Arthur, M. W. (2002). Promoting science-based prevention in communities. *Addictive Behavior, 27*, 951–976.

Hawley, S. R., Beckman, H., and Bishop, T. (2006). Development of an obesity prevention and management program for children and adolescents in a rural setting. *Journal of Community Health Nursing, 23*, 69–80.

Hinman, A. R. (2005). Financing vaccines in the 21st century: Recommendations from the National Vaccine Advisory Committee. *American Journal of Preventive Medicine, 29*, 71–75.

Hoagwood, K., Jensen, P. S., Feil, M., Vitiello, B., and Bhatara, V. S. (2000). Medication management of stimulants in pediatric practice settings: A national perspective. *Journal of Developmental and Behavioral Pediatrics, 21*, 322–331.

Holder, H. D., Gruenewald, P. J., Ponicki, W. R., Treno, A. J., Grube, J. W., Saltz, R. F., Voas, R. B., Reynolds, R., Davis, J., Sanchez, L., Gaumont, G., and Roeper, P. (2000). Effect of community-based interventions on high-risk drinking and alcohol-related injuries. *Journal of the American Medical Association, 284*, 2341–2347.

Hollingworth, W., Ebel, B. E., McCarty, C. A., Garrison, M. M., Christakis, D. A., and Rivara, F. P. (2006). Prevention of deaths from harmful drinking in the United States: The potential effects of tax increases and advertising bans on young drinkers. *Journal of Studies on Alcohol, 67*, 300–308.

Horwitz, S. M., Kelleher, K. J., Stein, R. E. K., Storfer-Isser, A., Youngstrom, E. A., Park, E. R., Heneghan, A. M., Jensen, P. S., O'Connor, K. G., and Hoagwood, K. E. (2007). Barriers to the identification and management of psychosocial issues in children and maternal depression. *Pediatrics, 119*, e208–e218.

Hutchinson, J. W., and Stafford, E. M. (2005). Changing parental opinions about teen privacy through education. *Pediatrics, 116*, 966–971.

Institute of Medicine. (2000). *To Err Is Human: Building a Safer Health System*. L. T. Kohn, J. M. Corrigan, and M. S. Donaldson (Eds.). Washington, DC: National Academy Press.

Institute of Medicine. (2001). *Crossing the Quality Chasm: A New Health System for the 21st Century*. Washington, DC: National Academy Press.

Institute of Medicine. (2004). *Patient Safety: Achieving a New Standard of Care*. P. Aspden, J. M. Corrigan, J. Wolcott, and S. M. Erickson (Eds.). Washington, DC: The National Academies Press.

Institute of Medicine. (2007a). *Ending the Tobacco Problem: A Blueprint for the Nation*. R. J. Bonnie, K. Stratton, and R. B. Wallace (Eds.). Washington, DC: The National Academies Press.

Institute of Medicine. (2007b). *Preventing Medication Errors*. P. Aspden, J. A. Wolcott, J. L. Bootman, and L. R. Cronenwett (Eds.). Washington, DC: The National Academies Press.

Jones, R. K., Purcell, A., Singh, S., and Finer, L. B. (2005). Adolescents' reports of parental knowledge of adolescents' use of sexual health services and their reactions to mandated parental notification for prescription contraception. *Journal of the American Medical Association, 293*, 340–348.

Kim, W. J., and The American Academy of Child and Adolescent Psychiatry Task Force on Workforce Needs. (2003). Child and adolescent psychiatry workforce: A critical shortage and national challenge. *Academic Psychiatry, 27*, 277–282.

Klitzner, T. S., and Chang, R.-K. R. (2003). Regionalization of pediatric cardiac services: From theory to practice. *Progress in Pediatric Cardiology, 18*, 43–47.

Knight, J. R., Shrier, L. A., Bravender, T. D., Farrell, M., Vander Bilt, J., and Shaffer, H. J. (1999). A new brief screen for adolescent substance abuse. *Archives of Pediatrics and Adolescent Medicine, 153*, 591–596.

Koerber, A., Crawford, J., and O'Connell, K. (2003). The effects of teaching dental students brief motivational interviewing for smoking cessation counseling: A pilot study. *Journal of Dental Education, 67*, 439–447.

Kolbe, L. J., Kann, L., and Collins, J. L. (1993). Overview of the Youth Risk Behavior Surveillance System. *Public Health Reports, 108*(Suppl. 1), 2–10.

LaBrie, J. W., Pedersen, E. R., Thompson, A. D., and Earleywine, M. (2007a). A brief decisional balance intervention increases motivation and behavior regarding condom use in high-risk heterosexual college men. *Archives of Sexual Behavior*, Epub, July 26.

LaBrie, J. W., Thompson, A. D., Huchting, K., Lac, A., and Buckley, K. (2007b). A group motivational interviewing intervention reduces drinking and alcohol-related negative consequences in adjudicated college women. *Addictive Behaviors, 32*, 2549–2562.

Lenhart, A., Madden, M., and Hitlin, P. (2005). *Teens and Technology: Youth Are Leading the Transition to a Fully Wired and Mobile Nation*. Washington, DC: Pew Internet and American Life Project.

Maccoby, E. E. (1984). Middle childhood in the context of the family. In W. A. Collins (Ed.). *Development During Middle Childhood: The Years from Six to Twelve* (pp. 184–239). Washington, DC: National Academy Press.

Markowitz, L. E., Dunne, E. F., Saraiya, M., Lawson, H. W., Chesson, H., and Unger, E. R. (2007). Quadrivalent human papillomavirus vaccine. Recommendations of the Advisory Committee on Immunization Practices (ACIP). *Morbidity and Mortality Weekly Report, 56,* RR-2.

McCormick, M. C., Shapiro, S., and Starfield, B. H. (1985). The regionalization of perinatal services: Summary of the evaluation of a national demonstration program. *Journal of the American Medical Association, 253,* 799–804.

McPherson, T. L., and Hersch, R. K. (2000). Brief substance use screening instruments for primary care settings: A review. *Journal of Substance Abuse Treatment, 18,* 193–202.

Middleman, A. B., Rosenthal, S. L., Rickert, V. I., Neinstein, L., Fishbein, D. B., and D'Angelo, L. (2006). Adolescent immunizations: A position paper of the Society for Adolescent Medicine. *Journal of Adolescent Health, 38,* 321–327.

Miranda, J., Duan, N., Sherbourne, C., Schoenbaum, M., Lagomasino, L., Jackson-Triche, M., and Wells, K. B. (2003). Improving care for minorities: Can quality improvement interventions improve care and outcomes for depressed minorities? Results of a randomized, controlled trial. *Health Services Research, 38*(2), 613–630.

Morreale, M. C., Stinnett, A. J., and Dowling, E. C. (Eds.). (2005). *Policy Compendium on Confidential Health Services for Adolescents* (2nd Ed.). Chapel Hill, NC: Center for Adolescent Health & the Law.

Murray, M. L., Thompson, M., Santosh, P. J., and Wong, I. C. K. (2005). Effects of the Committee on Safety of Medicine's advice on antidepressant prescribing to children and adolescents in the UK. *Drug Safety, 28,* 1151–1157.

Murray, T. H. (1996). *The Worth of a Child.* Berkeley: University of California Press.

National Institutes of Health Consensus Development Conference Statement. (2001, March). Diagnosis and management of dental caries throughout life. *Journal of Dental Education, 65*(10), 1162–1168.

National Research Council and Institute of Medicine. (2002). *Community Programs to Promote Youth Development.* J. Eccles and J. A. Gootman (Eds.). Washington, DC: National Academy Press.

National Research Council and Institute of Medicine. (2004). *Reducing Underage Drinking: A Collective Responsibility.* R. J. Bonnie and M. E. O'Connell (Eds.). Washington, DC: The National Academies Press.

Newacheck, P. W., Brindis, C. D., Cart, C. U., Marchi, K., and Irwin, C. E. (1999). Adolescent health insurance coverage: Recent changes and access to care. *Pediatrics, 104,* 195–202.

O'Brien, S. H., Holubkov, R., and Reis, E. C. (2004). Identification, evaluation, and management of obesity in an academic primary care center. *Pediatrics, 114,* e154–e159.

Ozer, E. M., Adams, S. H., Lustig, J. L., Gee, S., Garber, A. K., Gardner, L. R., Rehbein, M., Addison, L., and Irwin, C. E. (2005). Increasing the screening and counseling of adolescents for risky health behaviors: A primary care intervention. *Pediatrics, 115,* 960–968.

Praiss, I. L., Feller, I., and James, M. H. (1980). The planning and organization of a regionalized burn care system. *Medical Care, 18,* 202–210.

Quintos, J. B., and Castells, S. (2006). Management of metabolic syndrome in morbidly obese children and adolescents. *Pediatric Endocrinology Reviews, 3,* 564–570.

Rahdert, E. R. (Ed.). 1991. *The Adolescent Assessment/Referral System Manual* (DHHS Publication ADM 91-1735). Washington, DC: U.S. Department of Health and Human Services.

Rehab. (2007). *Free 24-Hour Text Service to Provide Helpline Information for Young People.* Available: http://www.rehab.ie/press/article.aspx?id=279 [February 7, 2008].

Riggs, S. R., and Alario, A. (1989). Adolescent substance use instructor's guide. In C. E. Dubé, M. G. Goldstein, D. C. Lewis, E. R. Myers, and W. R. Zwick (Eds.), *Project ADEPT Curriculum for Primary Care Physician Training* (pp. 1–57). Providence, RI: Brown University.

Rivara, F. P., Ebel, B. E., Garrison, M. M., Christakis, D. A., Wiehe, S. E., and Levy, D. T. (2004). Prevention of smoking-related deaths in the United States. *American Journal of Preventive Medicine, 27*(2), 118–125.

Rushton, J. L., Clark, S. J., and Freed, G. L. (2000). Pediatrician and family physician prescription of selective serotonin reuptake inhibitors. *Pediatrics, 105*, e82.

Rushton, J., Bruckman, D., and Kelleher, K. (2002). Primary care referral of children with psychosocial problems. *Archives of Pediatric and Adolescent Medicine, 156*, 592–598.

Sandmaier, M., Bell, A. D., Fox, H. B., McManus, M. A., and Wilson, J. E. (2007). *Under One Roof: Primary Care Models That Work for Adolescents*. Washington, DC: Incenter Strategies.

Schuchter, J., and Fairbrother, G. (2008). *Health Services Utilization among Adolescents from the 2005 NHIS.* An analysis of 2005 National Health Interview Survey data. Report to the Institute of Medicine Committee on Adolescent Health Care Services and Models of Care for Treatment, Prevention and Health Development. Available: http://www.cincinnatichildrens.org/assets/0/78/1067/1395/1833/1835/1849/1f9efa12-6777-48a1-9334-f9bddfc98616.pdf [March 19, 2008].

SexInfo. (2006). *A New Sexual Health Cell Phone Text Messaging Service for Young People in San Francisco.* Available: http://www.sextextsf.org [June 27, 2007].

Siegler, M. (1982). Sounding boards. Confidentiality in medicine—a decrepit concept. *New England Journal of Medicine, 307*, 1518–1521.

Society for Adolescent Medicine. (2003). *Health Guide for America's Teens.* Available: http://www.adolescenthealth.org/Health_Guide_for_Americas_Teens.pdf [February 5, 2008].

Spoth, R. L., Redmond, C., and Shin, C. (2001). Randomized trial of brief family interventions for general populations: Adolescent substance use outcomes 4 years following baseline. *Journal of Consulting and Clinical Psychology, 69*, 627–642.

Spoth, R. L., Redmond, C., Trudeau, L., and Shin, C. (2002). Longitudinal substance initiation outcomes for a universal preventive intervention combining family and school programs. *Psychology of Addictive Behaviors, 16*, 129–134.

Sulzbacher, S., Vallin, T., and Waetzig, E. Z. (2006). Telepsychiatry improves paediatric behavioral health care in rural communities. *Journal of Telemedicine and Telecare, 12*, 285–288.

Taubman, M. A., and Nash, D. A. (2006). The scientific and public-health imperative for a vaccine against dental caries. *Nature Reviews Immunology, 6*, 555–563.

U.S. Department of Health and Human Services. (2000). *Healthy People 2010* (2nd Ed.). Washington, DC: U.S. Government Printing Office.

U.S. Department of Health and Human Services. (2007). *21 Critical Health Objectives for Adolescents and Young Adults.* Available: http://www.cdc.gov/HealthyYouth/AdolescentHealth/NationalInitiative/pdf/21objectives.pdf [October 17, 2007].

U.S. Food and Drug Administration. (2007). *Medication Guide: Antidepressant Medicines, Depression and other Serious Mental Illnesses, and Suicidal Thoughts or Actions.* Available: http://www.fda.gov/cder/drug/antidepressants/antidepressants_MG_2007.pdf [January 31, 2008].

U.S. Preventive Task Force and Agency for Healthcare Research and Quality. (2004). *Screening for Family and Intimate Partner Violence.* Available: http://www.ahrq.gov/clinic/uspstf/uspsfamv.htm [May 27, 2008].

U.S. Preventive Task Force and Agency for Healthcare Research and Quality. (2007). *Screening for Chlamydial Infection*. Available: http://www.ahrq.gov/clinic/uspstf/uspschlm.htm [May 27, 2008].

Van Amstel, L. L., Lafleur, D. L., and Blake, K. (2004). Raising our HEADSS: Adolescent psychosocial documentation in the emergency room. *Academy of Emergency Medicine, 11*, 648–655.

Wentzel, K. R. (1991). Relations between social competence and academic achievement in early adolescence. *Child Development, 62*, 1066–1078.

Williams, J., Shore, S. E., and Foy, J. M. (2006). Co-location of mental health professionals in primary care settings: Three North Carolina models. *Clinical Pediatrics, 45*, 537–543.

Wissow, L. S., Gadomski, A., Roter, D., Larson, S., Brown, J., Zachary, C., Bartlett, E., Horn, I., Luo, X., and Wang, M. C. (2008). Improving child and parent mental health in primary care: A cluster-randomized trial of communication skills training. *Pediatrics, 121*, 266–275.

Young, T. L., and Ireson, C. (2003). Effectiveness of school-based telehealth care in urban and rural elementary schools. *Pediatrics, 112*, 1088–1094.

Zito, J. M., Safer, D. J., dosReis, S., Magder, L. S., Gardner, J. F., and Zarin, D. A. (1999). Psychotherapeutic medication patterns for youths with attention-deficit/hyperactivity disorder. *Archives of Pediatric and Adolescent Medicine, 153*, 1257–1263.

5

Preparing a Workforce to Meet the Health Needs of Adolescents

SUMMARY

- The current professional adolescent health care workforce is multidisciplinary.
- Existing adolescent health care training across disciplines fails to address many of the health needs of adolescents.
- The licensing, certification, and accreditation of programs for health care providers in disciplines and specialties that may serve adolescents are minimal, inconsistent, and insufficient in their inclusion of adolescent health content and competencies.
- Current adolescent health care training programs, including those that are high quality and interdisciplinary, are insufficient in number to prepare postgraduate health care professionals for roles in the academic sector.
- A few innovative discipline-specific and interdisciplinary adolescent health care training programs have been instrumental in defining curricular content, clinical practicums, and effective teaching modalities.

Adolescents are best served by providers with an understanding of their key developmental features and health issues. In short, *skills matter*. Therefore, critical to improving the health of adolescents in the United States is having a workforce prepared to address the complex needs of this age group. As Henry Kempe stated at the 1976 opening meeting of the Task Force on Pediatric Education, "All who care about children must care deeply about the education of those who provide their health services" (Cohen, 1984, p. 791). Education of the workforce is essential to the provision of health services for adolescents that are accessible, acceptable, appropriate, effective, and equitable in accordance with the framework set forth in Chapter 3. This chapter focuses on the contextual characteristic of provider skills and examines issues related to the adolescent health workforce.

At all levels of professional education, providers in all disciplines serving adolescents need to be equipped to work effectively with this age group. They must be attuned to the nature of adolescents' health problems, as well as have in their clinical repertoire a range of effective strategies for risk assessment, disease prevention, care coordination, treatment, and health promotion. Current evidence, some of which is presented in this chapter, suggests this is currently not the case—that is, the skills of many providers working with adolescents are inadequate. Whether providers report on their own perceptions of their competencies or adolescents describe the health services they have received, data reveal significant gaps in achieving the goal of a well-equipped workforce ready to meet the health needs of adolescents. In other words, too few health care providers in practice feel prepared to work with adolescents, even with regard to some of the most common health problems in this population, and the quality of services being provided has suffered as a result. Given the adolescent health issues and health service needs presented in Chapters 2, 3, and 4, an important goal for the training of health care providers is for all those who will offer health services for adolescents in their practices to enter the workforce equipped to work effectively with this age group.

This chapter begins by reviewing the composition of the current workforce providing adolescent health care services. It then examines gaps in the training of these providers and means that can be used to ensure their competence. The discussion turns next to some current models for training that show promise for imparting the knowledge and skills that need to be mastered by those who work with adolescents. Beyond basic-level training (i.e., educational programs for entry into a profession), specialists, educators, and scholars require advanced-level training that will prepare them to teach others entering the workforce and equip them to conduct research that will expand the evidence base supporting adolescent health care practice. The discussion therefore includes strategies for ensuring the training of adequate numbers of advanced-level adolescent specialists, educators, and scholars. The chapter then reviews challenges to training an adequate adolescent health care workforce. It should be noted that this chapter was not intended as a comprehensive review of education, training, and certification in the adolescent life stage for all health professionals (or the lack there of); rather, the focus is on the most important gaps and challenges in the preparation of the adolescent health workforce and current models that show promise in ensuring competency for these providers.

Advancing the competency and size of the adolescent health care workforce involves two critical questions. First, how can all levels of training in adolescent health—and in all pertinent disciplines—be of high quality? Second, what means can be used to expand the number of adolescent health specialists, educators, and scholars with the advanced teaching, leadership, and research skills necessary to work effectively in the salient educational and research settings?

COMPOSITION OF THE CURRENT WORKFORCE PROVIDING ADOLESCENT HEALTH SERVICES

The uniqueness of adolescent health problems—their social and behavioral origins, their developmental nature, and the multisystem needs involved—demands a multidisciplinary workforce. As articulated at the 1986 Health Futures of Youth conference, which created a 10-year agenda for protecting and promoting the health of adolescents, no one discipline has garnered the requisite knowledge and skills to address the complex health problems of this population (Blum and Smith, 1988). The array of health and social service providers that may be called upon to work with adolescents extends beyond dentists, physicians, nurses, nutritionists, psychologists, physician assistants, and social workers. Likewise, the requisite expertise and specialization reach well beyond pediatrics, family medicine, or other foci. Given the contexts in which adolescents live and the social nature of their health problems, the roles of those who work in juvenile justice, school health, mental health, reproductive health, substance use, and primary and secondary educational systems should be considered (Blum and Smith, 1988). Adolescents also seek out other specialists in the health care delivery system, such as dermatologists, chiropractors, and practitioners of alternative therapy. Moreover, the social nature of adolescent issues that are often embedded in multiple systems (family, school, community) means that public health interventions and case management (i.e., working within and across systems) play a key role in promoting the health of adolescents. Box 5-1 provides a comprehensive listing of the many types of providers considered part of the adolescent health care workforce.

It is essential to recognize that the diversity of the adolescent health care workforce extends beyond discipline or specialty. Cultural, racial, ethnic, socioeconomic, and geographic diversity are important as well, particularly with respect to reducing the disparities evident in a variety of health indica-

> **BOX 5-1**
> **Providers Involved in Health Care for Adolescents**
>
> **Professional and Related Occupations**
> - Chiropractors
> - Clinical laboratory technologists and technicians
> - Counselors
> - Dental hygienists
> - Dentists
> - Diagnostic-related technologists and technicians
> - Dieticians and nutritionists
> - Emergency medical technicians and paramedics
> - Health educators
> - Licensed practical and vocational nurses
> - Medical records and health information technicians
> - Optometrists
> - Pharmacists
> - Physician assistants
> - Physicians and surgeons
> - Podiatrists
> - Psychologists
> - Registered nurses
> - Social and human service assistants
> - Social workers
> - Speech–language pathologists
> - Support technicians for health diagnosing and treating practitioners
> - Therapists
>
> **Service Occupations**
> - Dental assistants
> - Home health aides
> - Medical assistants
> - Nursing aides, orderlies, and attendants
> - Personal and home care aides
> - Occupational therapists, assistants, and aides
> - Physical therapists, assistants, and aides
> - Receptionists and information clerks
>
> SOURCE: Bureau of Labor Statistics and U.S. Department of Labor (2007).

tors (e.g., rates of pregnancy, suicide, homicide, and substance use) among various subpopulations of adolescents, as described in Chapter 2.

Each discipline has differing pathways and levels at which basic education, specialization, and continuing education may and can occur. A half-century ago, pediatric medicine set the pace for creating a focus in the field of adolescent health. Considered the father of adolescent medicine, J. Roswell Gallagher first articulated the need for adolescent medicine as a subspecialty in pediatrics (Emans et al., 1998; Gallagher, 1957). Two decades later, in 1978, a taskforce of the American Academy of Pediatrics recommended that pediatric training in medicine take full responsibility for improving adolescent health services, stating, "The health needs of adolescents are being inadequately met" (Task Force on Pediatric Education, 1978, p. ix). Since then, the inadequacy of professional education in adolescent health has been the subject of increased attention among a number of other disciplines interacting with or specializing in health services for adolescents (Blum and Smith, 1988; Farrow and Saewyc, 2002). Critical questions have been raised regarding the adequacy of existing training programs, the articulation and inclusion of core competencies in adolescent health, and appropriate levels of expectations and requirements set by regulatory bodies (for licensure, certification, accreditation, and maintenance of licensure or certification) to ensure the adequacy of training at the individual and institutional levels (Blum and Smith, 1988).

This increased attention to adolescent health needs has prompted some positive developments. For example, the American Academy of Pediatric Dentistry first responded in 1986 by adopting adolescent-specific guidelines (American Academy of Pediatric Dentistry, 2005). With the stimulation of federal support through the Partnership in Program Planning for Adolescent Health (PIPPAH),[1] these guidelines were expanded in 2005 to include consideration of youth development, psychosocial concerns, eating disorders, and the transition to adult health services. Nonetheless, dentistry, like other disciplines outside of medicine, has yet to establish a substantive focus on workforce training that meets the specific needs of adolescents. PIPPAH goals such as promoting awareness about adolescent oral health within dentistry and integrating oral health with other professions' care for adolescents require adequate training of new oral health professionals. Yet there are currently no accreditation standards, nationally recognized curricula, faculty development guides, targeted web resources, texts, or other supporting materials for the training of general or pediatric dentists specifically in the care of this age group.

To meet the national need for providers equipped to work with adolescents, many more such providers will need to enter the workforce over the next decade. For example, considering just pediatricians who are certified in adolescent medicine, there is on average a ratio of 1 adolescent medicine

---

[1] Partnership in Program Planning for Adolescent Health: https://grants.hrsa.gov/webExternal/FundingOppDetails.asp?FundingCycleId=FC9AE007-1379-438E-8C70-2C29C340CE3A&ViewMode=EU&GoBack=&PrintMode=&OnlineAvailabilityFlag=&pageNumber=&version=&NC=&Popup.

physician to 105,000 adolescents in the United States. Seven states presently have no certified adolescent medicine specialists available. The current ratio is in dramatic contrast to the American Academy of Pediatrics' recommendation that 1 adolescent medicine specialist have the capacity to care for about 6,000 adolescents. Beyond the field of medicine (i.e., pediatrics, internal medicine, and family medicine), it is impossible to determine the size of today's workforce that specializes in adolescent health because no other discipline offers subspecialty board certification with this specific focus.

As noted above, ensuring a competent workforce for adolescent health care requires multiple levels of expertise, from generalist to educator/scholar. Translated into educational nomenclature, training in adolescent health may be acquired in basic or entry-level professional programs (e.g., M.D. program for physicians, A.D. or B.S.N. for nurses, D.D.S. or D.M.D. for dentists), in graduate school (e.g., master's, practice doctorate, D.Sc., or Ph.D. programs), or in postgraduate programs. Moreover, skills need to be maintained for the duration of professional practice through in service programs, certification courses, and continuing education offerings.

Using medicine as an example, a recent Institute of Medicine (IOM) report (2007), *Physicians for Public Health Careers,* addresses the training of physicians in that field. The report proposes three levels of providers, based on the breadth and depth of practice with certain population groups, the complexity of health issues being addressed, and the nature of the roles of the provider (e.g., primary care provider versus adolescent health educator). Building on this work of the IOM and that of Denninghoff and colleagues (2002), the committee identified three levels of providers necessary to ensure a qualified adolescent health care workforce:

- *Generalists*—professionals who serve populations that include adolescents and provide health care services for adolescents full- or part-time, even though they are not defined as adolescent health care providers or specialists (e.g., pediatric or family physicians; nurse practitioners; physician assistants; women's health care providers, such as gynecologists and midwives; general and pediatric dentists; psychologists; dieticians; and social workers).
- *Specialists*—professionals specializing in health services for adolescents, whether they do so for their entire career or as a change in specialty/focus at some point (e.g., adolescent or sports medicine specialists, adolescent nursing specialists, child and adolescent psychologists and psychiatrists, orthodontists, youth workers, school nurses). Primary care providers may provide services to adolescents in the capacity of either a generalist or a specialist, as defined above.
- *Educator and/or scholar*—professionals with recognized expertise

in adolescent health care who contribute to educating/training the future workforce of providers of such care and to the research/science of adolescent health services (e.g., academic faculty).

Finding: The current professional adolescent health care workforce is multidisciplinary.

GAPS IN THE TRAINING OF PROVIDERS

The prevailing notion among both health care providers and consumers is that all practitioners who work with adolescents have had the training to do so. Evidence strongly suggests that this is not the case. It has become increasingly clear that meeting this expectation is challenged by the complexities of adolescents' health needs and the U.S. health care system that delivers services to meet those needs, along with the struggles of educational programs in producing competent professionals with the required knowledge and skills. Identifying the gaps between providers' knowledge and skills and adolescents' health needs and standards for health care services that can meet those needs is essential if corrective action is to be taken.

Two sources of evidence point to the limitations and inadequacies of current training in adolescent health care: (1) surveys of health care providers' self-perceived competencies, and (2) evaluations of services provided, using, for example, chart reviews or patient reports.

Self-Perceived Inadequacies in Training

Health care providers' self-assessments of their competencies offer evidence of the limitations and inadequacies of their current training. Multiple disciplines have conducted surveys of graduates and professionals practicing in the field of adolescent health to determine their self-perceived competencies in meeting the physical, mental, and social health service needs of adolescents. Some of these surveys have been specific to certain disciplines, such as medicine (Biro et al., 1993; Blum, 1987; Cull et al., 2003; Emans et al., 1998; Klitsner et al., 1992; Korczak, MacArthur, and Katzman, 2006; Krol, 2004), nursing (Bearinger et al., 1992; Nerdahl et al., 1999; Saewyc et al., 2006), and nutrition (Hughes, 2003; Story et al., 2000). Others have examined competencies across multiple disciplines (Blum and Smith, 1988; Hellerstedt et al., 2000; Story et al., 2002). Some have encompassed child specialists, including pediatricians. On the other hand, some disciplines have yet to assess student and trainee preparation or self-perceived competencies specifically in adolescent care. For example, the American Dental Education Association's annual survey of graduating students queries senior students on their self-perceived preparation regarding 25 domains of practice, but does not distinguish adolescents from children. Nonetheless, the responses to this survey give some sense of how graduates perceive their competency in meeting the needs of adolescents: each year approximately 10 percent of respondents report that they are less than prepared in the field of pediatric dentistry (which includes routine care of adolescents), and slightly more than half report that they are unprepared to deliver orthodontic services (which are provided most frequently to adolescents) (Chmar et al., 2007; Weaver, Haden, and Valachovic, 2002a,b, 2004; Weaver et al., 2005). There is a similar lack of information on how other child specialists (e.g., child psychologists and psychiatrists) perceive their competency with particular respect to adolescent health needs. Further detailed investigation into the adequacy of the training of child specialists in relation to adolescent health is needed.

Generally, surveys aimed at determining self-perceived competencies in adolescent health solicit self-reports from respondents drawn from the rosters of professional organizations whose members are likely to have had adolescents in their practice populations (e.g., the American Academy of Pediatrics, National Association of Pediatric Nurse Practitioners, American Dietetic Association, American School Health Association). Respondents to these surveys typically are asked to identify their self-perceived levels of competency in dealing with a host of common adolescent health problems. In addition, they are often asked about the frequency with which they observe these problems in their practice, as well as their interest in further education in the area.

Although the topics or health issues included in these self-report surveys vary somewhat by discipline, common themes emerge. Frequently self-assessed areas of inadequacy include oral health (Krol, 2004), sexual and reproductive health (Hellerstedt et al., 2000; Klitsner et al., 1992), eating and weight problems, psychological problems, substance use (Klitsner et al., 1992; Story et al., 2000, 2002), sports medicine, violence, and psychological assessment (Emans et al., 1998). To take one disciplinary example (Saewyc et al., 2006), more than 25 percent of 520 nurses who reported working with adolescents identified low levels of knowledge/skills in 14 of 28 common health issues among adolescents, including depression, eating disorders, and violence; more than half reported low levels of knowledge of issues affecting more vulnerable populations—those who are in the foster care system, homeless, or gang-affiliated. Nurses' self-perceived competence in working with lesbian, gay, bisexual, and transgender[2] (LGBT) adoles-

---

[2]The group referred to as "lesbian, gay, bisexual, and transgender" sometimes also encompasses the term "questioning" and is commonly referred to by the acronym LGBT (or GLBT) or LGBTQ (or GLBTQ). For the purposes of this report, the identifier "lesbian, gay, bisexual, and transgender" or LGBT is used.

cents had not improved over a decade (Bearinger et al., 1992), and comfort in counseling about pregnancy options had declined.

Evaluation of Services Provided

The development of standards or guidelines for the delivery of adolescent health services makes it possible both to assess the gaps between what is expected and what is observed in the provision of such services and to take appropriate corrective action (typically through training). Several standards or guidelines for the delivery of child and adolescent health services are available to practitioners. Examples include *Bright Futures: Guidelines for Health Supervision of Infants, Children and Adolescents* (Green, 1994), produced by the Maternal and Child Health Bureau within the Health Resources and Services Administration, Department of Health and Human Services (DHHS); the American Academy of Pediatrics' *Health Supervision Guidelines* (Stein, 1997); *The Clinician's Handbook of Preventive Services* (U.S. Department of Health and Human Services, 1994); the *Guide to Clinical Preventive Services*, developed by the U.S. Preventive Services Task Force (1996); the *Clinical Guideline on Adolescent Oral Health Care* of the American Academy of Pediatric Dentistry (2005); and the American Medical Association's Guidelines for Adolescent Preventive Services (GAPS) (Elster and Kuznets, 1994).

Since the mid-1990s, a number of studies have examined the extent to which such standards and guidelines for adolescent health care have been adopted and put into routine use. The most widely evaluated have been GAPS, whose implementation has been assessed in managed care and other group practice arrangements, as well individual private practices. On the basis of physician self-report surveys, Ozer and colleagues (1998) concluded that managed care settings were more conducive than other practice arrangements to systematic and widespread implementation of GAPS, although routine incorporation of the guidelines still fell below expected thresholds even in those settings. Klein and colleagues (2001) assessed the implementation of GAPS in community and migrant health centers, using practitioner and adolescent reports as well as chart reviews. They found that system-level policies were instrumental in the adoption of practice standards for adolescent health services, facilitated by provider training, resource materials, and administrative reinforcement. Despite these successful mechanisms, however, provision of preventive services to adolescents still fell short of the guidelines, particularly in psychosocial and behavioral areas. Using chart reviews to assess providers' adherence to the GAPS recommendations for comprehensive psychosocial assessment of adolescents, Blum and colleagues (1996) derived similar findings. Providers with high levels of experience in adolescent health who were working in adolescent-focused community clinics incorporated the greatest number of prescribed screening questions into their protocols. Adherence to the recommended guidelines for preventive services corresponded to the extent of training in adolescent health (e.g., through fellowship programs). In contrast, those in private practice who served clients of all ages (who were also less likely to have received specialized adolescent health training) were the least likely to use the GAPS protocols, particularly in addressing adolescents' psychosocial health issues and concerns.

Finding: Existing adolescent health care training across disciplines fails to address many of the health needs of adolescents.

MEANS OF ENSURING THE COMPETENCE OF THE WORKFORCE

Multiple sources of evidence pointing to deficits in knowledge and skills among the workforce serving adolescents raise the question of what competencies are necessary to provide quality health services for adolescents, and of these, which are common across disciplines and unique to particular disciplines. In 2004, Hoge and colleagues published a summary of stakeholder consensus on recommended best practices for improving workforce education, in this case specific to behavioral rather than adolescent health. The first of 16 recommendations posits that "education and training is competency-based" (Hoge et al., 2004, p. 94).

Essential knowledge and skills in adolescent health are key to developing providers' abilities to deliver quality health care services to this age group. Practitioners are expected to synthesize developmental theories and interdisciplinary knowledge about adolescent health with discipline-specific research and wisdom regarding practice in the delivery of health care services. Moreover, the breadth of biopsychosocial knowledge required to provide effective care for adolescents continues to expand at a rapid pace. Beyond knowledge and skills for direct service delivery, each provider needs to acquire skills for collaboration with an interdisciplinary team that typically functions within a complex, multifaceted health care delivery system.

Requisite knowledge and skills, or competencies, serve as guideposts for designing and ensuring adequate training and continual education for all health professionals. In the context of the present discussion, competencies are tangible criteria that have four primary purposes: (1) defining scope of practice, (2) providing guidance for curricular development and evaluation of learner outcomes, (3) establishing standards by which an individual's acquisition of knowledge and skills can be assessed (e.g., for purposes of licensure or credentialing) and the quality of an educational institution can be measured (for purposes of accreditation) (Astroth, Garza, and Taylor, 2004), and (4) serving as a standard against which the quality of clinical services can be compared (i.e., whether the services provided reflect specific competencies of the provider) (Blum et al., 1996). Some of the literature on competencies (particularly in the areas of youth development, behavioral health, and child/adolescent psychiatry) examines the usefulness of and need for competencies in defining scope of practice and guiding the entry-level training required for employment or certification in certain disciplines and specialties.

Competencies are typically categorized into broad areas or domains considered fundamentally necessary for providers who, in the present context, deliver care to adolescents. Within each competency domain, expectations for knowledge and skill acquisition differ according to the discipline and level of the professional (i.e., generalist, specialist, educator/scholar). In terms of curricular development, the teaching of competencies can be ordered such that each level builds on the knowledge and skills learned previously. The continual assessment of competencies acquired can serve as a measure of learning and readiness for practice.

Many competencies in adolescent health cut across all or most disciplines, whereas others vary in accordance with a specific disciplinary perspective or scope of practice, being tailored to certain roles or types of providers (Astroth, Garza, and Taylor, 2004; Beresin and Mellman, 2002; Denninghoff et al., 2002; Hoge, Huey, and O'Connell, 2004; Hoge et al., 2002; Shelton, 2003). At the 1986 Health Future of Youth conference, the *Study Group Report on Training of Health Professions in Adolescent Health Care* defined five broad components of entry-level training considered to be "baseline knowledge, skills and attitudes necessary for all who work with youth" (Blum and Smith, 1988, p. 46S): (1) growth and development, (2) psychological and physical morbidities, (3) communications and problem solving, (4) community services, and (5) attitudes. While each of these components might be applicable across the life span, the study group described special concerns for each within the context of adolescents and their environments.

Training at the specialist level prepares professionals for leadership roles, particularly in education and clinical services focused primarily on adolescents. Specialist training builds on the core knowledge and skills defined for entry-level professionals. The Health Future study group's report briefly outlined priorities for specialist training, but only for five disciplines: medicine, nursing, nutrition, psychology, and social work (Blum and Smith, 1988). Since the publication of that report, only one discipline/specialty—pediatrics—has identified elements of curriculum required for board certification in an adolescent medicine subspecialty. Some disciplines have worked toward specific standards for practice. For example, standards for pediatric nursing are currently being developed jointly by the Society for Pediatric Nursing and the National Association of Pediatric Nurse Practitioners (personal communication with the American Academy of Nursing's Expert Panel for Child, Adolescent, and Family Nursing, November 10, 2007). Overall, however, there continues to be a lack of clarity and consistency regarding the requisite knowledge and skills that make up competencies in adolescent health within each discipline and at various provider levels (generalist, specialist, and educator/scholar).

Areas or domains of competency common across disciplines reflect the behavioral and contextual characteristics presented in Chapter 1 and discussed throughout this report. For example, health and health behavior need to be understood within pertinent social contexts (*context matters*); segments of the adolescent population have unique health needs (*need matters*); and adolescence is characterized by significant and dramatic developmental changes (*development matters*). Other domains of competency applicable to all disciplines relate more to the delivery of services, paralleling the underlying assumptions that families are partners in adolescents' health and their use of health services (*family matters*); that achieving optimal health for adolescents requires public health interventions involving integration and coordination of individual- and population-focused services (*community matters*); and that the availability, nature, and content of health services for adolescents are profoundly affected by financing systems and related policies (*money matters*, and *policy matters*). With respect to financing, currently only one federal agency in the United States—the Maternal and Child Health Bureau within DHHS—offers training grants focused solely on adolescent health. Annually, it commits $2.64 million to the support of seven interdisciplinary Leadership Education in Adolescent Health (LEAH) programs housed in seven universities nationwide (described below). Given that there are almost 42 million adolescents aged 10–19 in the United States (U.S. Census Bureau, 2006), this means that each year the federal government invests approximately 6 cents per adolescent in training specialists and educators/scholars in the skills required to teach tomorrow's adolescent health care providers.

In summary, the extant literature, though quite limited, describes domains of competency that vary by discipline. Some competencies relate specifically to the health and service needs of adolescents, while others focus more on the delivery of services within interdisciplinary health care settings and on larger contextual issues. Greater consistency is needed in the delineation of domains of competency, and greater clarity is needed regarding required competencies at the various levels of training. Meeting these needs is the next step in ensuring an adequate workforce trained to meet the health needs of adolescents.

Finding: The licensing, certification, and accreditation of programs for health care providers in disciplines and specialties that may serve adolescents are minimal, inconsistent, and insufficient in their inclusion of adolescent health content and competencies.

CURRENT MODELS FOR TRAINING SPECIALISTS AND EDUCATORS/SCHOLARS

Nearly three decades ago, leaders in the field of adolescent health, using a variety of models and strategies, began making concerted efforts to expand and improve professional training for those who might eventually work with adolescents. Models for such training, as well as curricular emphases and teaching modalities, vary according to the range of competencies delineated above. Beyond the competencies that need to be taught in basic educational programs for all those entering a health profession (e.g., B.S.N. for nursing, M.P.A. and M.D. for medicine, D.D.S. and D.M.D. for dentistry, Ph.D. for psychology), models for adolescent health training range from formal 1- to 5-year advanced degree programs (e.g., M.S., M.A., M.S.W., Ph.D.) to postgraduate subspecialty fellowship programs. Additionally, once these competencies have been incorporated into the core requirements in basic and specialty programs, they must continue to be assessed in an ongoing, reinforcing manner through recertification or maintenance-of-certification programs.

Models for Formal Training Programs

Interdisciplinary Adolescent Health Programs

In 1977 the Maternal and Child Health Bureau began funding the interdisciplinary LEAH programs with the specific goal of preparing leaders in the field of adolescent health. The intent was to create a cadre of adolescent health specialists and educators/scholars who in turn would advance clinical practice, research, and the training of an expanded workforce by assuming leadership roles in the academic and public health sectors. The seven programs funded initially were required to include five disciplines in their leadership training: medicine, nursing, nutrition, psychology, and social work. Typically, only one new fellow in each discipline matriculates in each of 5 years in each of the seven programs. Of the major health disciplines discussed throughout this report, only dentistry is excluded from the programs. The intensity and duration of training within each program vary by discipline, ranging from several months to 3 years (required for a pediatric subspecialty in adolescent medicine). Fellows are expected to advance their knowledge and skills in clinical care of adolescents while developing their research and teaching capacity for work in the field of adolescent health.

Since the mid-1970s, the LEAH programs have competed every 5 years for new awards that support faculty and fellows across the five disciplines. Today support continues for training in the five disciplines in each of the seven funded programs. The funding level for each program has remained almost stationary over the 30-year period, with an annual total of $2,640,000 being dedicated to support for the seven programs.

As noted above, the LEAH programs are the only educational programs supported by federal funds specifically targeting adolescent health. In addition, a few other interdisciplinary training programs for various specialties and educator/scholar levels focused on adolescent health are supported by federal funds, although these funds do not target adolescent health training. For example, the Centers for Disease Control and Prevention (CDC) currently supports Prevention Research Centers (PRCs) housed in schools of medicine and public health nationwide. However, only 6 of the 33 currently funded PRCs emphasize adolescent-related issues in their research and training; only one to two research fellows are in training in each of these 6 programs. Moreover, PRC training is not clinically focused.

Likewise, 3 years ago CDC launched an initiative focused on health protection research. Although the request for proposals for this CDC initiative did not target adolescent health, one of the three funded programs (at the University of Minnesota School of Nursing) has this emphasis. Currently, 18 pre- and postdoctoral trainees in medicine, nursing, nutrition, and psychology receive support from this CDC-funded program.

Discipline-Specific Programs and Certification for Specialists and Educators/Scholars

Single-discipline training programs far outnumber interdisciplinary programs in adolescent health. Adolescent medicine is not a primary discipline like, for example, pediatrics; therefore, options include adolescent medicine subspecialties in pediatric, family, and internal medicine, as well as master's and clinical and research doctorates focused on adolescent health in the areas of nutrition, nursing, psychology, public health, and social work, to name but a few. Unquestionably, medicine has led the other disciplines in defining training requirements and establishing a certification process for adolescent health care.

Postresidency fellowship programs for those subspecializing in adolescent medicine Training programs in adolescent medicine for physicians were established in the 1960s. These programs require training in comprehensive inpatient and outpatient services while also encompassing psychosocial competencies.

Postgraduate fellowship training in adolescent medicine follows completion of an accredited residency in pediatrics, internal medicine, or family medicine. The required length of the training varies by specialty: 2 years for internal and family medicine and 3 years for pediatrics. After completion of an accredited fellowship program, a board certification exam must be taken and passed. In addition, the American Board of Pediatrics requires all subspecialty candidates to show evidence of scholarly achievement. The first certification exam in adolescent medicine in pediatrics was administered in 1994, and yielded 209 board-certified pediatricians with a subspecialty in adolescent medicine; today more than 500 pediatricians have been certified in this subspecialty (Althouse and Stockman, 2007). According to the American Board of Medical Specialties, 170 certificates in adolescent medicine were issued from 1996 to 2006 in internal medicine (39) and family medicine (131) (American Board of Medical Specialties, 2007). Together, then, approximately 700 pediatricians and internal and family medicine physicians have been certified in adolescent medicine. The first 16 fellowship programs for a subspecialty in adolescent medicine were accredited in 1998 by the Accreditation Council on Graduate Medical Education; currently there are 26 such accredited programs nationwide.

Limited data exist on the characteristics of physicians who are board-certified in adolescent medicine, yet several trends warrant noting. According to the American Board of Pediatrics, the American Board of Family Medicine, and the American Board of Internal Medicine, from 2004 to 2005 the number of pediatrician, family medicine physician, and internal medicine physician fellows in adolescent medicine (i.e., pursuing subspecialty certification) decreased by 10 percent, from 74 to 66. In 2006, 66 pediatricians, family medicine physicians, and internal medicine physicians enrolled in an adolescent medicine fellowship; only 17 percent were male. Just as pediatrics in general has seen an increase in the proportion of women entering the field, the proportion of females in training for a subspecialty in adolescent medicine has increased to a high of 83 percent; the reasons for this change remain unclear (Althouse and Stockman, 2007). Particularly concerning is the lack of interest in the adolescent medicine subspecialty among pediatricians. In 2005, of 866 first-time candidates applying for the general pediatrics examination who indicated an interest in one of the 16 subspecialty areas offered by the American Board of Pediatrics, only 1.4 percent cited adolescent medicine, which was fifteenth among the 16 subspecialties (ahead only of medical toxicology) (Althouse and Stockman, 2007).

Master's or doctoral degrees focused on adolescent health The level at which various disciplines in fields other than medicine specialize, in this case in adolescent health, varies. Specialization typically occurs in master's or doctoral programs. Such is the case, for example, in nursing, nutrition, psychology, and social work. Just as in medicine, providers who seek a focus in adolescent health are likely to be drawn from the child, family, adult, and public health arenas. University programs offering degrees with an emphasis or major in related areas such as these likely offer a set of courses that focus on various content related to adolescent health. Practicum options provide opportunities for a variety of clinical experiences with adolescents, including those in public health settings. Although there are no uniform requirements or competencies for such training as there are for fellowships in adolescent medicine, adolescent health courses generally include content covering some or all of the competencies identified above.

In contrast to the defined criteria for board certification in the subspecialty of adolescent medicine for physicians (e.g., length and content of fellowship training, adolescent medicine exam), such a set of requirements has been articulated for no other discipline except psychology. To receive board certification as a clinical child and adolescent psychologist, one must obtain a doctoral degree from an accredited program, be licensed or certified for independent practice as a psychologist, and complete a specialty training program accredited by the American Psychological Association. All eligible psychologists also must have completed an approved internship and 1 year of supervised practice, with an additional year of work focused primarily on children and adolescents, or have completed a postdoctoral residency program in clinical child and adolescent psychology. The Academy of Clinical Child and Adolescent Psychology is a member of the American Board of Professional Psychology, which has a 60-year history of overseeing standards and processes for certification.[3]

Continuing education The competencies that are incorporated into the core requirements and certification in basic and specialty programs may continue to be assessed in an ongoing, reinforcing manner through recertification or maintenance-of-certification programs. For example, members of the American Board of Medical Specialties have established core requirements to monitor and maintain necessary competencies for specialty medical certification, called Maintenance of Certification™ (Miller, 2005).

Summary Certification criteria set by boards of professional academies for the disciplines of both medicine and psychology provide standards for

---
[3] See http://www.clinicalchildpsychology.net/27610/index.html.

training that have been instrumental in defining curricular content, clinical practicums for educational programs, and continuing education that prepare specialists or educators/scholars in the field of adolescent health. Although some other disciplines offer options for specializing in adolescent health, the lack of certification for providers and accreditation at the programmatic level means there is no uniformity in curricular expectations and offerings across programs for this specialty. Articulating sets of competencies tailored to each discipline and offering accreditation (at the institutional level) and certification (at the individual level) would lead to consistency of training in adolescent health among disciplines, and could be instrumental in ensuring an adequate workforce of specialists and educators/scholars prepared to teach others and conduct research to inform practice in the field.

Innovative Strategies for Training in Adolescent Health

Several innovative teaching strategies can contribute to ensuring a competent adolescent health workforce. Some of these strategies are aimed at directly improving clinical practice through either hands-on training or distance learning, while others are designed to equip educators/trainers with up-to-date content and effective teaching approaches. Some examples are described in this section.

One strategy involves using adolescents as simulated patients to teach health care providers across multiple disciplines and at various levels (e.g., medicine and nursing students, medical residents, nurse practitioners, pharmacy students). For example, Brown and colleagues (2005) piloted a program, designed for residents and medical students, aimed at developing skills in the core competency of communication related specifically to mental health issues. The program consisted of lectures followed by practice sessions using adolescents as simulated patients. Those in training, as well as the simulated patients, reacted positively to the experience, concluding that it was an effective approach for teaching interviewing skills to address even complex patient issues. Hardoff and Schonmann (2001) likewise recommended the use of adolescents as simulated patients, employing role-play exercises to develop communication skills. Those who have implemented training using adolescent simulated patients advise that faculty collaborate with high schools and college units having drama departments to identify adolescent actors (Schultz and Marks, 2007).

The availability of online, Internet-based train-the-trainer programs has significantly increased the likelihood that teachers and faculty will be better equipped to teach clinicians in adolescent health. Online resources also make it possible to reach more diverse and geographically dispersed groups of providers who work with adolescents. A group consisting primarily of physicians, representing 11 European countries and under the direction of Pierre-Andre Michaud, an adolescent medicine specialist from the University of Lausanne, Switzerland, designed an easy-to-use, up-to-date curriculum, including content, teaching strategies, tools for educators/trainers, and evaluation methods (Michaud et al., 2004). Called EuTEACH (European Training in Effective Care and Health), this online resource is a flexible curriculum with 17 thematic modules on topics ranging from adolescent development to youth advocacy.[4]

In the United States, Lawrence Neinstein, a physician who has authored a leading textbook on adolescent health, created an online curriculum each section of which includes background, cases, questions and answers, and web links, plus references. The curriculum is designed for both teachers and service providers.[5] Intended as a source of supplemental instruction, the interactive website, while not exhaustive, addresses common adolescent health topics including puberty, communication, confidentiality, sexuality, medical problems, dermatology, eating disorders, and substance use.

The National Adolescent Health Information Center (NAHIC), located at the University of California, San Francisco, offers another online resource.[6] Guided by a team of nationally renowned adolescent health researchers and with funding from the Maternal and Child Health Bureau, NAHIC offers a variety of resources and tools for adolescent health care providers and educators/scholars, including fact sheets, reports synthesizing research data, and guides for program development. It also includes a broad range of curriculum tools, including a sample syllabus that can be adapted for different disciplines and courses, recommended reading materials, data sources, suggested assignments, case studies, links to other useful resources, and sample presentations. Examples of unit topics include violence, mental health and suicide, sexuality/teen pregnancy/sexually transmitted infections, and community interventions.

The Rocky Mountain Public Health Education Consortium (RMPHEC)[7] is another source for adolescent health training curriculum. RMPHEC's mission is to improve the health status of and eliminate health disparities among women, children, and families, including those with special health needs. An online course on adolescent health is provided to increase the knowledge, skills, and capacity of public health professionals, paraprofessionals, organizations, and systems in the Rocky Mountain and surrounding states and tribes within the region.

---

[4] See http://www.euteach.com.
[5] See http://www.usc.edu/student-affairs/Health_Center/adolhealth.
[6] See http://nahic.ucsf.edu.
[7] See http://services.tacc.utah.edu/rmphec/index.asp.

Pediatrics in Practice[8] offers online continuing medical education courses based on the American Academy of Pediatrics' guidelines for providing health supervision of infants, children, and adolescents (Green and Palfrey, 2002). The program, called Bright Futures, includes courses focused on health promotion and faculty development. Interactive health promotion modules cover such topics as health, partnership, communication, education, and cultural competency, while teaching modules impart strategies designed to enhance instruction in the health promotion curriculum.

Finally, in 1996 the Office of Adolescent Health within the Maternal and Child Health Bureau launched PIPPAH, a collaborative of adolescent-related professional associations whose scope includes adolescents and their families. Partnering organizations include the American Academy of Pediatrics, the American College of Prevention Medicine, the American Bar Association, CityMatCH, the Healthy Teen Network, the National Association of County and City Health Officials, the National Conference on State Legislatures, and the National Institute for Health Care Management. PIPPAH is dedicated to improving the health of adolescents through system-level strategic organization, program development, and collaboration. One mission of this initiative is the training of health care providers through the creation of online toolkits, policy briefs, tip sheets, and a listing of recommended resources.[9] An example of a product resulting from this initiative is the continuing education online course available through the American Nurses Association.[10]

Findings:

- *Current adolescent health care training programs, including those that are high quality and interdisciplinary, are insufficient in number to prepare postgraduate health care professionals for roles in the academic sector.*
- *A few innovative discipline-specific and interdisciplinary adolescent health care training programs have been instrumental in defining curricular content, clinical practicums, and effective teaching modalities.*

CHALLENGES TO TRAINING A COMPETENT WORKFORCE

A number of factors impede progress toward ensuring a competent adolescent health workforce. Some come into play at the individual level

---

[8]See http://www.pediatricsinpractice.org.
[9]See http://www.socialworkers.org/pippah/about.asp.
[10]See http://nursingworld.org/mods/archive/mod4/ceah1.htm.

and affect both the number and competencies of providers; others exert their influence at the institutional or systemwide level.

Attitudes and Economics

As noted above, the number of providers seeking a career in adolescent health is inadequate to meet the needs of the adolescent population. Deterrents to entering the field are both attitudinal and economic. Many providers avoid working with adolescents because they are uncomfortable with addressing the complex biopsychosocial issues faced by this age group; this discomfort is attributable primarily to providers' lack of relevant training and preparation (Conard et al., 2003; Golden et al., 2001; Kaslow et al., 2004; Nerdahl et al., 1999; Remschmidt and Belfer, 2005). As for economic disincentives, adolescent health practitioners tend to have among the lowest levels of remuneration across disciplines because so many of their encounters with patients are focused on *process* more than *procedure*, thereby garnering less reimbursement (Golden et al., 2003; Kim and American Academy of Child and Adolescent Psychiatry Task Force on Workforce Needs, 2003; Rickert, 2003). In the case of medicine, as noted above, specialization in adolescent health requires 3 years of additional training following completion of residency (e.g., in pediatrics or family medicine). While the subspecialty certification in adolescent medicine helps to ensure physicians' readiness to address the wide range of health issues confronting adolescents, the postponement of entry into the workforce beyond residency status can serve as a disincentive (Althouse and Stockman, 2007; Jay, 2007).

Educational Priorities

A number of unmet challenges within educational systems make it difficult to ensure competency in adolescent health among providers at all levels—generalist, specialist, and educator/scholar. Educators raise the question of what curricular content can be eliminated to allow for the addition of content on adolescent health. As a result, classroom lectures, textbooks, and overall curricular plans often neglect adolescent health content, instead moving from childhood to adulthood with little attention to the unique concerns and needs of the adolescent population. Coupled with the likelihood that licensure exams will not test in the area of adolescent health and accrediting bodies will not require this competency (with the exception of pediatric medicine and child and adolescent psychology as detailed above), there is little external incentive to shift curriculum to include a strong adolescent health focus.

Inconsistency or Lack of an Adolescent Focus in the Criteria of Regulatory Bodies

Requirements for licensure and certification of health care providers and accreditation of entry-level, graduate, and postgraduate/fellowship programs vary significantly by discipline, state, and governing regulatory body/accreditation council or board. Moreover, requisite levels of education for licensure can range from baccalaureate to doctoral degrees. In nursing, for example, one can take a registered nurse licensure exam after completing a 2-year associate's degree or a 4-year baccalaureate degree. This variation makes it difficult to provide an overall picture of the consistency with which health care providers are expected to be competent in the array of knowledge and skills needed to work with adolescents. For example, in their effort to summarize core competencies for physicians in general and for psychiatric specialists in particular, Beresin and Mellman (2002) identified six national organizations involved in residency education, training, accreditation, and certification that have input on the question of what is essential.

Another example that speaks to the variation in requirements is drawn from the field of counseling for drug and alcohol use and mental health counseling. Kerwin and colleagues (2006) examined state requirements for U.S. providers in these specialties and found two distinct training models. For drug and alcohol counselors, expectations include formal curricular plans; in contrast, an apprentice model guides the training of mental health counselors. Along with these differing training expectations, certification requirements vary from state to state.

As a further example, current dental education accreditation standards require no adolescent-specific content. Adolescents are cited only in a general competency requirement that graduates be prepared to provide dental services appropriate to "the child, adolescent, adult, and geriatric patient" (Commission on Dental Accreditation, 2007, p. 15). Similarly, there are no unique or specific accreditation requirements for specialty training programs in pediatric dentistry that focus on adolescents. Rather, adolescents are expressly included with children in the definition of the specialty and in each of the clinical competency requirements for the target population (Commission on Dental Accreditation, 1998).

SUMMARY

At the individual, institutional, and systemwide levels, certain impediments challenge the ability to ensure an adequately prepared workforce ready to meet the often complex biopsychosocial needs of adolescents. Elsewhere in this report, additional challenges have been discussed. Together, these challenges have a considerable impact on adolescents' access to quality health services, which is determined in part by the competencies of health care providers (as outlined in Chapter 3). Adolescents are best served by those with an understanding of their key developmental features and health issues. The responsibility for adequately equipping health care providers with the essential knowledge and skills needed to work with adolescents rests with educational programs. Yet evidence from providers reporting on their own self-assessed competencies in adolescent health, as well as data gathered from chart reviews and patient reports, reveals that educational programs are falling far short of fulfilling this responsibility. Another goal is to create a critical mass of specialists and educators/scholars in a variety of disciplines who can educate a diverse group of providers to meet the health needs of diverse groups of adolescents. Ensuring an adequate workforce requires the support and sustainment of a specialty in adolescent health that has the potential to produce educators/scholars.

REFERENCES

Althouse, L. A., and Stockman, J. A. (2007). Pediatric workforce: A look at adolescent medicine data from the American Board of Pediatrics. *Journal of Pediatrics, 150,* 100.e2–102.e2.

American Academy of Pediatric Dentistry. (2005). *Guidelines on Adolescent Oral Health Care.* Available: http://www.aapd.org/media/Policies_Guidelines/G_Adoleshealth.pdf [November 12, 2007].

American Board of Medical Specialties. (2007). *Moving Forward Together.* Evanston, IL: American Board of Medical Specialties.

Astroth, K. A., Garza, P., and Taylor, B. (2004). Getting down to business: Defining competencies for entry-level youth workers. *New Directions for Youth Development, 104,* 25–37.

Bearinger, L. H., Wildey, L., Gephart, J., and Blum, R. W. (1992). Nursing competence in adolescent health: Anticipating the future needs of youth. *Journal of Professional Nursing, 8,* 80–86.

Beresin, E., and Mellman, L. (2002). Competencies in psychiatry: The new outcomes-based approach to medical training and education. *Harvard Review of Psychiatry, 10,* 185–191.

Biro, F. M., Siegel, D. M., Parker, R. M., and Gillman, M. W. (1993). A comparison of self-perceived clinical competencies in primary care residency graduates. *Pediatric Research, 34,* 555–559.

Blum, R. (1987). Physicians' assessment of deficiencies and desire for training in adolescent care. *Journal of Medical Education, 62,* 401–407.

Blum, R., and Smith, M. (1988). Training of health professionals in adolescent health care. Study group report. *Journal of Adolescent Health Care, 9,* 46S–50S.

Blum, R. W., Beuhring, T., Wunderlich, M., and Resnick, M. D. (1996). Don't ask, they won't tell: Health screening of youth. *American Journal of Public Health, 86,* 1767–1772.

Brown, R., Doonan, S., and Shellenberger, S. (2005). Using children as simulated patients in communication training for residents and medical students: A pilot program. *Academic Medicine: Journal of the Association of American Medical Colleges, 80,* 1114–1120.

Bureau of Labor Statistics and U.S. Department of Labor. (2007). *Career Guide to Industries, 2006–2007 Edition, Health Care*. Available: http://www.bls.gov/oco/cg/cgs035.htm [September 13, 2007].

Chmar, J. E., Harlow, A. H., Weaver, R. G., and Valachovic, R. W. (2007). Annual ADEA survey of dental school seniors, 2006 graduating class. *Journal of Dental Education, 71*, 1228–1253.

Cohen, M. I. (1984). The Society for Behavioral Pediatrics: A new portal in a rapidly moving boundary. *Pediatrics, 73*, 791–798.

Commission on Dental Accreditation. (1998). *Accreditation Standards for Advanced Specialty Education Programs in Pediatric Dentistry*. Chicago, IL: American Dental Association.

Commission on Dental Accreditation. (2007). *Standards for Dental Education Programs*. Chicago, IL: American Dental Association.

Conard, L. E., Fortenberry, D., Blythe, M., and Orr, D. P. (2003). Pharmacists' attitudes toward and practices with adolescents. *Archives of Pediatric and Adolescent Medicine, 157*, 361–365.

Cull, W. L., Yudkowsky, B. K., Shipman, S. A., Pan, R. J., and American Academy of Pediatrics. (2003). Pediatric training and job market trends: Results from the American Academy of Pediatrics third-year resident survey, 1997–2002. *Pediatrics, 112*, 787–792.

Denninghoff, K. R., Knox, L., Cunningham, R., and Partain, S. (2002). Emergency medicine: Competencies for youth violence prevention and control. *Academic Emergency Medicine, 9*, 947–956.

Elster, A. B., and Kuznets, N. (1994). *Guidelines for Adolescent Preventive Services (GAPS): Recommendations and Rationale*. Chicago, IL: American Medical Association.

Emans, S. J., Bravender, T., Knight, J., Frazer, C., Luoni, M., Berkowitz, C., Armstrong, E., and Goodman, E. (1998). Adolescent medicine training in pediatric residency programs: Are we doing a good job? *Pediatrics, 102*, 588–595.

Farrow, J. A., and Saewyc, E. M. (2002). Work group III: Identifying effective strategies and interventions for improving adolescent health at the individual level. *Journal of Adolescent Health, 31*, 226–229.

Gallagher, J. R. (1957). The adolescent and pediatric education. *Pediatrics, 19*, 937–939.

Golden, N. H., Seigel, W. M., Fisher, M., Schneider, M., Quijano, E., Suss, A., Bergeson, R., Seitz, M., and Saunders, D. (2001). Emergency contraception: Pediatricians' knowledge, attitudes, and opinions. *Pediatrics, 107*, 287–292.

Golden, N. H., Katzman, D. K., Kreipe, R. E., Stevens, S. L., Sawyer, S. M., Rees, J., Nicholls, D., and Rome E. (2003). Eating disorders in adolescents: Position paper of the Society for Adolescent Medicine. *Journal of Adolescent Health, 33*, 496–503.

Green, M. (Ed.). (1994). *Bright Futures: Guidelines for Health Supervision of Infants, Children, and Adolescents*. Washington, DC: National Center for Education in Maternal and Child Health, Georgetown University.

Green, M., and Palfrey, J. (2002). *Bright Futures: Guidelines for Health Supervision of Infants, Children, and Adolescents* (2nd Revised Ed.). Washington, DC: National Center for Education in Maternal and Child Health, Georgetown University.

Hardoff, D., and Schonmann, S. (2001). Training physicians in communication skills with adolescents using teenage actors as simulated patients. *Medical Education, 35*, 206–210.

Hellerstedt, W. L., Smith, A. E., Shew, M. L., and Resnick, M. D. (2000). Perceived knowledge and training needs in adolescent pregnancy prevention: Results from a multidisciplinary survey. *Archives of Pediatrics and Adolescent Medicine, 154*, 679–684.

Hoge, M. A., Jacobs, S., Belitsky, R., and Migdole, S. (2002). Graduate education and training for contemporary behavioral health practice. *Administration and Policy in Mental Health, 29*, 335–357.

Hoge, M. A., Huey, L. Y., and O'Connell, M. J. (2004). Best practices in behavioral health workforce education and training. *Administration and Policy in Mental Health*, 32, 91–106.
Hughes, R. (2003). Public health nutrition workforce composition, core functions, competencies and capacity: Perspectives of advanced-level practitioners in Australia. *Public Health Nutrition*, 6(6), 607–613.
Institute of Medicine. (2007). *Training Physicians for Public Health Careers*. Washington, DC: The National Academies Press.
Jay, S. M. (2007). The pediatric subspecialty of adolescent medicine-Help wanted! *Journal of Pediatrics*, 150, A2.
Kaslow, N. J., Borden, K. A., Collin, F. L., Forrest, L., Illfelder-Kaye, J., Nelson, P. D., Rallo, J. S., Vasquez, M. J. T., and Willmuth, M. E. (2004). Competencies conference: Future directions in education and credentialing in professional psychology. *Journal of Clinical Psychology*, 60, 699–712.
Kerwin, M. E., Walker-Smith, K., and Kirby, K. C. (2006). Comparative analysis of state requirements for the training of substance abuse and mental health counselors. *Journal of Substance Abuse Treatment*, 30, 173–181.
Kim, W. J., and American Academy of Child and Adolescent Psychiatry Task Force on Workforce Needs. (2003). Child and adolescent psychiatry workforce: A critical shortage and national challenge. *Academic Psychiatry*, 27, 277–282.
Klein, J. D., Allan, M. J., Elster, A. B., Stevens, D., Cox, C., Hedberg, V. A., and Goodman, R. A. (2001). Improving adolescent preventive care in community health centers. *Pediatrics*, 107, 318–327.
Klitsner, I. N., Borok, G. M., Neinstein, L., and MacKenzie, R. (1992). Adolescent health care in a large multispecialty prepaid group practice. Who provides it and how well are they doing? *The Western Journal of Medicine*, 156, 628–632.
Korczak, D. J., MacArthur, C., and Katzman, D. K. (2006). Canadian pediatric residents' experience and level of comfort with adolescent gynecological health care. *Journal of Adolescent Health*, 38, 57–59.
Krol, D. M. (2004). Educating pediatricians on children's oral health: Past, present, and future. *Pediatrics*, 113, e487–e492.
Michaud, P. A., Stronski, S., Fonseca, H., Macfarlane, A., and EuTEACH Working Group. (2004). The development and pilot testing of a training curriculum in adolescent medicine and health. *Journal of Adolescent Health*, 35, 5157.
Miller, S. H. (2005). American Board of Medical Specialties and reposition for excellence in lifelong learning: Maintenance of certification. *The Journal of Continuing Education in the Health Professions*, 25, 151–156.
Nerdahl, P., Berglund, D., Bearinger, L. H., Saewyc, E., Ireland, M., and Evans, T. (1999). New challenges, new answers: Pediatric nurse practitioners and the care of adolescents. *Journal of Pediatric Health Care*, 13, 183–190.
Ozer, E. M., Brindis, C. D., Millstein S. G., Knopf, D. K., and Irwin, C. E., Jr. (1998). *America's Adolescents: Are They Healthy?* San Francisco: University of California, National Adolescent Health Information Center.
Remschmidt, H., and Belfer, M. (2005). Mental health care for children and adolescents worldwide: A review. *World Psychiatry*, 4, 147–153.
Rickert, V. (2003). Crossing the threshold. *Journal of Adolescent Health*, 33, 134–137.
Saewyc, E. M., Bearinger, L. H., McMahon, G., and Evans, T. (2006). A national needs assessment of nurses providing health care to adolescents. *Journal of Professional Nursing*, 22, 304–313.

Schultz, K. K., and Marks, A. (2007). Community-based collaboration with high school theatre students as standardized patients. *American Journal of Pharmaceutical Education, 17*, 29.

Shelton, D. (2003). The clinical practice of juvenile forensic psychiatric nurses. *Journal of Psychosocial Nursing and Mental Health Services, 41*, 42–53.

Stein, M. (Ed.). (1997). *Health Supervision Guidelines* (3rd Ed.). Elk Grove Village, IL: American Academy of Pediatrics.

Story, M. T., Neumark-Sztainer, D. R., Ireland, M., and Evans, T. (2000). Adolescent health and nutrition: A survey of perceived knowledge and skill competencies and training interests among dietitians working with youth. *Journal of the American Dietetic Association, 100*, 362–364.

Story, M. T., Neumark-Sztainer, D. R., Sherwood, N. E., Holt, K., Sofka, D., Trowbridge, F. L., and Barlow, S. E. (2002). Management of child and adolescent obesity: Attitudes, barriers, skills, and training needs among health care professionals. *Pediatrics, 110*, 210–214.

Task Force on Pediatric Education. (1978). *Report on the Future of Pediatric Education*. Elk Grove Village, IL: American Academy of Pediatrics.

U.S. Census Bureau. (2006). *National Population Estimates for the 2000s. Estimates by Age, Sex, Race, and Hispanic Origin: January 1, 2006*. Available: http://www.census.gov/popest/national/asrh/2005_nat_res.html [November 6, 2007].

U.S. Department of Health and Human Services. (1994). *The Clinician's Handbook of Preventive Services: Put Prevention into Practice*. Alexandria, VA: International Medical Publishers.

U.S. Preventive Services Task Force. (1996). *Guide to Clinical Preventive Services* (2nd Ed.). Baltimore, MD: Williams and Wilkins.

Weaver, R. G., Haden, N. K., and Valachovic, R. W. (2002a). Annual ADEA survey of dental school seniors: 2001 graduating class. *Journal of Dental Education, 66*, 1209–1222.

Weaver, R. G., Haden, N. K., and Valachovic, R. W. (2002b). Annual ADEA survey of dental school seniors: 2002 graduating class. *Journal of Dental Education, 66*, 1388–1404.

Weaver, R. G., Haden, N. K., and Valachovic, R. W. (2004). Annual ADEA survey of dental school seniors: 2003 graduating class. *Journal of Dental Education, 68*, 1004–1027.

Weaver, R. G., Chmar, J. E., Haden, N. K., and Valachovic, R. W. (2005). Annual ADEA survey of dental school seniors: 2004 graduating class. *Journal of Dental Education, 69*, 595–619.

6

Health Insurance Coverage and Access to Adolescent Health Services

SUMMARY

- More than 4 million adolescents aged 10–18 are medically uninsured. Uninsured rates are higher among the poor and near poor, racial and ethnic minorities, and noncitizens than among the general adolescent population.
- As is true for all Americans, medically uninsured adolescents are less likely to have a regular source of primary care and use medical and dental care less often compared with those who have insurance.
- The majority of medically uninsured adolescents aged 10–18 are eligible for public coverage but not yet enrolled. Their parents say they would enroll their children in public programs, but many do not know their children are eligible.
- Having health insurance does not ensure adolescents' access to affordable, high-quality services given problems associated with high out-of-pocket cost-sharing requirements, limitations in benefit packages, and low provider reimbursement levels. For example, the current system for financing health insurance coverage leads to underinvestments in disease prevention and treatment in some areas that are particularly problematic for adolescents.

The availability, nature, and content of health services for adolescents are profoundly affected by the ability to pay for those services through public and private health insurance. Fundamentally, *money matters*, and *policies matter* with respect to financing systems. This chapter focuses on these two contextual characteristics. It examines the extent to which adolescents have adequate insurance coverage for the health services they need; the emphasis is on financing issues and the public policies that relate to health insurance coverage. The discussion addresses limitations of the current financing system for adolescent health services with respect to both the lack of health insurance coverage and shortcomings of the coverage for adolescents who are insured.

LACK OF HEALTH INSURANCE COVERAGE

As is true for all Americans, adolescents who are medically uninsured often receive care late in the development of a health problem or not at all. As a result, they are at higher risk for hospitalization for conditions amenable to timely outpatient care and for missed diagnoses of serious and even life-threatening conditions (Institute of Medicine, 2002a). As discussed in Chapter 2, some conditions (e.g., injuries, asthma) are particularly important in the adolescent population, and without timely care, frequently lead to unnecessary hospitalization. Additionally, dental care accounts for only 4.4 percent of total U.S. health expenditures for the general population, but accounts for 29.2 percent of health expenditures among those aged 6–17 compared with 37.3 percent for all other ambulatory health services (Cohen et al., 1996). This section examines how a lack of health insurance relates to limitations in adolescents' access to needed health services, reviews disparities in insurance coverage and eligibility for adolescents, and describes some approaches that could be used to address these issues.

Access

Those who lack health insurance are much more likely to go without health care than the insured (Institute of Medicine, 2001). The Institute of Medicine (IOM) has presented important evidence that being medically uninsured has a negative effect on health-related outcomes and chronic conditions among adults. The IOM study included a review of research investigating the health of working adults with and without health insurance (Institute of Medicine, 2002a). In a follow-up to that study, the IOM examined the impact of uninsurance on families, children, and adolescents. In this IOM study and other research, it was found that adolescents who lack health insurance coverage have worse access to needed health services than those who have coverage, although barriers remain for insured adolescents as well, as discussed later in this chapter (Callahan and Cooper, 2005; Ford, Bearman, and Moody, 1999; Institute of Medicine, 2002b; Klein et al., 2006; Lieu, Newacheck, and McManus, 1993; National Adolescent Health Information Center, 2005; Newacheck et al., 1999; Shenkman, Youngblade, and Nackashi, 2003; Yu et al., 2001). Gaps in insurance coverage, particularly for mental health and dental services, also appear to cause access problems (Olson, Tang, and Newacheck, 2005).

Table 6-1 shows how access to care differs between adolescents who are medically insured and uninsured along a number of different dimensions: failure to get needed medical care because of cost, delays in getting needed care because of cost, failure to get needed prescription drugs because of cost, the absence of a usual source for health care, and failure to see a physician in the past year (tabulations based on data from the 2004–2005 National Health Interview Survey).[1] For each measure, the medically uninsured are worse off than those with public or private coverage. For example, 13 percent of those aged 10–18 who were uninsured failed to get needed medical care and 11 percent to get needed prescription drugs because of cost, compared with 2.6 percent and 4.3 percent, respectively, for those with public coverage and 1.1 percent and 2.1 percent, respectively, for those with private coverage. Similarly, almost half of the medically uninsured in this age group lacked a usual source of care, and 41 percent had not seen a physician during the past year, compared with 6.6 and 14.4 percent, respectively, for those with public coverage and 3.6 and 11.8 percent, respectively, for those with private coverage. The discrepancy between levels of access to care enjoyed by the medically insured and uninsured is the greatest for those with poor health. Those with multiple risk factors can suffer quite severe limitations in access to care. Thus, 16.1 percent of uninsured adolescents aged 10–18 who reported fair or poor health status failed to get medical care because of cost in 2004–2005, compared with 5.3 percent of their counterparts covered by public insurance (tabulations based on data from the U.S. National Health Interview Survey, 2004–2005).

According to the 2004 Medical Expenditure Panel Survey, three-fourths (76.4 percent) of U.S. adolescents aged 13–20 had dental coverage from either private (55.7 percent) or public (23.6 percent) sources. This represents a significant increase in coverage subsequent to enactment of the State Children's Health Insurance Program (SCHIP), with public dental coverage increasing for eligible children and adolescents by 73 percent between 1996 and 2004 (from 12.0 to 20.7 percent). However, the disparity between services provided to medically insured and uninsured adolescents is typi-

---

[1] Insurance status is defined as of the time of the survey. Public coverage includes Medicaid, the State Children's Health Insurance Program (SCHIP), and other state coverage, while private coverage includes employer-sponsored and nongroup coverage.

TABLE 6-1 Indicators of Access to Care Among Adolescents Aged 10–18 by Coverage Status

Indicator of Access	Adolescents with Public Coverage[a] Percent	Std. Error	Adolescents with Private Coverage[b] Percent	Std. Error	Uninsured Adolescents Percent	Std. Error
Failed to get needed medical care because of cost	2.6	0.3	1.1	0.1	13.3	0.8
Delayed getting medical care because of cost	4.1	0.4	2.4	0.2	17.2	0.9
Failed to get needed prescription drugs because of cost	4.3	0.5	2.1	0.2	11.2	1.1
No usual source of care	6.6	0.6	3.6	0.3	41.3	1.8
No physician visit in the past year	14.4	0.8	11.8	0.5	40.6	1.9

[a] Includes Medicaid, State Children's Health Insurance Program, and other state coverage.
[b] Includes employer-sponsored insurance and nongroup insurance.
SOURCE: Tabulations from the 2004–2005 National Health Interview Survey.

cally greater for dental care than for medical care because of the structure of dental coverage. Based on the National Survey of America's Families, it is estimated that 42 percent of uninsured adolescents aged 11–17 failed to make recommended dental visits in a year, a rate three times higher than that for their privately insured counterparts. These uninsured adolescents were also 2.4 times more likely to miss recommended dental visits than medical health maintenance visits (Yu et al., 2002).

At all ages, those with private health insurance coverage access more dental care than those who are uninsured, even in the absence of a dental benefit plan. The federal Medical Expenditure Panel Survey found that among those aged 13–20, those with no health insurance were half as likely to make a dental visit in a year as those with private coverage (27.5 percent compared with 57.5 percent) (Manski and Brown, 2007). In contrast, having publicly financed coverage is far less predictive of making a dental visit, as children and adolescents with public coverage were only modestly more likely to do so than those who were uninsured (34.1 percent compared with 27.5 percent). Having dental coverage further increases the likelihood of receiving dental care. Among children and adolescents under age 18, more than half (55.6 percent) of those with no insurance did not make a preventive dental visit in a year, while only half as many who had medical coverage (27.7 percent) and a third as many with both medical and dental coverage (19.9 percent) went without preventive dental care (Kenney, McFeeters, and Yee, 2005).

Many adolescents fall through the cracks in the insurance system because of gaps in both public and private coverage (Collins et al., 2006, 2007). More than 4 million individuals aged 10–18 have no health insurance coverage whatsoever, according to recent census data (tabulations based on data from the 2005 Current Population Survey).[2] It is striking to note that if those aged 19–24 are included, this figure rises to more than 12 million.

Disparities in Coverage by Selected Population Characteristics

For adolescents, medically uninsured rates are higher for those with lower income, for Hispanics (and to a lesser extent for African Americans) compared with whites, and for noncitizens compared with citizens (see Figure 6-1) (tabulations in this section are based on data from the 2005 Current Population Survey). Uninsured rates are also higher for those in

---

[2]These estimates have been adjusted for the underreporting of public coverage on the Current Population Survey.

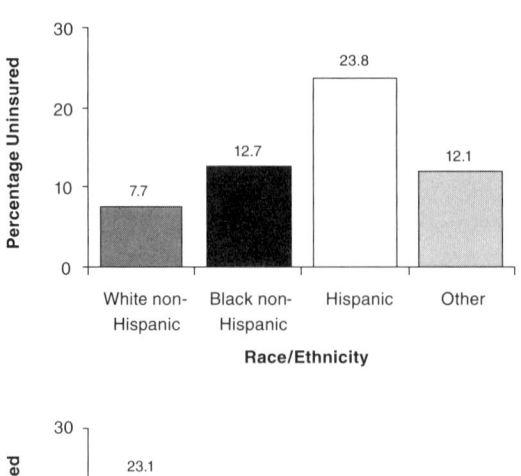

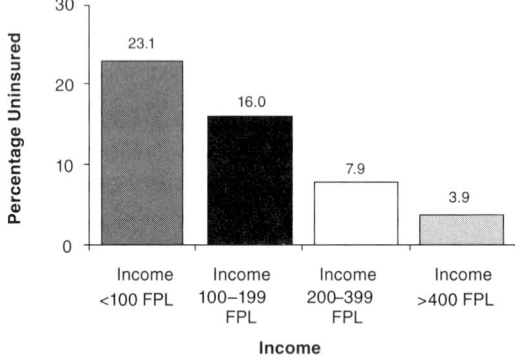

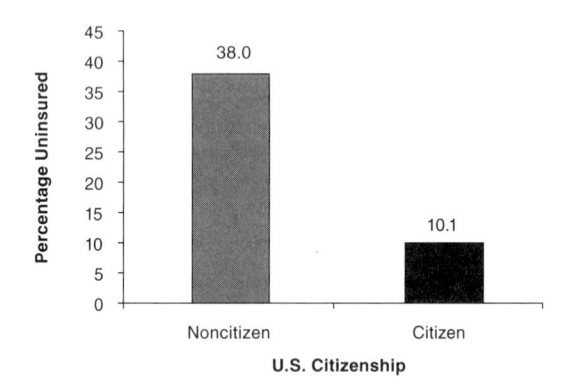

FIGURE 6-1 Uninsured rates among adolescents aged 10–18 by race/ethnicity, income, and U.S. citizenship, 2004. Data reflect adjustments for the underreporting of public coverage.
NOTE: FPL = federal poverty level.
SOURCE: Tabulations based on data from the 2005 Annual Social and Economic Supplement to the Current Population Survey.

health insurance units with nonworking or self-employed adults or only those employed by small firms.[3]

Not only do low-income adolescents have higher uninsured rates compared with higher-income adolescents, but almost half (44.4 percent) of all uninsured adolescents have family incomes below the federal poverty level. Uninsured adolescents are diverse in terms of their race/ethnicity: 40.1 percent are white, 17.0 percent are African American, 35.8 percent are Hispanic, and 7.0 percent are in the "other race" category. Despite having much higher uninsured rates, noncitizens constitute less than one-fifth (17.3 percent) of uninsured adolescents (tabulations from the 2005 Current Population Survey).

Medically uninsured rates are substantially lower for adolescents in families that include at least one adult employed by a large firm (defined as more than 100 employees). For example, across the entire 10–18 age group, those in families with at least one adult working for a large firm were less than half as likely to be medically uninsured as those in families with all adults working for smaller firms—a differential driven by the much higher rate of employer-sponsored coverage in the large-firm category (tabulations from the 2005 Current Population Survey).

Older adolescents (aged 19–24) who are full-time students are much less likely to lack insurance coverage than those in the same age group who are part-time students or are not students (tabulations from the 2005 Current Population Survey). This differential is likely to be driven by full-time students' greater access to both insurance coverage provided through colleges and employer-sponsored coverage from their parents.

Although fewer adolescents have dental than medical coverage, disparities in coverage by age, income, race, parental education, sex, and special-needs conditions are similar. In the aggregate, 22.1 percent of the population under age 17 is estimated to have no dental coverage based on the National Survey of Children's Health. Highest rates of a lack of dental coverage are reported among children and adolescents who also lack medical coverage (79.3 percent), foreign-born Hispanics (66.8 percent), those who live in households in which the highest educational attainment is less than high school (36.0 percent), and those in poverty (27.8 percent) (Liu et al., 2007). Rates of a lack of dental coverage among adults are higher (34.2 percent, based on data from the Medical Expenditure Panel Survey) than those among the adolescent population, primarily because public dental coverage is generally unavailable to adults, yet these disparities

---

[3]Health insurance units (HIUs) reflect the unit that would be used to determine eligibility for both private and public coverage. HIUs encompass the members of a nuclear family who could be considered eligible for a family health insurance policy. The terms "families" and "health insurance units" are used interchangeably in this chapter.

persist (Manski and Brown, 2007). As evidence has grown that maternal oral health profoundly impacts children's oral health and may affect birth outcomes as well, a number of states have recently added dental benefits to their adult Medicaid programs for pregnant women.

Findings:

- More than 4 million adolescents aged 10–18 are medically uninsured. Uninsured rates are higher among the poor and near poor, racial and ethnic minorities, and noncitizens than among the general adolescent population.
- As is true for all Americans, medically uninsured adolescents are less likely to have a regular source of primary care and use medical and dental care less often compared with those who have insurance.

Eligibility for Coverage for Adolescents

Although those aged 19–24 lie outside the age range covered in this report, it is striking to note that eligibility for public coverage is lower for this group than for those aged 18 and under (Brindis, Morreale, and English, 2003; Cohen Ross, Cox, and Marks, 2007; Fox, Limb, and McManus, 2007b). Currently, the majority of states offer health and dental coverage under Medicaid and SCHIP for almost all children with family incomes below 200 percent of the federal poverty level (Cohen Ross, Cox, and Marks, 2007).[4] In contrast, most individuals aged 19–24 qualify for public coverage only if they meet narrow categorical eligibility standards (e.g., pregnancy, disability, Temporary Assistance for Needy Families Program). While some states have extended Medicaid coverage to adolescents who are leaving the foster care system, many who leave foster care become uninsured (English, Morrreale, and Larsen, 2003; English, Stinnett, and Dunn-Georgiou, 2006). Similarly, a study of SCHIP enrollees in 10 states found that two-thirds of disenrollees aged 18 or older were uninsured 6 months after they disenrolled from the program, a much higher proportion than that found among younger disenrollees (Kenney et al., 2005).

In addition, individuals aged 19–24 are less likely than those aged 10–18 to qualify for employer-based medical coverage (Collins et al., 2006). This is the case because of restrictions under private plans requiring that individuals over age 18 be full-time college students to qualify for employer-

---

[4]As of July 2006, 41 states and the District of Columbia had income thresholds of 200 percent of the federal poverty level or above for citizen children and certain groups of immigrant children.

based coverage through a parent, and because many in this age range who are employed are not offered employer-sponsored coverage (Clemans-Cope and Garrett, 2006). Moreover, the employment-based coverage that is available to those aged 19–24 may not be affordable (especially for those who are low-income), or for those in good health and lacking chronic health problems, it may not be perceived as providing benefits that outweigh the costs. For those who lack access to employer-sponsored insurance, finding affordable coverage in the nongroup insurance market may be difficult; this is particularly true for those who have health problems. Similarly, the nongroup dental insurance market offers plans that are typically limited in services, payment levels, or participating providers.

The medically uninsured are concentrated at the upper end of the 19–24 age range, as fully 4.5 million individuals aged 22–24 and 3.6 million aged 19–21 lack coverage, compared with a total of 4.4 million aged 10–18 (tabulations in this section are based on data from the 2005 Annual Social and Economic Supplement to the Current Population Survey). Likewise, uninsured rates increase over this age range, with the largest jump—from 15.3 to 30.5 percent, an increase of about 100 percent—occurring between the 17–18 and 19–21 age groups. Uninsured rates reach 36.6 percent among those aged 22–24. These high uninsured rates among those aged 19–24 are a function of lower reliance on both public and private coverage—29.1 percent of those aged 10–13 have Medicaid/SCHIP coverage and 56.6 percent employer-sponsored insurance, compared with 9.5 percent and 42.2 percent, respectively, of those aged 22–24. As indicated above, young adults are much less likely than adolescents aged 18 and under to qualify for both public and private coverage.

Addressing the Problem of Medically Uninsured Adolescents

Many poor adolescents, particularly those between the ages of 10 and 18, are medically uninsured despite being eligible for Medicaid or SCHIP coverage. Tabulations in this section are based on data from the 2005 Annual Social and Economic Supplement to the Current Population Survey and Urban Institute estimates of eligibility for Medicaid and SCHIP. As described in more detail below, knowledge barriers and problems associated with the Medicaid and SCHIP enrollment processes appear to deter participation in public programs among these uninsured adolescents. Overall, 65 percent of all uninsured adolescents (aged 10–18)—more than 2.8 million individuals—appear to be eligible for Medicaid or SCHIP coverage. More than 80 percent of uninsured adolescents living below 200 percent of the federal poverty level are eligible. As adolescents reach age 19, their eligibility for Medicaid/SCHIP coverage decreases significantly. Eligibility overall is much higher among younger relative to older adolescents who are uninsured: eligibility rates are 65 percent, 62 percent, and 67 percent among adolescents aged 10–13, 14–16, and 17–18, respectively, compared with 20 and 12 percent, respectively, among those aged 19–21 and 22–24.

Enrollment in public coverage appears to improve access to care relative to being uninsured for adolescents aged 18 and under (Dick et al., 2004; Kenney, 2007; Klein et al., 2007). In the three studies referenced here and previously described dental studies, enrollment in public coverage increased the likelihood of having a usual source of care and of receiving preventive care. In addition, Klein and colleagues (2007) found that the extent to which confidential care and preventive counseling were provided to adolescents increased following enrollment in public coverage. Both they and Kenney (2007) also found that enrollment in public coverage reduced unmet health care needs among adolescents.

Together, Medicaid and SCHIP could address nearly two-thirds of the uninsured problem among those aged 10–18 and 84 percent of the problem among those in low-income families in this age group (defined as having an income below 200 percent of the federal poverty level). The bulk of the remaining low-income uninsured adolescents aged 10–18 who do not qualify for Medicaid or SCHIP coverage are legal immigrants who are ineligible for coverage because they have not been in the country for more than 5 years; are undocumented immigrants and qualify only for emergency Medicaid, which is very limited in scope; live in the nine states that have income thresholds below 200 percent of the federal poverty level; or do not live in selected California counties or states that have targeted insurance coverage initiatives with state or local funds. Access to employer-sponsored coverage is also very limited among noncitizen children (Ku and Matani, 2001; Ku and Waidmann, 2003; Schur and Feldman, 2001). Therefore, reducing uninsurance among noncitizen adolescents will likely require expanding Medicaid and SCHIP coverage to more immigrant children.

More than 80 percent of all low-income parents say they would enroll their uninsured adolescents aged 13–17 in Medicaid/SCHIP if told the adolescents were eligible (see Figure 6-2). Therefore, policies aimed at increasing awareness of Medicaid and SCHIP among families whose adolescents could qualify for public coverage hold promise for being successful (Kenney, Haley, and Tebay, 2004). However, just 43 percent of parents of low-income uninsured adolescents believed their adolescents were eligible for coverage, a much lower proportion than found for younger children (Kenney, Haley, and Tebay, 2004). Moreover, 40 percent believed that the Medicaid and SCHIP application processes were easy, a figure again lower than that for parents of younger children (Kenney, Haley, and Tebay, 2004). Thus, increasing participation in Medicaid/SCHIP among adolescents may require targeted outreach and enrollment efforts aimed specifically at families with adolescents.

HEALTH INSURANCE COVERAGE AND ACCESS 275

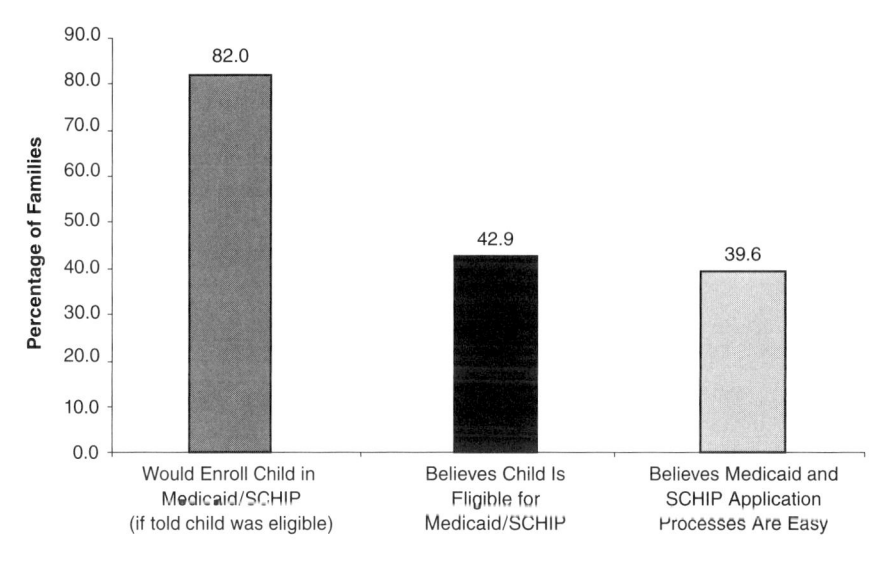

FIGURE 6-2 Awareness and perceptions of Medicaid/State Children's Health Insurance Program among low-income families with uninsured adolescents aged 13–17.
SOURCES: Tabulations are based on the Centers for Disease Control and Prevention, National Center for Health Statistics, State and Local Area Integrated Telephone Survey, National Survey of Children with Special Health Care Needs, 2001.

Although those aged 19–24 are beyond the primary focus of this report, it is useful to compare their uninsured problem with that of younger adolescents. Only a small fraction of the uninsured in this older age group—just 20 percent of those aged 19–21 and 12 percent of those aged 22–24—appear to be eligible for public coverage. Moreover, among the uninsured living below the poverty line aged 19–21 and 22–24, respectively, just 36 and 23 percent meet the requirements for Medicaid/SCHIP eligibility. In addition, very few uninsured in these age groups with incomes between 100 and 200 percent of the federal poverty level are eligible for Medicaid/SCHIP coverage.

Therefore, substantially reducing uninsurance among those aged 19–24 will require more than increasing participation in existing Medicaid and SCHIP programs. One approach would be to require that employer-based insurance plans cover dependents up to age 23 or higher. For example, new laws that became effective in 2006 in New Jersey and Colorado require group health plans to cover more dependents up to ages 30 and age 25, respectively (Collins et al., 2006). A number of private health insurance programs have developed specialized benefit packages for this age group (Brindis et al., 2007). Massachusetts, for example, has addressed this problem by providing private coverage for those aged 19–25.

In addition, expanding school-based health insurance coverage to more full- and part-time students through mandates or other incentives could reduce uninsurance among the more than 7 million medically uninsured (Collins et al., 2006). However, greatly reducing uninsurance among poor and near-poor adolescents in this age group will likely require an expansion of eligibility for public coverage since many of these individuals would not have access to affordable group or nongroup insurance coverage. Under current law, states can expand Medicaid eligibility up to age 21 and receive federal matching payments to help cover those costs. Further expansions would require changes in federal statute or waivers.

Finding: The majority of medically uninsured adolescents aged 10–18 are eligible for public coverage but not yet enrolled. Their parents say they would enroll their children in public programs, but many do not know their children are eligible.

SHORTCOMINGS OF EXISTING COVERAGE

Having health insurance coverage does not ensure adolescents' access to the health services they need. Following an overview of existing health insurance coverage for adolescents, this section reviews four particular shortcomings of the coverage provided: inadequate coverage of preventive, sexual and reproductive health, mental health and substance abuse treatment, and dental services; access problems related to high cost sharing or lack of provider participation; lack of incentives to invest in preventive and chronic care services; and limited confidentiality policies for adolescents receiving health services. A fifth shortcoming of health insurance coverage related to access to quality health care was discussed in Chapter 3.

Overview of Existing Sources of Health Insurance for Adolescents

Adolescents receive health insurance coverage from three sources: Medicaid, SCHIP, and private insurers. Benefits and cost-sharing arrangements vary across these sources, as described below.

Medicaid

Medicaid provides very generous coverage for services needed by adolescents. For adolescents up to age 21, the Early and Periodic Screening, Diagnostic, and Treatment (EPSDT) mandate, which requires coverage of periodic screenings as well as all federally allowable diagnostic and treatment services found to be necessary as a result of a screen, is intended to ensure that Medicaid benefits for preventive, sexual and reproductive health, mental health and substance abuse treatment, and dental services are comprehensive. In addition, these services should not require any cost sharing for adolescents in families with incomes below 100 percent of the federal poverty level, although—with the exception of preventive, family planning, and emergency services—cost sharing can be as much as 10 percent of the service cost for those in families with incomes up to 150 percent of the federal poverty level and as much as 20 percent for those in families with higher incomes (Solomon, 2007). However, there is no research documenting states' use of the EPSDT benefit to cover the diagnostic and treatment services needed by adolescents and no research on how authorization decisions are made by either managed care organizations or state utilization review staff.

State Children's Health Insurance Program (SCHIP)

SCHIP, which covers adolescents up to age 19, is often more restrictive than Medicaid in the 36 states that have elected to operate separate SCHIP programs modeled after private coverage. Most of these states use their state employees' benefit plans as their benchmark. However, 10 of the 36 states offer Medicaid look-alike coverage with EPSDT provisions, and 6 offer enhanced coverage for specialty services through wrap-around benefits (Fox, Levtov, and McManus, 2003). Under SCHIP, states may impose premiums or require copayments or coinsurance, but they may not impose cost-sharing requirements for preventive services, and total cost sharing may not exceed 5 percent of a family's income. Research on state coverage policies is limited in that, with the exception of mental health, substance abuse treatment, and dental services, it does not provide information on the details of coverage. Neither does it offer a current assessment of the extent to which any of the benefits are actually authorized.

Private Health Insurance

Adolescents with private health insurance are likely to have less comprehensive coverage than those with public insurance. Although benefit packages in employer-sponsored health plans have become broader in the past few decades, benefit limits, cost-sharing requirements, and condition and treatment exclusions have generally narrowed the amount of coverage. Yet there is little current information on the benefit restrictions applicable to most services important to adolescents or even on the availability of preventive and certain reproductive services. In addition, information on cost-sharing requirements, except for basic health services, is generally lacking—a significant gap in knowledge given that high annual family deductibles and service copayments or coinsurance for both in- and out-of-network services often present substantial financial barriers, particularly for adolescents seeking services on their own. Moreover, there is no literature on the actual authorization of services that require prior approval.

Coverage of Adolescent-Specific Health Services

Insured adolescents experience particular shortcomings in the coverage of certain health services, most notably preventive services, sexual and reproductive health services, mental health and substance abuse treatment, and dental services. Although access to services is dependent on multiple variables, such as provider availability and transportation, coverage of benefits is an essential first step to ensuring that adolescents receive the services they require. This section details those issues.

Preventive Services

Medicaid Under Medicaid, states are required to cover EPSDT screening services but have discretion in establishing periodicity schedules, as well as the required content of visits. A recent study found that in 2006, only 33 states required annual screenings for adolescents; the remaining 18 required screenings every other year or even less frequently (Fox, Limb, and McManus, 2007a). In addition, states' directives with respect to anticipatory guidance, a federally required component of the screening service, vary widely, with only 50 percent of states stipulating such guidance on nutrition and fewer than 40 percent on substance abuse (Fox, Limb, and McManus, 2007a). An earlier study found that in 2000, screening requirements for conditions and behavior relevant to adolescence—hypertension, physical abuse, alcohol use, contraception use, depression, eating disorders, obesity, risky sexual practices, school problems, substance abuse, and tobacco use—were not stipulated in the vast majority of states. The largest proportion (40 percent) required screening for hypertension (McNulty and Covert, 2001).

For older adolescents/young adults over age 19, preventive, screening, and diagnostic services are an optional Medicaid benefit. In 2004, only 35 states covered this benefit, although usually without copayments (Kaiser Commission on Medicaid and the Uninsured, 2004b). Information on the scope of coverage and its appropriateness for this age group is not available. A separate study found that in 2003, 48 states provided some level of immunization coverage for those over age 18, but only 32 covered all the immunizations recommended by the Advisory Committee on Immunization

Practices (Rosenbaum et al., 2003). Nominal cost sharing was required by 27 states (Rosenbaum et al., 2003).

SCHIP Under SCHIP, states operating separate benefit programs are federally required to provide preventive care and immunizations without cost sharing, but states have broader discretion in the frequency and content of preventive health visits than they do under Medicaid. Unfortunately, little has been written on the content of preventive services for adolescents covered by SCHIP. A 2003 study by the Maternal and Child Health Policy Research Center (MCHPRC) found that nearly all states covered annual preventive visits for adolescents aged 12–19 (Fox, Limb, and McManus, 2003), but little is known about the required content of these visits.

Private insurers Current information on the availability of coverage for annual preventive care services for privately insured adolescents is not available since large-scale surveys, such as the Kaiser/Health Research and Educational Trust (HRET) Survey and the Bureau of Labor Statistics' National Compensation Survey, ask only about well-baby visits and adult preventive care. Neither is there current information on immunizations. Research by the MCHPRC found that in 1999, preventive exams were covered by almost all commonly sold health maintenance organization (HMO) and preferred provider organization (PPO) plans, yet while two-thirds of these plans covered adolescents through age 21, few provided any specifics about the periodicity of preventive care visits. Monetary limits on preventive care visits, usually $200, were included in 15 percent of plans. Immunizations, like preventive care, were covered by almost all plans, but in close to 40 percent of plans, that coverage did not extend through age 21. Cost sharing was required in almost 90 percent of plans for preventive visits and almost three-quarters of plans for immunizations, most often in the form of a $10 copayment (Fox, McManus, and Reichman, 2002).

Sexual and Reproductive Health Services

Medicaid Medicaid's mandatory EPSDT benefit should ensure that adolescents up to age 21 have coverage for sexual and reproductive health services, including gynecological exams, screening for sexually transmitted infections (STIs), family planning counseling, contraceptives, and pregnancy-related services. In 15 states that have Medicaid family planning waivers, including California and New York, adolescents can receive confidential Medicaid-financed family planning services without regard to parental income. Of significance, however, male adolescents are eligible for such services in only 7 of these 15 states (Fox, Limb, and McManus, 2007b). In addition, cost sharing is prohibited for family planning services, and states are required to allow enrollees to receive those services from any participating Medicaid provider, even if that provider is not part of an enrollee's managed care network. One study found that all states covered oral contraceptives and gynecological exams, but that only about two-thirds covered STI screening and family planning counseling (Schwalberg et al., 2001).

SCHIP Although states with separate SCHIP programs are not subject to any federal requirements to cover sexual and reproductive health services or to limit cost sharing for these services, the sparse research available suggests that the majority of states are providing adolescents most, if not all, sexual and reproductive health services without significant cost-sharing requirements. Combined findings from two studies showed that all states with separate SCHIP programs covered gynecological exams, almost always including a family planning counseling service; all states covered STI screening; and all but four states covered the most commonly used prescription contraceptives (Gold and Sonfield, 2001; Fox, Limb, and McManus, 2003). Cost sharing was required in about half of the states for physician visits and prescription drugs, but the amounts were generally minimal—$3 to $5 (Fox, Limb, and McManus, 2003).

Private insurers It would appear that the vast majority of privately insured adolescents have coverage for at least certain sexual and reproductive health services. Findings from a survey of employees' benefits in small, medium, and large firms suggest that almost all privately insured adolescents have coverage for annual gynecological exams and about 90 percent for oral contraceptives (The Kaiser Family Foundation and Health Research and Educational Trust, 2004). Less is known about private health insurance coverage for STI screening, family planning counseling, and pregnancy-related services. However, a 2001 survey of benefits offered by small, medium, and large employers found that on average, fewer than 40 percent covered chlamydia screening (Bondi et al., 2006), and the MCHPRC's 1999 study found that fewer than 20 percent of private plans covered pregnancy-related services for pregnant dependent adolescents, and fewer than 30 percent covered family planning counseling (Fox, McManus, and Reichman, 2003). Cost-sharing information for reproductive services is unavailable.

Mental Health and Substance Abuse Treatment Services

While the affordability of health care in general is an important issue for adolescents, the affordability of mental health and substance abuse treatment is particularly problematic. The availability of those services has long suffered from bias and stigma against persons with such disorders, which traditionally have resulted in higher patient cost sharing, lower benefits, and more limited networks than is the case for any other medical conditions. Box 6-1 provides an overview of the financing of mental health and substance abuse treatment services.

Medicaid All mental health and substance abuse treatment services needed by adolescents—including outpatient care, inpatient care, intensive community-based services, and even residential services—should be available under EPSDT. For older adolescents, Medicaid coverage is more variable and more commonly available for mental health services than for substance abuse treatment. In 2003, according to a national survey conducted by the Substance Abuse and Mental Health Services Administration, all states covered outpatient mental health services, such as counseling and medication management, and all covered inpatient mental health services, but only about 80 percent provided coverage for substance abuse treatment on an outpatient or inpatient basis (Robinson et al., 2003). Partial hospitalization and other intensive outpatient services were covered by 45 states for mental health conditions but by only 25 states for substance abuse conditions, while residential treatment services were covered for mental health treatment in 30 states and for substance abuse treatment in just 15 states (Robinson et al., 2003). The literature does not provide detail on states' scope of coverage, nor does it reveal much about cost sharing for these services.

SCHIP States are not federally required to cover either mental health or substance abuse treatment services under separate SCHIP programs, but all states have opted to provide SCHIP coverage for both inpatient and outpatient services. While EPSDT-like coverage or wrap-around benefits in 15 states provide comprehensive mental health and substance abuse coverage, the extent of coverage available to adolescents in the remaining states varies widely and is sometimes more restrictive for substance abuse treatment than for mental health services. As revealed in the MCHPRC study, adolescents in the 36 states with separate SCHIP programs in 2003 would be subject to a limit of 30 outpatient visits in a quarter of states for mental health services and in a third of states for substance abuse treatment. For inpatient care, adolescents would find mental health coverage limited to a 30-day maximum in almost a third of states and substance abuse coverage limited either to 30 days or to detoxification only in almost 40 percent of states. Partial hospitalization would be expressly covered in three-quarters of states for mental health treatment and in just over half of states for substance abuse treatment, but generally only as a conversion benefit[5] (which

---

[5] If partial hospitalization is available as a conversion benefit, an individual may receive those services instead of inpatient services. Usually, the conversion is one inpatient day for two partial hospitalization visits.

BOX 6-1
Overview of Financing of Mental Health and Substance Abuse Treatment Services

For several decades in the twentieth century, mental health specialty services were funded and organized by public mental health authorities predominantly at the state level. Even as general medical care became increasingly the domain of commercial insurance and Medicaid/Medicare in the second half of the century, the specialty mental health care system was strongly influenced by the public mental health system. However, the last 30 years saw mental health advocates push successfully for access to Social Security Income enrollment, expanded Medicaid benefits, housing support, and other federal and state social insurance programs for persons with mental disorders. These programs greatly increased the integration of persons with these disorders into services and the community, but also made policy and financing for mental health services a small component of much larger programs, such as Medicaid. Today, although mental health services across all programs are funded at a higher level than at any time in the past, mental health advocates are increasingly less able to influence policy with the needs of adolescents affected by mental disorders in mind because of the size and scope of these larger programs. This trend is likely to continue as the numbers of public mental health institutions and spending on public mental health specialty services diminish (Nutt and Hogan, 2005).

The affordability of mental health care for adolescents is modulated by the complex patchwork of public and private payors that constitute the putative health care system in the United States. The resulting inequities and inadequacies in health care delivery for children and families generally and adolescents in particular are extensively documented. These inequities and inadequacies are exacerbated for adolescents with mental disorders seeking care because of higher levels of patient cost sharing for such care, more limited benefits, greater demand for health care management, and bias against adolescents with mental disorders as compared with those with other disorders. Although these factors are historical remnants of the placement of adolescents with mental disorders in public institutions, their persistence today means there are considerable barriers to affordable mental health care for many adolescents. For example, out-of-pocket costs for health care for adolescents with common mental disorders are higher than for those with other common medical problems.

A variety of efforts over the past two decades have been aimed at lowering cost barriers to mental health services for both adolescents and others with mental disorders. These include expansions of adolescents' eligibility for Medicaid and the State Children's Health Insurance Program (SCHIP) to levels equal to those for younger children; Early and Periodic Screening, Diagnostic, and Treatment (EPSDT) screening recommendations for Medicaid-eligible adolescents; legislative parity initiatives for non–Employee Retirement Income Security Act (ERISA) commercial insurance plans in several states; and the elimination of custody relinquishment in some states for Medicaid reimbursement in intensive settings. In addition, the use of Social Security Income eligibility for Medicaid enrollment for many severely affected adolescents has expanded. Recently, some states have improved Medicaid reimbursement for primary care mental health services. Unfortunately, many financial barriers to effective mental health care remain.

might be available on a case-by-case basis in other states). Residential treatment would be covered in about three-quarters of states for both mental heath and substance abuse conditions. Two states, however, would impose an annual cap of $6,000 or $8,000 on substance abuse treatment but not on mental health care. In addition, several states would impose a limit of 30 visits or 30 days of inpatient care for mental health and substance abuse services combined, further limiting coverage for adolescents with co-occurring conditions (Fox, Levtov, and McManus, 2003).

The MCHPRC study found that cost sharing for some types of mental health and substance abuse treatment services was required in most of the 36 separate SCHIP programs, but was usually nominal. About a third required cost sharing for outpatient services—usually a $5 copayment—but one state required coinsurance amounting to 50 percent of the service cost. About a quarter of states required cost sharing for inpatient care, with $25 being the average charge, but two states required significant coinsurance (Fox, Levtov, and McManus, 2003).

Private insurers Almost all privately insured adolescents appear to have coverage for mental health services, while a somewhat smaller proportion have coverage for substance abuse treatment, although typically with limits on outpatient visits or inpatient days. According to the 2006 Kaiser/HRET Survey, it is likely that 97 percent of adolescents insured under employer-sponsored plans have mental health benefits, but that as many as two-thirds face an annual maximum of 30 outpatient visits and 30 or fewer inpatient days (The Kaiser Family Foundation and Health Research and Educational Trust, 2006). In fact, more than a third of plans limit coverage to 20 or fewer visits, and 10 percent limit coverage to 10 or fewer inpatient days (The Kaiser Family Foundation and Health Research and Educational Trust, 2006). An earlier study found that benefit limits imposed under behavioral health plans are more likely to affect children and adolescents than adults, particularly for those with chronic mood disorders or psychoses (Peele, Lave, and Kelleher, 2002).

With respect to substance abuse treatment, a survey of employees' benefits in small, medium, and large firms found that in 2003, almost 90 percent of adolescents covered under employer-based plans would have had coverage for outpatient treatment and almost 95 percent for inpatient treatment, but always with visit or day limits and sometimes with inpatient benefits limited to detoxification (U.S. Bureau of Labor Statistics, 2005). The only information on benefit limits is from the earlier MCHPRC study, which found that 20 outpatient visits and 30 inpatient days were the most common limits (U.S. Bureau of Labor Statistics, 2005).

The MCHPRC study also found that benefit limits were often combined for mental health and substance abuse treatment services. Two-thirds of plans imposed coverage exclusions for conditions such as personality disorders, conduct disorders, behavior disorders, attention-deficit hyperactivity disorder, impulse control disorder, chronic conditions, self-inflicted injuries, emotional disorders, and eating disorders, as well as conditions that do not improve within a short period of time. In addition, more than half of plans excluded specific types of treatment, such as family counseling, services not for evaluation and crisis intervention, psychological testing, and behavior modification (U.S. Bureau of Labor Statistics, 2005).

Dental Services

Medicaid Comprehensive dental services, including regular dental examinations and necessary services related to the relief of pain, restoration of teeth, and maintenance of dental health, are required services for all adolescents up to age 21 through the EPSDT benefit. Upon turning 21, dental coverage for Medicaid beneficiaries is provided by their state Medicaid plan as an optional service. Currently only 9 states provide coverage for reasonably comprehensive preventive and restorative dental services for those over age 21, while 15 states provide coverage for only emergency relief of pain and infection, and 7 have no dental Medicaid benefit of any kind for those over age 21 (Edelstein, Schneider, and Laughlin, 2007). Copayments for covered adult dental services are required in 25 states, but the specific amounts are not available (Kaiser Commission on Medicaid and the Uninsured, 2004a).

SCHIP States are not federally required to cover dental services under separate SCHIP programs. Nonetheless, all states but one currently include some level of dental coverage in their state plans for children and adolescents. Because dental coverage is optional, there is no consistent access to dental services in some states through SCHIP. For example, Colorado and Delaware did not include a dental benefit in their plans until years after establishing medical coverage programs; Texas and Utah dropped their dental coverage only to reinstate it later; Georgia and other states have intermittently considered eliminating dental coverage; and Tennessee provides medical but not dental coverage to adolescents from families with income levels targeted by the SCHIP program. In addition, states vary considerably in the extent of dental coverage offered because the original SCHIP legislation does not define dental coverage. SCHIP plans therefore vary considerably in their dental service limits, including treatment frequencies, materials, procedures, and ages. They also vary considerably in the extent of coverage. Six states (Colorado, Florida, Michigan, Montana, New York, and Texas) have imposed caps of less than $1,000 per year on dental benefits, thereby significantly limiting the utility of this benefit for many adolescents. Others have imposed higher dollar caps and copayment requirements that impede access to dental services for adolescents from targeted working-poor families.

The American Dental Association (Edelstein, Schneider, and Laughlin, 2007) reports that 19 states have elected to cover dental services for all SCHIP beneficiaries through separate SCHIP plans, 8 through combination separate SCHIP and Medicaid plans, and 21 through Medicaid expansion or expansion look-alike designs. Medicaid expansion states are required to provide comprehensive EPSDT dental benefits to adolescents through age 19. All 27 states with full or partial separate dental plans cover basic diagnostic, preventive, and reparative services with minor exceptions, but a high proportion of these states do not cover prosthodontic (6 states), periodontic (7 states), and orthodontic services (14 states).

Private insurers About half of privately insured adolescents are likely to have coverage for dental services through employer-sponsored plans (The Kaiser Family Foundation and Health Research and Educational Trust, 2006; U.S. Bureau of Labor Statistics, 2006). Unfortunately, the scope of dental benefits is not documented in either of the referenced surveys, nor is cost-sharing information available.

Cost Sharing and Provider Participation

Out-of-pocket cost sharing, particularly in private plans, may deter individuals and families from seeking needed care. When families face high deductibles and copayments, they may be reluctant to attend to ongoing health care needs, leading to an increase in unmet needs (Buntin et al., 2005; Newhouse, 2004; Newhouse and the Insurance Experiment Group, 1993). Over the last decade, deductibles and out-of-pocket cost-sharing requirements have increased in private plans (Glied and Remler, 2005; Mercer Health and Benefits, 2007). Between 2003 and 2005, the share of firms that offered employees a high-deductible health insurance plan rose from 5 to 20 percent (The Kaiser Family Foundation and Health Research and Educational Trust, 2005).

Historically, public policies have been designed to keep out-of-pocket cost sharing in public programs low, although higher cost sharing is permitted under SCHIP than under Medicaid, and the Deficit Reduction Act of 2005 permitted more cost sharing in Medicaid. To date, no published study has examined the effects on adolescents of different copayment schedules in public programs.

In addition, having benefits with low cost sharing on paper does not always translate into access to services because providers may be unwilling to offer services under that type of insurance coverage. This is a particular concern for Medicaid programs, whose provider reimbursement levels are well below market rates in many service areas (Tang, 2001; Zuckerman et al., 2004). Research suggests that physicians' participation in Medicaid and SCHIP is higher in states that pay them more (Berman et al., 2002). Just two-thirds of all physicians have no limits on the number of Medicaid and SCHIP patients they will see (Tang, Yudkoswky, and Davis, 2003), and Medicaid patients have become increasingly concentrated at fewer and fewer physicians' offices (Cunningham and May, 2006).

In addition, despite the availability of relatively generous mental health and substance abuse benefits for publicly insured adolescents, an abundant literature documents significant access difficulties due to multiple factors, including shortages and maldistribution of providers (Kim, 2003; Koppelman, 2004; New Freedom Commission on Mental Health, 2003; Thomas and Holzer, 1999; U.S. Department of Health and Human Services, 1999), waiting lists for services, and lack of transportation (Semansky and Koyanagi, 2004). Separate capitation arrangements for behavioral health services may present an additional barrier to the receipt of needed services. A number of studies have found that adolescents enrolled in behavioral health carve-out plans receive fewer inpatient services but more residential, outpatient, and other community-based services; these studies did not assess whether this substitution is appropriate to meet the adolescents' needs (Burns et al., 1999; Libby et al., 2002; Stroul et al., 1998).

Investment in Preventive and Chronic Care Services

Prevention and sustained, effective treatment for chronic physical, dental, and mental health problems were identified as key elements of health services for adolescents earlier in this report. However, the current health care financing system, with its fragmented coverage for the nonelderly, does not offer strong incentives to invest in prevention or to treat chronic health problems adequately. Individuals rarely maintain the same insurance coverage over their life span (Herring, 2006). Private insurance plans, which remain the norm, are built around employer-based coverage provided on a voluntary basis, which is not necessarily affordable or even available. Eligibility for public coverage varies across states and with age, family circumstances and income, and health status (Centers for Medicaid and Medicare Services, 2005a,b).

Thus, individuals' insurance coverage changes when they experience any of a number different events, such as a birthday; a job change for themselves, their spouse, or a parent; marriage; divorce; disability; or a change in family income. Since individuals switch insurance coverage over the course of their lives, any investments made by a given insurer that yield health care savings down the road will not necessarily result in a payoff to that insurer.

In addition, some preventive investments may not yield health care savings but may instead produce savings in other areas, such as the criminal justice system. Given these externalities, the current health care financing system leads to lower investments in prevention than would occur under alternative financing arrangements.

For Medicaid-insured adolescents, reimbursement policies are not structured to support the delivery of comprehensive preventive services. Only 33 states, for example, pay for annual preventive visits for adolescents (Fox, Limb, and McManus, 2007a). Moreover, risk reduction counseling services to address such issues as family problems, sexual practices and contraceptives, and injury prevention are reimbursed in only about half of states (Fox, Limb, and McManus, 2007a). Restrictions on billing for two services on the same day are also an impediment to the delivery of comprehensive preventive services. While a billing mechanism does exist that allows a provider to be reimbursed for a well-adolescent visit and the provision of additional health counseling, only 7 Medicaid agencies expressly allow the practice, while 18 explicitly deny it (Fox, Limb, and McManus, 2007a).

Insurer Policies on Confidential Adolescent Health Services

Payment policies utilized by third-party payors compromise the delivery of confidential services to adolescents, even in states that have laws allowing minors to consent on their own to certain sensitive services. The managed care practice of sending documents to the primary insured party (usually a parent) undermines the ability of providers to deliver truly confidential services to adolescents and has a particularly strong impact on adolescents' receipt of behavioral and sexual and reproductive health services (Gudeman, 2003). These documents, known as explanations of benefits (EOBs), usually detail the services delivered and any outstanding cost-sharing payment that is owed. This practice is universal among private payors and is also used by managed care companies delivering services to adolescents enrolled in Medicaid and SCHIP, even in the absence of cost-sharing requirements, as no state has included a prohibition against sending EOBs in its managed care contracts (Brindis et al., 1999).

> **Finding:** *Having health insurance does not ensure adolescents' access to affordable, high-quality services given problems associated with high out-of-pocket cost-sharing requirements, limitations in benefit packages, and low provider reimbursement levels. For example, the current system for financing health insurance coverage leads to underinvestments in disease prevention and treatment in some areas that are particularly problematic for adolescents.*

SUMMARY

Approximately one in nine adolescents (11.5 percent) aged 10–18 lack insurance coverage. Many adolescents are uninsured despite being eligible for Medicaid or SCHIP coverage. Those who are without coverage are less likely to have a usual source of care and to receive health services and more likely to have unmet health needs. However, adolescents who have coverage experience difficulty gaining access to the services they need because of a combination of limits in benefits packages, cost-sharing requirements, lack of access to providers, and unavailability of confidential health services. These problems are particularly acute with respect to preventive, sexual and reproductive health, mental health and substance abuse treatment, and dental services.

REFERENCES

Berman, S., Dolins, J., Tang, S., and Yudkowsky, B. (2002). Factors that influence the willingness of private primary care pediatricians to accept more Medicaid patients. *Pediatrics, 110*, 239–248.

Bondi, M. A., Harris, J. R., Atkens, D., French, M. E., and Umland, B. (2006). Employer coverage of clinical preventive services in the United States. *American Journal of Health Promotion, 20*, 214–222.

Brindis, C., Kirkpatrick, R., Macdonald, T., VanLandeghem, K., and Lee, S. (1999). *Adolescents and the State Children's Health Insurance Program: Healthy Options for Meeting the Needs of Adolescents.* Washington, DC: Association of Maternal and Child Health Programs and San Francisco: University of California, Policy Information and Analysis Center for Middle Childhood and Adolescence and National Adolescent Health Information Center.

Brindis, C. D., Morreale, M. C., and English A. (2003). The unique health care needs of adolescents. *Future of Children, 13*, 117–135.

Brindis, C. D., Hair, E. C., Cochran, S., Cleveland, K., Valderrama, L. T., and Park, M. J. (2007). Increasing access to program information: A strategy for improving adolescent health. *Maternal and Child Health Journal, 11*, 27–35.

Buntin, M. B., Damberg, C., Haviland, A., Lurie, N., Kapur, K., and Marquis, M. S. (2005). *Consumer-Directed Health Plans: Implications for Health Care Quality and Cost.* Report Prepared for the California HealthCare Foundation. Santa Monica: RAND.

Burns, B. J., Teagle, S. E., Schwartz, M., Angold, A., and Holtzman, A. (1999). Managed behavioral health care: A Medicaid carve-out for youth. *Health Affairs, 18*, 214–225.

Callahan, S. T., and Cooper, W. O. (2005). Uninsurance and health care among young adults in the United States. *Pediatrics, 116*, 88–95.

Centers for Disease Control and Prevention, National Center for Health Statistics. (2001). *State and Local Area Integrated Telephone Survey, National Survey of Children with Special Health Care Needs, 2001.* Available: http://www.cdc.gov/nchs/data/series/sr_02/sr02_136.pdf [August 15, 2008].

Centers for Medicaid and Medicare Services. (2005a). *Low-Cost Health Insurance for Families and Children. Insure Kids Now!* Available: http://www.cms.hhs.gov/LowCostHealthInsFamChild/02_InsureKidsNow.asp#TopOfPage [June 5, 2007].

Centers for Medicaid and Medicare Services. (2005b). *Medicaid Eligibility.* Available: http://www.cms.hhs.gov/MedicaidEligibility/ [June 5, 2007].

Clemans-Cope, L., and Garrett, B. (2006). *Changes in Employer-Sponsored Health Insurance Sponsorship, Eligibility, and Participation: 2001 to 2005.* Washington, DC: Kaiser Commission on Medicaid and the Uninsured.

Cohen, J. W., Machlin, M. S., Zuvekas, S. H., Stagnitti, M. N., and Thorpe, J. M. (1996). *Research Findings #12: Health Care Expenses in the United States 1996.* Rockville, MD: Agency for Healthcare Research and Quality.

Cohen Ross, D., Cox, L., and Marks, C. (2007). *Resuming the Path to Health Coverage for Children and Parents: A 50-state Update on Eligibility Rules, Enrollment and Renewal Procedures, and Cost-Sharing Practices in Medicaid and SCHIP in 2006.* Washington, DC: Kaiser Commission on Medicaid and the Uninsured.

Collins, S. R., Schoen, C., Kriss, J. L., Doty, M. M., and Mahato, B. (2006). *Rite of Passage? Why Young Adults Become Uninsured and How New Policies Can Help* (updated May 24, 2006). New York: Commonwealth Fund.

Collins, S. R., Schoen, C., Kriss, J. L., Doty, M. M., and Mahato, B. (2007). *Rite of Passage? Why Young Adults Become Uninsured and How New Policies Can Help* (updated August 8, 2007). New York: Commonwealth Fund.

Cunningham, P., and May, J. (2006). *Medicaid Patients Increasingly Concentrated among Physicians.* Tracking Report No. 16. Washington, DC: Center for Studying Health System Change.

Dick, A. W., Brach, C., Allison, R. A., Shenkman, E., Shone, L. P., Szilagyi, P. G., Klein, J. D., and Lewit, E. M. (2004). SCHIP's impact in three states: How do the most vulnerable children fare? *Health Affairs, 23,* 63–75.

Edelstein, B. L., Schneider, D., and Laughlin, R. J. (2007). *SCHIP Dental Performance over the First 10 Years: Findings from the Literature and a New ADA Survey.* Chicago, IL: American Dental Association.

English, A., Morreale, M. C., and Larsen, J. (2003). Access to health care for youth leaving foster care: Medicaid and SCHIP. *Journal of Adolescent Health, 32,* 53–69.

English, A., Stinnett, A. J., and Dunn-Georgiou, E. (2006). *Health Care for Adolescents and Young Adults Leaving Foster Care: Policy Options for Improving Access.* Chapel Hill, NC, and San Francisco, CA: Center for Adolescent Health and the Law and Public Policy Analysis and Education Center for Middle Childhood, Adolescent and Young Adult Health.

Ford, C. A., Bearman, P. S., and Moody, J. (1999). Foregone health care among adolescents. *Journal of the American Medical Association, 282,* 2227–2234.

Fox, H. B., McManus, M. A., and Reichman, M. B. (2002). *Private Health Insurance for Adolescents: Is It Adequate?* Washington, DC: Maternal and Child Health Policy Research Center.

Fox, H. B., Levtov, R. G., and McManus, M. A. (2003). *Eligibility, Benefits, and Cost Sharing in Separate SCHIP Programs.* Washington, DC: Maternal and Child Health Policy Research Center.

Fox, H. B., Limb, S. J., and McManus, M. A. (2003). *Separate SCHIP Programs: Generous Coverage for Children with Special Needs in Most States.* Washington, DC: Maternal and Child Health Policy Research Center.

Fox, H. B., McManus, M. A., and Reichman, M. B. (2003). Private health insurance for adolescents: Is it adequate? *Journal of Adolescent Health, 32*(Suppl. 6), 12–24.

Fox, H. B., Limb, S. J., and McManus, M. A. (2007a). *Preliminary Thoughts on Restructuring Medicaid to Promote Adolescent Health.* Washington, DC: Incenter Strategies for the Advancement of Adolescent Health.

Fox, H. B., Limb, S. J., and McManus, M. A. (2007b). *The Public Health Insurance Cliff for Older Adolescents.* Fact Sheet—No. 4. Washington, DC: Incenter Strategies for the Advancement of Adolescent Health.

Glied, S., and Remler, D. (2005). *The Effect of Health Savings Accounts on Health Insurance Coverage.* Issue Brief. New York: The Commonwealth Fund.

Gold, R. B., and Sonfield, A. (2001). Reproductive health services for adolescents under the State Children's Health Insurance Program. *Family Planning Perspectives, 33,* 81–87.

Gudeman, R. (2003). *Adolescent Confidentiality and Privacy under the Health Insurance Portability and Accountability Act.* San Francisco, CA: National Center for Youth Law.

Herring, B. (2006). *Suboptimal Coverage of Preventive Care Due to Expected Turnover among Private Insurers.* Working Paper. Atlanta, GA: Emory University.

Institute of Medicine. (2001). *Coverage Matters: Insurance and Health Care.* Washington, DC: National Academy Press.

Institute of Medicine. (2002a). *Care Without Coverage: Too Little, Too Late.* Washington, DC: National Academy Press.

Institute of Medicine. (2002b). *Health Insurance Is a Family Matter.* Washington, DC: National Academy Press.

Kaiser Commission on Medicaid and the Uninsured. (2004a). *Medicaid Benefits: Online Database. Benefits by Service: Dental Services (October 2004).* Available: http://www.kff.org/medicaid/benefits/service.jsp?gr=offandnt=onandso=0andtg=0andyr=2andcat=6andsv=6 [April 15, 2007].

Kaiser Commission on Medicaid and the Uninsured. (2004b). *Medicaid Benefits: Online Database. Benefits by Service: Diagnostic, Screening, and Preventive Services (October 2004).* Available: http://www.kff.org/medicaid/benefits/service.jsp?gr=offandnt=onandso=0andtg=0andyr=2andcat=7andsv=8 [April 15, 2007].

The Kaiser Family Foundation and Health Research and Educational Trust. (2004). *Employer Health Benefits 2004 Annual Survey.* Washington, DC: The Kaiser Family Foundation.

The Kaiser Family Foundation and Health Research and Educational Trust. (2005). *Employer Health Benefits: 2005 Summary of Findings.* Washington, DC: The Kaiser Family Foundation.

The Kaiser Family Foundation and Health Research and Educational Trust. (2006). *Employer Health Benefits 2006 Annual Survey.* Washington, DC: The Kaiser Family Foundation.

Kenney, G. (2007). The impacts of SCHIP on children who enroll: Findings from ten states. *Health Services Research, 42,* 1520–1543.

Kenney, G., Haley, J., and Tebay, A. (2004). *Awareness and Perceptions of Medicaid and SCHIP Among Low-Income Families with Uninsured Children: Findings from 2001.* Princeton, NJ, and Washington, DC: Mathematica Policy Research, Inc., and The Urban Institute.

Kenney, G. M., McFeeters, J. R., and Yee, J. Y. (2005). Preventive dental care and unmet dental needs among low-income children. *American Journal of Public Health, 95,* 1360–1366.

Kenney, G., Trenholm, C., Dubay, L., Kim, M., Moreno, L., Rubenstein, J., Sommers, A. S., Zuckerman, S., Black, W., Blavin, F., and Ko, G. (2005). *The Experiences of SCHIP Enrollees and Disenrollees in 10 States: Findings from the Congressionally Mandated SCHIP Evaluation.* Princeton, NJ, and Washington, DC: Mathematica Policy Research, Inc., and The Urban Institute.

Kim, W. J. (2003). Child and adolescent psychiatry workforce: A critical shortage and national challenge. *Academic Psychiatry, 27,* 277–282.

Klein, J. D., Shenkman, E., Brach, C., Shone, L. P., Col, J., Schaffer, V. A., Dick, A. W., VanLandeghem, K., and Szilagyi, P. G. (2006). Prior health care experiences of adolescents who enroll in SCHIP. *Journal of Health Care for the Poor and Underserved, 17,* 789–807.

Klein, J. D., Shone, L. P., Szilagyi, P. G., Bayorska, A., Wilson, K., and Dick, A. W. (2007). Impact of the State Children's Health Insurance Program on adolescents in New York. *Pediatrics, 119,* 809–811.

Koppelman, J. (2004). *The Provider System for Children's Mental Health: Workforce Capacity and Effective Treatment*. Washington, DC: National Health Policy Forum.

Ku, L., and Matani, S. (2001). Left out: Immigrants' access to health care and insurance. *Health Affairs, 20*, 247–257.

Ku, L., and Waidmann, T. (2003). *How Race/Ethnicity, Immigration Status, and Language Affect Health Insurance Coverage, Access to Care and Quality of Care Among the Low-Income Population*. Kaiser Commission on Medicaid and the Uninsured. Available: http://www.kff.org/uninsured/upload/How-Race-Ethnicity-Immigration-Status-and-Language-Affect-Health-Insurance-Coverage-Access-to-and-Quality-of-Care-Among-the-Low-Income-Population.pdf [September 26, 2007].

Libby, A. M., Cuellar, A., Snowden, L. R., and Orton, H. D. (2002). Substitution in a Medicaid mental health carve out: Services and costs. *Journal of Health Care Finance, 28*, 11–23.

Lieu, T. A., Newacheck, P. W., and McManus, M. A. (1993). Race, ethnicity, and access to ambulatory care among U.S. adolescents. *American Journal of Public Health, 83*, 960–965.

Liu, J., Probst, J. C., Martin, A. B., Wang, J. Y., and Salina, C. F. (2007). Disparities in dental insurance coverage and dental care among U.S. children: The National Survey of Children's Health. *Pediatrics, 119*, S12–S21.

Manski, R. J., and Brown, E. (2007). *Dental Use, Expenses, Private Dental Coverage, and Changes, 1996 and 2004*. MEPS Chartbook No. 17. Rockville, MD: Agency for Healthcare Research and Quality.

McNulty, M., and Covert, C. (2001). *Financing Preventive Services for Low-Income Adolescents: A State Medicaid Policy Study*. Rochester, NY: University of Rochester School of Medicine.

Mercer Health and Benefits. (2007). *2006 National Survey of Employer-Sponsored Health Plans—Survey Highlights*. New York: Mercer Health and Benefits.

National Adolescent Health Information Center. (2005). *A Health Profile of Adolescent and Young Adult Males*. San Francisco: University of California.

New Freedom Commission on Mental Health. (2003). *Achieving the Promise: Transforming Mental Health Care in America. Final Report*. DHHS Pub. No. SMA-03-3832. Rockville, MD: U.S. Department of Health and Human Services.

Newacheck, P. W., Brindis, C. D., Cart, C. U., Marchi, K., and Irwin, C. E., Jr. (1999). Adolescent health insurance coverage: Recent changes and access to care. *Pediatrics, 104*, 195–202.

Newhouse, J. P. (2004). Consumer-directed health plans and the rand health insurance experiment. *Health Affairs, 23*, 107–113.

Newhouse, J. P., and Insurance Experiment Group. (1993). *Free for All? Lessons from the RAND Health Insurance Experiment*. Cambridge, MA: Harvard University Press.

Nutt, P., and Hogan, M. (2005). Downsizing best practices: A 12-year study of change in a state mental health system. *New Research in Mental Health, 16*, 209–221.

Olson, L. M., Tang, S.-F., and Newacheck, P. W. (2005). Children in the United States with discontinuous health insurance coverage. *New England Journal of Medicine, 353*, 382–391.

Peele, P. B., Lave, J. R., and Kelleher, K. J. (2002). Exclusions and limitations in children's behavioral health care coverage. *Psychiatric Services, 53*, 591–594.

Robinson, G., Kaye, N., Bergman, D., Moreaux, M., and Baxter, C. (2003). *State Profiles of Mental Health and Substance Abuse Services in Medicaid*. Rockville, MD: U.S. Department of Health and Human Services, Substance Abuse and Mental Health Services Administration, Center for Mental Health Services.

Rosenbaum, S., Stewart, A., Cox, M., and Lee, A. (2003) *The Epidemiology of U.S. Immunization Law: Medicaid Coverage of Immunization for Non-Institutionalized Adults*. Washington, DC: Center for Health Services Research and Policy, George Washington University.

Schur, C. L., and Feldman, J. 2001. *Running in Place: How Job Characteristics, Immigrant Status, and Family Structure Keep Hispanics Uninsured*. New York: The Project HOPE Center for Health Affairs and the Commonwealth Fund.

Schwalberg, R., Zimmerman, B., Mohamadi, L., Giffen, M., and Anderson Mathis, S. (2001). *Medicaid Coverage of Family Planning Services: Results of a National Survey*. Washington, DC: The Kaiser Family Foundation.

Semansky, R., and Koyanagi, C. (2004). Obtaining child mental health services through Medicaid: The experience of parents in two states. *Psychiatric Services, 55*, 24–25.

Shenkman, E., Youngblade, L., and Nackashi, J. (2003). Adolescents' preventive care experiences before entry into the State Children's Health Insurance Program. *Pediatrics, 112*, e533–e541.

Solomon, J. (2007). *Cost-Sharing and Premiums in Medicaid. What Rules Apply?* Washington, DC: Center on Budget and Policy Priorities.

Stroul, B. A., Pires, S. A., Armstrong, M. I., and Meyers, J. C. (1998). The impact of managed care on mental health services for children and their families. *The Future of Children, 8*, 119–133.

Tang, S.-F. (2001). *Medicaid Reimbursement Survey, 2001: 50 States and the District of Columbia*. Elk Grove Village, IL: American Academy of Pediatrics, Division of Health Policy Research.

Tang, S.-F., Yudkoswky, B. K., and Davis, J. C. (2003). Medicaid participation by private and safety-net pediatricians, 1993 and 2000. *Pediatrics, 112*, 368–372.

Thomas, C. R., and Holzer, C. E. (1999). National distribution of child and adolescent psychiatrists. *Journal of the American Academy of Child and Adolescent Psychiatry, 38*, 9–16.

U.S. Bureau of Labor Statistics. (2005). *National Compensation Survey: Employee Benefits in Private Industry in the United States, 2003*. Bulletin 2577. Washington, DC: U.S. Department of Labor.

U.S. Bureau of Labor Statistics. (2006). *National Compensation Survey: Employee Benefits in Private Industry in the United States, March 2006*. Summary 06-05. Washington, DC: U.S. Department of Labor.

U.S. Department of Health and Human Services. (1999). *Mental Health: A Report of the Surgeon General—Executive Summary*. Rockville, MD: U.S. Department of Health and Human Services, Substance Abuse and Mental Health Services Administration, Center for Mental Health Services, National Institutes of Health, National Institute of Mental Health.

Yu, S. M., Bellamy, H. A., Schwalberg, R. H., and Drum, M. A. (2001). Factors associated with use of preventive dental and health services among U.S. adolescents. *Journal of Adolescent Health, 29*, 395–405.

Yu, S. M., Bellamy, H. A., Kogan, M. D., Dunbar, J. L., Schwalberg, R. H., and Schuster, M. A. (2002). Factors that influence receipt of recommended preventive pediatric health and dental care. *Pediatrics, 110*, e73–e81.

Zuckerman, S., McFeeters, J., Cunningham, P., and Nichols, L. (2004). Changes in Medicaid physician fee, 1998–2003: Implications for physician participation. *Health Affairs, 23*, Web Exclusive. Available: http://content.healthaffairs.org/cgi/content/full/hlthaff.W4.374/DC1 [October 13, 2008].

7

Overall Conclusions and Recommendations

According to the World Health Organization (1995, p. 3), "One of the most important commitments a country can make for future economic, social, and political progress and stability is to address the health and development needs of its adolescents." Adolescence is a time of major transition between childhood and adulthood. It is a period when significant physical, psychological, and behavioral changes occur and when young people develop many of the habits, behaviors, and relationships they will carry into their adult lives. The health system has a crucial role to play in promoting healthful behavior and preventing disease during adolescence.

The National Academies' Board on Children, Youth, and Families formed the Committee on Adolescent Health Care Services and Models of Care for Treatment, Prevention, and Healthy Development, with funding from The Atlantic Philanthropies, in May 2006 to study adolescent health and the adolescent health system. This committee was asked to explore the following issues:

- **Features of Quality Adolescent Health Services.** What does the evidence base suggest constitutes high-quality health care and health promotion services for adolescent populations? What do parents, community leaders, and adolescents themselves perceive to be essential features of such services?
- **Approaches to the Provision of Adolescent Health Services.** What are the strengths and limitations of different service models in addressing adolescent health care needs? What lessons have been learned in efforts to promote linkages and integration among ado-

lescent health care, health promotion, and adolescent development services? What service approaches show significant promise in offering primary care as well as prevention, treatment, and health promotion services for adolescents with special health care needs and for selected adolescent populations?
- **Organizational Settings and Strategies.** What organizational settings, finance strategies, and communication technologies promote engagement with, access to, and use of health services by adolescents? Are there important differences in the use and outcomes of different service models among selected adolescent populations on the basis of such characteristics as social class, urbanicity, ethnicity, gender, sexual orientation, age, special health care needs, and risk status?
- **Adolescent Health System Supports.** What policies, mechanisms, and contexts promote high-quality health services for adolescents? What innovative strategies have been developed to address such concerns as decision making, privacy, confidentiality, consent, and parental notification in adolescent health care settings? What strategies help adolescents engage with and navigate the health care system, especially those at significant risk for health disorders in such areas as sexual and reproductive health, substance use, mental health, violence, and diet? What barriers impede the optimal provision of adolescent health services?
- **Adolescent Health Care Providers.** What kinds of training programs for health care providers are necessary to improve the quality of health care for adolescent populations?

CHALLENGES, LIMITATIONS, AND SUCCESSES

The committee was challenged in addressing the above issues because (1) the relevant data and scientific literature are limited in a number of key areas; (2) a broad diversity of profiles characterizes adolescents aged 10–19 in the United States; (3) the health status of adolescents is defined by multiple measures, including not only traditional measures of mortality and morbidity, but also behavioral characteristics; (4) health services for adolescents comprise a series of individual services delivered in myriad settings and through varied institutional structures, with limited common goals and no coherent, organizing system; (5) evaluation of health services for adolescents has been limited, and there is no agreed-upon set of standards within the field of adolescent health with which to evaluate the success of individual programs or compare services and service models; and (6) information on issues related to the adolescent health workforce, such as competency requirements for health professionals who work with adolescents, is difficult to obtain.

To carry out this study in the face of these challenges, the committee:

- Conducted a comprehensive review of the existing evidence on the health status of adolescents.
- Examined the current health system as it relates to the care of adolescents—health services available to adolescents, the settings where they receive these services, how the services are delivered and by whom. To this end, the committee:
  - reviewed the existing literature.
  - visited programs that provide a range of adolescent health services.
  - commissioned papers on a number of the issues the committee was asked to address.
  - conducted public workshops with invited expert speakers to solicit additional information on these issues.
  - interviewed both adolescents and health care providers.

The committee then applied its collective expertise and experience to consolidate and deliberate upon this wide range of information. In its deliberations, the committee identified important areas of emphasis for adolescent health services, as well as behavioral and contextual characteristics that require attention in the design of these services; agreed upon standards of service quality; and made an assessment of the gaps between these standards and the current range of services available to adolescents. The committee also reviewed the training needs and current requirements for providers of adolescent health services and identified deficits in these areas. In addition, it examined health insurance alternatives for adolescents and assessed the extent to which public and private financing options meet adolescents' health service needs.

As a result of these efforts, the committee formulated many findings that are highlighted throughout this report. In this final chapter, these findings are summarized and consolidated into seven overall conclusions. These conclusions serve in turn as the basis for the committee's eleven recommendations, directed to both public and private entities, for investing in, strengthening, and improving the system of health services for adolescents.

SUMMARY FINDINGS AND OVERALL CONCLUSIONS

Adolescent Health Status

Adolescents aged 10–19 make up a significant portion of the total U.S. population—14 percent (42 million) in 2006. The health of adolescents can be defined by traditional measures (mortality rates, incidence of disease, and prevalence of chronic conditions). A more complex and complete picture of adolescent health status, however, also encompasses the prevalence of various leading adolescent behaviors and health outcomes, as well as health indicators that may adversely affect health status in adulthood.

An analysis of the 21 Critical Health Objectives for ages 10–24, a subset of the Centers for Disease Control and Prevention's (CDC's) Healthy People 2010, highlights how little progress has been made in the overall health status of adolescents since the year 2000. Of the 21 objectives—which encompass a broad range of concerns, from reducing deaths, reducing suicides, and increasing mental health treatment to increasing seat belt use, reducing binge drinking, and reducing weapon carrying—the only ones that have shown improvement for adolescents since 2000 are behaviors leading to unintentional injury, pregnancy, and tobacco use. Negative trends include increased mortality due to motor vehicle crashes related to alcohol, increased obesity/overweight, and decreased physical activity.

Certain groups of adolescents have particularly high rates of comorbidity, defined as the simultaneous occurrence of two or more diseases, health conditions, or risky behaviors. These adolescents are particularly vulnerable to poor health. Moreover, specific groups of adolescents—such as those who are poor; in the foster care system; homeless; in families that have recently immigrated to the United States; lesbian, gay, bisexual, or transgender; or in the juvenile justice system—may have higher rates of chronic health problems and may engage in more risky behavior as compared with the overall adolescent population. These adolescents may have especially complex health issues that often are not addressed by the health services and settings they use. Furthermore, members of racial and ethnic minorities are becoming a larger portion of the overall U.S. adolescent population. And because minority racial or ethnic status is closely linked to poverty and a lack of access to quality health services, the number of adolescents experiencing significant disparities in access to quality health services can be expected to increase as well.

> Overall Conclusion 1: Most adolescents are thriving, but many engage in risky behavior, develop unhealthful habits, and experience physical and mental health conditions that can jeopardize their immediate health and contribute to poor health in adulthood.

Features of Quality Adolescent Health Services

The committee was asked to consider what features constitute high-quality adolescent health services. The provision of such services is dependent on successful interactions between adolescents and health service settings and systems, and achieving this requires a multifaceted approach. The committee was guided by two basic frameworks in its data collection, review of the evidence, and deliberations on various dimensions of adolescent health status and health services. The first of these frameworks focuses on behavioral and contextual characteristics that influence how adolescents interact with the health system, and the second on the objectives of adolescent health services. Neither framework alone is sufficient to explain significant variations in adolescent health outcomes; rather, they complement each other and, in tandem, provide a more complete picture of the features of the health system that should be improved in order to provide adolescents high quality care and thus help to improve their health status.

Framework 1: Behavioral and Contextual Characteristics

Certain sets of behavioral and contextual characteristics, listed below, matter for adolescents in the ways they approach and interact with health care services, providers, and settings. When these characteristics are addressed in the design of health services for adolescents, those services can offer high-quality care that is particularly attuned to the needs of this age group. These characteristics helped frame the chapters of this report and, where relevant and supported by the evidence, are reflected in the committee's recommendations.

- **Development matters.** Adolescence is a period of significant and dramatic change spanning the physical, biological, social, and psychological transitions from childhood to young adulthood. This dynamic state influences both the health of young people and the health services they require.
- **Timing matters.** Adolescence is a critical time for health promotion. Many health problems and much of the risky behavior that underlies later health problems begin during adolescence. Prevention, early intervention, and timely treatment improve health status for adolescents and prepare them for healthy adulthood; such services also decrease the incidence of many chronic diseases in adulthood.
- **Context matters.** Social context and such factors as income, geography, and cultural norms and values can profoundly affect the health of adolescents and the health services they receive.

- **Need matters.** Some segments of the adolescent population, defined by both biology and behavior, have health needs that require particular attention in health systems.
- **Participation matters.** Effective health services for young people invite adolescents and their families to engage with clinicians.
- **Family matters.** At the same time that adolescents are growing in their autonomy, families continue to affect adolescents' health and overall well-being and to influence what health services they use. Young people without adequate family support are particularly vulnerable to risky behavior and poor health and therefore often require additional support in health service settings.
- **Community matters.** Good health services for adolescents encompass population-focused as well as individual and family services since the environment in which adolescents live, as well as the supports they receive in the community, are important.
- **Skill matters.** Young people are best served by providers who understand the key developmental features, health issues, and overall social environment of adolescents.
- **Money matters.** The availability, nature, and content of health services for adolescents are affected by such financial factors as public and private health insurance, the amount of funding invested in special programs for adolescents, and the support available for adequate training programs for providers of adolescent health services.
- **Policy matters.** Policies, both public and private, can have a profound effect on adolescent health services. Carefully crafted policies are a foundation for strong systems of care that meet a wide variety of individual and community needs.

Framework 2: Objectives of Health Services for Adolescents

Research from various sources and the experiences of adolescents and health care providers, health organizations, and research centers suggest the importance of designing health services that can attract and engage adolescents, create opportunities to discuss sensitive health and behavioral issues, and offer high-quality care as well as guidance for health promotion and disease prevention. Consistent with these findings and views, a variety of national and international organizations have defined critical elements of health systems that would improve adolescents' access to appropriate services, highlighted design elements that would improve the quality of those services, and identified ways to foster patient–provider relationships that can lead to better health for adolescents.

The World Health Organization has identified five characteristics that constitute objectives for responsive adolescent health services:

- **Accessible.** Policies and procedures ensure that services are broadly accessible.
- **Acceptable.** Policies and procedures consider culture and relationships and the climate of engagement.
- **Appropriate.** Health services fulfill the needs of all young people.
- **Effective.** Health services reflect evidence-based standards of care and professional guidelines.
- **Equitable.** Policies and procedures do not restrict the provision of and eligibility for services.

These five objectives provided the committee with a valuable framework for assessing the use, adequacy, and quality of adolescent health services; comparing the extent to which different services, settings, and providers meet the health needs of young people in the United States; identifying the gaps that keep services from achieving these objectives; and recommending ways to close these gaps.

Approaches to the Provision of Adolescent Health Services and Organizational Settings and Strategies

The committee was asked to explore the range of approaches to the provision of adolescent health services and elucidate their respective strengths and limitations. In doing so, the committee was to highlight efforts aimed at promoting linkages and integration among adolescent health care, health promotion, and adolescent development services, and at offering primary care, prevention, treatment, and health promotion services for adolescents with special health care needs and for selected subpopulations. This study was also focused on settings and strategies that influence the use and outcomes of different services by the diverse adolescent population.

Adolescents receive both primary care and specialty care services. They receive these services in various settings, including private physician and dentist offices, community outpatient departments, school-based health centers, emergency departments, and even mobile vans, and from various providers, including doctors, nurse practitioners, dentists, psychologists, and social workers.

Evidence shows that while private office-based primary care services are available to most adolescents, those services depend significantly on fee-based reimbursement and are not always accessible, acceptable, appropriate, or effective for some adolescents, particularly those who are uninsured or underinsured. Such young people often have difficulty gaining access to mainstream primary care services; require additional support in order to connect with health care providers; and may rely extensively on such safety-net settings as hospital-, community-, and school-based health centers for their primary care. For example, adolescents are the age group most likely to depend on emergency departments for routine health care. Indeed, evidence shows that for some adolescents, safety-net settings may be more accessible, acceptable, appropriate, effective, and equitable than mainstream services. This may be especially so for more vulnerable populations of uninsured or underinsured adolescents. Although an extensive literature on the quality of school-based health services for adolescents is available, few studies have examined the quality of other safety-net primary care services, such as those that are hospital- or community-based, on which so many adolescents depend.

Evidence also shows that existing specialty services in the areas of mental health, sexual and reproductive health, oral health, and substance abuse treatment are not accessible to most adolescents, nor do they always meet the needs of many adolescents who receive care in safety-net settings. Even when such services are accessible, many adolescents may not find them acceptable because of concerns that confidentiality is not fully ensured, especially in such sensitive domains as substance use or sexual and reproductive health.

In general, the committee found that some existing models of primary and specialty care services for adolescents reflect one or more of the five objectives of accessibility, acceptability, appropriateness, effectiveness, and equity. However, none of these models have been demonstrated to possess all five of these characteristics.

> **Overall Conclusion 2:** Many current models of health services for adolescents exist. There is insufficient evidence to indicate that any one particular approach to health services for adolescents achieves significantly better results than others.

Furthermore, the committee found that the various settings, services, and providers used by adolescents often are not coordinated with each other, and the result is barriers to and gaps in care. In some areas, such as the organization of mental health services for adolescents, the system of services is in substantial disarray because of financing barriers, eligibility gaps, and both confidentiality and privacy concerns—all of which can hamper transitions across care settings.

> **Overall Conclusion 3:** Health services for adolescents currently consist of separate programs and services that are often highly fragmented,

poorly coordinated, and delivered in multiple public and private settings.

The committee also found that many adolescent health services and settings take a limited, problem-oriented approach and focus on care for certain health conditions or specific issues, thus failing to meet the broader needs and behavioral challenges that characterize adolescence. Because of this narrow focus, many providers of health services are poorly equipped to foster disease prevention and health promotion for adolescents. This is especially true in the areas of mental health, oral health, and substance abuse, as well as services that address sexual behavior and reproductive health.

Overall Conclusion 4: Health services for adolescents are poorly equipped to meet the disease prevention, health promotion, and behavioral health needs of all adolescents. Instead, adolescent health services are focused mainly on the delivery of care for acute conditions, such as infections and injuries, or special care addressing specific issues, such as contraception or substance abuse.

Adolescent Health System Supports

The committee was asked to explore the policies and mechanisms of support that promote high-quality health services for adolescents, as well as the barriers that impede optimal service provision. In doing so, the committee considered issues related to privacy and confidentiality, as well as health insurance.

Privacy and Confidentiality

Concerns about privacy and confidentiality may be a significant aspect of many adolescents' interactions with health services. During screening and assessment, for example, sensitivity to stigma and bias may affect the adolescent patient's willingness to trust and communicate with health professionals or return for follow-up care. As well, while professional guidelines for the practice of adolescent medicine stress the importance of privacy and confidentiality in interactions with adolescent patients, parents frequently receive information about their children's health services. Many medical professionals recognize the importance of parents' involvement in their adolescent children's health care decisions. At the same time, however, privacy concerns influence adolescents' willingness to seek services at all, their choice of provider, their candor in giving a health history, their willingness to accept specific services, and other important aspects of access to care. The committee found evidence showing that confidentiality increases the acceptability of services and the willingness of adolescents to seek them, especially for issues related to sexual behavior, reproductive health, mental health, and substance use. The committee concluded that existing state and federal policies generally protect the confidentiality of adolescents' health information when they are legally allowed to consent to their own care, and that it is critical that any efforts to improve health systems for adolescents ensure continued consent and confidentiality for adolescents seeking care.

Health Insurance

The committee found that financial support for health services is fundamental to promoting adolescents' engagement with, access to, and use of these services. More than 5 million adolescents aged 10–18 are uninsured. Uninsured rates are higher among the poor and near poor, racial and ethnic minorities, and noncitizens. As is true for all Americans, uninsured adolescents are less likely to have a regular source of primary care and use medical and dental care less often than those who have insurance. Having health insurance, however, does not ensure adolescents' access to affordable, high-quality services given current shortages of health care providers and problems associated with high out-of-pocket cost-sharing requirements, limitations in benefit packages, and low provider reimbursement levels, especially in areas that involve counseling or case management of multiple health conditions. For example, the current system of health insurance coverage is often limited or nonexistent for treatment and prevention in areas that are particularly problematic for adolescents, such as obesity, intentional and unintentional injury, mental health, dental care, and substance abuse. Furthermore, uninsured adolescents aged 10–18 who are eligible for public coverage often are not enrolled either because their parents do not know they are eligible or because complexities of the enrollment processes deter participation.

> **Overall Conclusion 5: Large numbers of adolescents are uninsured or have inadequate health insurance, which can lead to a lack of access to regular primary care, as well as limited behavioral, medical, and dental care. One result of such barriers and deficits is poorer health.**

Adolescent Health Care Providers

The committee was asked to consider the elements of health provider training necessary to improving the quality of health services for adolescent populations. The committee found that whether providers report on their own perceptions of their competencies or adolescents describe the care they have received, data reveal significant gaps in the achievement of a well-equipped and appropriately trained workforce ready to meet the health needs of adolescents. At all levels of professional education, health care providers in every discipline serving adolescents should receive specific and detailed education in the nature of adolescents' health problems and have in their clinical repertoire a range of effective ways to treat and prevent disease in this age group, as well as to promote healthy behavior and lifestyles within a developmental framework. Evidence suggests this currently is not the case.

Overall Conclusion 6: Health care providers working with adolescents frequently lack the necessary skills to interact appropriately and effectively with this age group.

Research Needs

Developing a clear definition of adolescent health status is a critical step in delivering health services and forming health systems that can respond appropriately to the specific needs of adolescents. Moreover, the ability to understand and characterize health status within this definition is dependent on available data, particularly that related to adolescent behavior. Those concerned with the health of adolescents—health practitioners, policy makers, and families—would benefit from ready access to high-quality and more precise data that would aid in better understanding the consequences of health-influencing behaviors for the health status of adolescents.

Overall Conclusion 7: The characterization of adolescents and their health status by such traditional measures as injury and illness does not adequately capture the developmental and behavioral health of adolescents of different ages and in diverse circumstances.

This report proposes several approaches to improving health systems for adolescents to make services more accessible, acceptable, appropriate, effective, and equitable. Such improvements are particularly important to support healthy development for those adolescents who are more vulnerable to poor health or unhealthful habits and risky behavior because of their demographic characteristics or other circumstances. As noted above, however, limited evidence is available on health outcomes associated with alternative service approaches. Therefore, the committee attempted to identify areas in which research could yield knowledge that would support quality improvements in the organization and delivery of health services for adolescents. For example, the evidentiary base currently does not support the formulation of performance standards and operational criteria that would make it possible to compare the strengths and limitations of different service delivery models in meeting the needs of all adolescents, as well as specific subpopulations. In particular, few evaluations provide insight into the validity and reliability of screening tools and counseling techniques for the most vulnerable groups of adolescents. Efforts to improve the knowledge base on the provision of services to these groups should therefore be a major priority in efforts to improve health services and the quality of care for adolescents.

LOOKING AHEAD: RECOMMENDATIONS

The committee's ultimate goal in this report is to synthesize contemporary issues in adolescent health and to examine strengths and deficiencies in the health system that responds to these issues. The report also provides a framework for identifying key objectives of a high-quality system of health services for all adolescents in the United States, with particular attention to those who engage more heavily in risky behavior or who face major barriers in gaining access to health services.

Based on the overall conclusions presented above and reflecting the need for a multifaceted approach to fostering successful interactions between adolescents and health service settings and systems, the committee makes eleven recommendations, directed to both public and private entities, for investing in, strengthening, and improving health services for adolescents. These recommendations embody many of the behavioral and contextual characteristics—development, timing, context, need, participation, family, community, skill, money, and policy—that the committee explored in its evidence review. If acted upon in a coordinated and comprehensive manner, the following recommendations should improve the accessibility, acceptability, appropriateness, effectiveness, and equity of health services delivered to adolescents.

Primary Health Care

Recommendation 1: Federal and state agencies, private foundations, and private insurers should support and promote the development and use of a coordinated primary health care system that strives to improve health services for all adolescents.

Carrying out this recommendation would involve federal and state agencies, private foundations, and private insurers working with local primary care providers to coordinate services between primary and specialty care services. It would also entail providing opportunities for primary care services to interact with health programs for adolescents in multiple safety-net settings, such as schools, hospitals, and community health centers.

Recommendation 2: As part of an enhanced primary care system for adolescents, health care providers and health organizations should focus attention on the particular needs of specific groups of adolescents who may be especially vulnerable to risky behavior or poor health because of selected population characteristics or other circumstances.

Implementing this recommendation would involve focusing explicit attention on issues of access, acceptability, appropriateness, effectiveness, and equity of health services for an increasingly racially and ethnically diverse population of adolescents and for selected adolescent groups, such as those who are poor; in the foster care system; homeless; in families that have recently immigrated to the United States; lesbian, gay, bisexual, or transgender; or in the juvenile justice system.

Recommendation 3: Providers of adolescent primary care services and the payment systems that support them should make disease prevention, health promotion, and behavioral health—including early identification, management, and monitoring of current or emerging health conditions and risky behavior—a major component of routine health services.

For this recommendation to be realized, providers of adolescent primary care services would need to give attention to the coordination and management of the specialty services young people often need. They would coordinate screening, assessment, health management, and referrals to specialty services. They would also monitor behavior that increases risk in such areas as injury, mental health, oral health, substance use, violence, eating disorders, sexual activity, and exercise. Performance measures for these services would need to be incorporated into criteria used for credentialing, pay-for-performance incentives, and quality measurement. And perhaps most important, payment systems would need to finance such services and activities.

Public Health System

Recommendation 4: Within communities—and with the help of public agencies—health care providers, health organizations, and community agencies should develop coordinated, linked, and interdisciplinary adolescent health services.

To effect this recommendation, health care providers across communities would need to work together to encourage rapid and coordinated services through collocation or participation in regional planning and action groups organized by managed care plans, large group networks, health professional associations, or public health agencies. Beyond direct patient services, primary care providers and providers of mental health/substance abuse, reproductive, nutritional, and oral health services would have to establish public and private programs in a region for managing referrals; coordinating electronic patient information; and staffing adolescent call centers and regional services to communicate directly with adolescents, their families, and various providers. In addition, the particular health needs of adolescents, especially the most vulnerable populations, would need to be addressed in the development of electronic health records. Such records offer a significant opportunity to ensure coordinated care, as well as to provide adolescent-focused patient portals, messaging and reminder services, and electronic personalized health education services to improve interventions. An overarching principle in the implementation of this recommendation is that adolescents should be asked to give explicit consent for the sharing of information about them, a point addressed in the committee's next recommendation.

Privacy and Confidentiality

Recommendation 5: Federal and state policy makers should maintain current laws, policies, and ethical guidelines that enable adolescents who are minors to give their own consent for health services and to receive those services on a confidential basis when necessary to protect their health.

To implement this recommendation, federal and state policy makers would need to examine the variations among states in the age of consent for care for adolescents and consider the impact of such variations on adolescents' access to and use of services that are essential to protecting their health (e.g., services for contraception, sexually transmitted infections/HIV, mental health, and substance use). A balance is needed between maintaining the confidentiality of information and records regarding care for which adolescent minors are allowed to give their consent, and encouraging the involvement of parents and families in the health services received by adolescents whenever possible, both supporting and respecting their role and importance in adolescents' lives and health care.

Adolescent Health Care Providers

Recommendation 6: Regulatory bodies for health professions in which an appreciable number of providers offer care to adolescents should incorporate a minimal set of competencies in adolescent health care and development into their licensing, certification, and accreditation requirements.

To implement this recommendation, regulatory bodies would need to use national meetings of specialists and educators/scholars within relevant disciplines to define competencies in adolescent health. They would also have to require professionals who serve adolescents in health care settings to complete a minimum amount of education in basic areas of adolescent development, health issues unique to this life stage, and a life course framework that encourages providers to focus on helping their adolescent patients develop healthful habits that can be carried forward into their adult lives. Finally, agencies that fund training programs would have to adhere to the requirements of the regulatory bodies (i.e., with regard to accreditation, licensure, and certification, and to maintenance of licensure or certification where appropriate), and content on adolescent health would have to be mandatory in all relevant training programs.

> Recommendation 7: Public and private funders should provide targeted financial support to expand and sustain interdisciplinary training programs in adolescent health. Such programs should strive to prepare specialists, scholars, and educators in all relevant health disciplines to work with both the general adolescent population and selected groups that require special and/or more intense services.

To effect this recommendation, public and private funders would need to ensure that professionals who serve adolescents in health care settings are trained in how to relate to adolescents and gain their trust and cooperation; how to develop strong provider–patient relationships; and how to identify early signs of risky and unhealthful behavior that may require further assessment, intervention, or referral. Also essential to the training of these professionals is knowing how to work with more vulnerable adolescents, such as those who are in the foster care system; homeless; in families that have recently immigrated to the United States; lesbian, gay, bisexual, or transgender; or in the juvenile justice system. Important as well is to increase the number of Leadership Education in Adolescent Health programs that train health professionals in adolescent medicine, psychology, nursing, social work, and nutrition, and to enhance the program by adding dentistry.

Health Insurance

> Recommendation 8: Federal and state policy makers should develop strategies to ensure that all adolescents have comprehensive, continuous health insurance coverage.

Federal and state legislatures and governments should consider the following options for implementing this recommendation: require states to provide Medicaid or other forms of health insurance coverage for especially vulnerable or underserved groups of adolescents, particularly those who are in the juvenile justice and foster care systems, and support states in meeting this requirement; design and implement Medicaid and State Children's Health Insurance Program policies to increase enrollment and retention of eligible but uninsured adolescents; and improve incentives for private health insurers to provide such coverage (e.g., by requiring school-based coverage and allowing nongroup policies tailored to adolescents). Note that while these options would increase insurance coverage among adolescents, broader health care reform efforts would be required to ensure universal coverage. A consequence of allowing more segmentation in nongroup health insurance policies across age groups could be increased costs for older adults if younger, healthier adults are removed from the risk pool. In addition, expanding access to and election of coverage among poor adolescents would be necessary to increase the rates of insured adolescents.

Recommendation 9: Federal and state policy makers should ensure that health insurance coverage for adolescents is sufficient in amount, duration, and scope to cover the health services they require. Such coverage should be accessible, acceptable, appropriate, effective, and equitable.

Public and private health plans, including self-insured plans, should consider several options for carrying out this recommendation. First, they could see that benefit packages cover at a minimum the following key services for adolescents: preventive screening and counseling, at least on an annual basis; case management; reproductive health care that includes screening, education, counseling, and treatment; assessment and treatment of mental health conditions, such as anxiety disorders and eating disorders, and of substance abuse disorders, including those comorbid with mental health conditions; and dental services that include prevention, restoration, and treatment. Second, they could ensure coverage for mental health and substance abuse services at primary or specialty care sites that provide integrated physical and mental health care, and require Medicaid to cover mental health rehabilitation services. Third, they could make certain that providers are reimbursed at reasonable, market-based rates for the adolescent health services they provide. Finally, they could ensure that out-of-pocket cost sharing (including mental health and other health services) is set at levels that do not discourage receipt of all needed services.

Research Agenda

Recommendation 10: Federal health agencies and private foundations should prepare a research agenda for improving adolescent health services that includes assessing existing service models, as well as developing new systems for providing services that are accessible, acceptable, appropriate, effective, and equitable.

Federal health agencies should consider a number of options for carrying out this recommendation. First, they could identify performance standards and operational criteria that could be used to compare the strengths and limitations of different models of health service delivery in meeting the needs of all young people, as well as specific groups. In developing such standards and criteria, an effort should be made to translate the features of accessibility, acceptability, appropriateness, effectiveness, and equity into clear standards and ways to measure their achievement. Second, they could determine the effectiveness (not just the efficacy) of selected mental health, behavioral, and developmental interventions for adolescents. This research should be aimed at identifying individual, environmental, and other contextual factors that significantly affect the likelihood of establishing, operating, and sustaining effective interventions in a variety of service settings. Third, they could assess and compare the health status (defined by selected population characteristics and other circumstances) and health outcomes of young people who receive care through different service models and in different health settings, as well as of those who are difficult to reach and serve. Fourth, they could identify effective ways to reach more underserved and vulnerable adolescents with appropriate and accessible health services. Such research might also consider how to integrate the features of accessibility, acceptability, appropriateness, effectiveness, and equity into the primary care environment for all adolescents, as well as into the training of providers who interact with adolescents. Finally, they could evaluate the validity and reliability of various screening tools and counseling techniques for selected groups of adolescents.

Monitoring Progress

Recommendation 11: The Federal Interagency Forum on Child and Family Statistics should work with federal agencies and, when possible, states to organize and disseminate data on the health and health services, including developmental and behavioral health, of adolescents. These data should encompass adolescents generally, with subreports by age, selected population characteristics, and other circumstances.

To implement this recommendation, federal agencies would need to adopt consistent age brackets that cluster data by ages 10–14 and 15–19 and consistent identifiers of socioeconomic status, geographic location, gender, and race and ethnicity. Also needed are consistent identifiers of specific vulnerable adolescent populations, including those in the foster care system; those who are homeless; those who are in families that have recently immigrated to the United States; those who are lesbian, gay, bisexual, or transgender; and those in the juvenile justice system. Important as well is to track emerging disparities in access to and utilization of health services, with attention to specific components of health care, such as screening, assessment, and referral, as well as an emphasis on racial and ethnic differences. Finally, longitudinal studies are needed on the effects of both health-promoting and health-compromising behaviors that often emerge in the second decade of life and continue into adulthood.

CLOSING THOUGHTS

While the gaps and problems in the health services used by young people discussed in this report are not unique to this age group, a compelling case can be made for improving health services and systems both to support the healthy development of adolescents and to enhance their transitions from childhood to adolescence and from adolescence to adulthood. Current interest in restructuring the way health care is delivered and financed in the United States—and defining the content of care itself more broadly—is based on a growing awareness that existing health services and systems for virtually all Americans have important and costly shortcomings. In the midst of these discussions, the distinct deficits faced by adolescents within the health system deserve particular attention. Their developmental complexities and risky behavior, together with the need to extend their care beyond the usual disease- and injury-focused services, are key considerations in any attempt to reform the nation's chaotic health care system—especially if adolescents are to benefit. Even if the larger systemic issues of access to the health system were resolved, more would likely need to be done to achieve better health for adolescents during both the adolescent years and the transition to adulthood.

REFERENCE

World Health Organization, United Nations Population Fund, and United Nations Children's Fund. (1995). *Action for Adolescent Health: Towards a Common Agenda*: *Recommendations from a Joint Study Group*. Available: http://www.who.int/child_adolescent_health/documents/frh_adh_97_9/en/index.html [May 28, 2008].

Appendix A

Acronyms

AAFP	American Academy of Family Physicians
AAP	American Academy of Pediatrics
ABPP	American Board of Professional Psychology
ACOG	American College of Obstetricians and Gynecologists
ADD	attention-deficit disorder
ADHD	attention-deficit hyperactivity disorder
AIDS	acquired immunodeficiency syndrome
APA	American Psychological Association
AUDIT	Alcohol Use Disorders Identification Test
BMI	body mass index
BYC	Broadway Youth Center
CBT	cognitive-behavioral therapy
CCM	Chronic Care Model
CDC	Centers for Disease Control and Prevention
CSAT	Center for Substance Abuse Treatment
DATOS	Drug Abuse Treatment Outcome Study
DAWN	Drug Abuse Warning Network
DHHS	U.S. Department of Health and Human Services
DHWP	Department of Health and Wellness Promotion
DOD	Department of Defense
DSM-IV	*Diagnostic and Statistical Manual*, 4th edition

EHR	electronic health record
EOB	explanations of benefits
EPSDT	Early Periodic Screening, Diagnosis, and Treatment
ERISA	Employee Retirement Income Security Act
GAIN	Global Appraisal of Individual Need
GAPS	Guidelines for Adolescent Preventive Services
GED	General Educational Development
GLBTQ	gay, lesbian, bisexual, transgender, or questioning
HIT	health information technology
HIV	human immunodeficiency virus
HMO	health maintenance organization
HPV	human papillomavirus
HRSA	Health Resources and Services Administration
IMG	integrated medical group
IOM	Institute of Medicine
IPA	Independent Practice Association Physician Group
IT	information technology
LEAH	Leadership Education in Adolescent Health
LGBT	lesbian, gay, bisexual, or transgender
LSU	Louisiana State University
MCHB	Maternal and Child Health Bureau
MCHPRC	Maternal and Child Health Policy Research Center
MEPS	Medical Expenditure Panel Survey
MET/CBT	motivational enhancement therapy/cognitive-behavioral therapy
NAHIC	National Adolescent Health Information Center
NAS	National Academy of Sciences
NHAMCS	National Hospital Ambulatory Medical Care Survey
NHANES	National Health and Nutrition Examination Survey
NHDS	National Hospital Discharge Survey
NHIS	National Health Interview Survey
NIAAA	National Institute on Alcohol Abuse and Alcoholism
NIDA	National Institute on Drug Abuse
NRC	National Research Council
NSDUH	National Survey on Drug Use and Health
NSFG	National Survey of Family Growth
NSSATS	National Survey of Substance Abuse Treatment Services

NVSS	National Vital Statistics System
OTA	Office of Technology Assessment
OYD	Office of Youth Development
PIPPAH	Partnership in Program Planning for Adolescent Health
POSIT	Problem Oriented Screening Instrument for Teenagers
PRC	Prevention Research Center
PTSD	post-traumatic stress disorder
SAM	Society of Adolescent Medicine
SAMHSA	Substance Abuse and Mental Health Services Administration
SCHIP	State Children's Health Insurance Program
SCORM	Shared Content Object Reference Model
SPEEK	Sinai Peers Encouraging Empowerment through Knowledge
SSI	Supplemental Security Income
STI	sexually transmitted infection
TANF	Temporary Aid to Needy Families
TB	tuberculosis
TEDS	Treatment Episode Data Set
WHO	World Health Organization
YDI	Youth Development Institute
YRBS	Youth Risk Behavior Survey

Appendix B

Harris Interactive Omnibus Survey Questions

BASE: 12- TO 18-YEAR-OLDS

The next few questions are about health care. Health care includes services provided by a doctor, nurse or other health care provider. It includes checkups, "well" visits, school physicals, or medical care when you are sick or injured.

Q1. Which of the following best describes what you do to get health care from a doctor or other health care provider?

1. I always have my parent or guardian help me get health care services.
2. I usually have my parent or guardian help me get health care services.
3. I rarely have my parent or guardian help me get health care services—only in special situations.
4. I usually have my friends help me get health care services.
5. I always get health care services by myself—I don't get help from family or friends.
6. None of these.

BASE: 12- TO 18-YEAR-OLDS

Q2. What does your parent or guardian usually do to help you get health care from a doctor or other health care provider? Please check all that apply.

1. Pays for all or part of the health care.
2. Helps in scheduling appointments.
3. Helps find the right doctor or health care provider.
4. Drives me or takes me to the doctor's office, hospital or other health care office.
5. Gives me advice on when I should see a doctor or other health care provider.
6. None of these.

BASE: 12- TO 18-YEAR-OLDS

Q3. Which of the following ever prevent you from getting health care? Please check all that apply.

1. It costs too much.
2. I have no health insurance.
3. It is too hard to get to appointments that fit my schedule.
4. I have no way to get to appointments.
5. I am not sure the visits are private or confidential.
6. The medical staff does not understand my ethnic or cultural background.
7. The medical staff is not interested in listening to my concerns.
8. I will not be treated with respect.
9. I am worried that my parents will find out information I don't want them to know.
10. Something else.
11. Nothing prevents me from getting health care.

BASE: SELECTED MORE THAN ONE RESPONSE IN Q3

Q4. What is the main thing that prevents you from getting health care? [DISPLAY ONLY RESPONSES SELECTED IN Q3]

1. It costs too much.
2. I have no health insurance.
3. It is too hard to get to appointments that fit my schedule.
4. I have no way to get to appointments.

5 I am not sure the visits are private or confidential.
6 The medical staff does not understand my ethnic or cultural background.
7 The medical staff is not interested in listening to my concerns.
8 I will not be treated with respect.
9 I am worried that my parents will find out information I don't want them to know.
10 Something else.

BASE: 12- TO 18-YEAR-OLDS

Q5. How interested are you in using email, text messaging or other technology to get health information, be reminded of medical appointments, or speak with a health care provider?

1 Not at all interested.
2 Somewhat interested.
3 Fairly interested.
4 Very interested.
5 Extremely interested.

BASE: 12- TO 18-YEAR-OLDS

Q6. What would you most like to change about your health care to make it more helpful to you? Please include medical, dental, or mental health care services.

Appendix C

Biographical Sketches of Committee Members and Staff

Robert S. Lawrence, MD *(Chair)*, is the Center for a Livable Future Professor and Professor of Environmental Health Sciences, Health Policy, and International Health at The Johns Hopkins University Bloomberg School of Public Health. Dr. Lawrence is a graduate of Harvard College and Harvard Medical School, and trained in internal medicine at the Massachusetts General Hospital in Boston. He served for 3 years as an epidemic intelligence service officer at the Centers for Disease Control, U.S. Public Health Service. Dr. Lawrence is a Master of the American College of Physicians and a Fellow of the American College of Preventive Medicine, and a member of the Institute of Medicine, the Association of Teachers of Preventive Medicine, the American Public Health Association, and Physicians for Human Rights. From 1970 to 1974, he was a member of the faculty of medicine at the University of North Carolina at Chapel Hill, where he helped develop a primary health care system funded by the Office of Economic Opportunity. In 1974, he was appointed as the first director of the Division of Primary Care at Harvard Medical School, where he subsequently served as Charles S. Davidson Associate Professor of Medicine and Chief of Medicine at the Cambridge Hospital until 1991. From 1991 to 1995, he was director of Health Sciences at the Rockefeller Foundation. From 1984 to 1989, Dr. Lawrence chaired the U.S. Preventive Services Task Force of the Department of Health and Human Services; he served on the successor Preventive Services Task Force from 1990 to 1995. He currently serves as a consultant to the Task Force on Community Preventive Services at the Centers for Disease Control and Prevention (CDC). Dr. Lawrence has participated in human rights investigations on behalf of Physicians for Human Rights

(PHR) and other human rights groups in Chile, Czechoslovakia, Egypt, El Salvador, Guatemala, Kosovo, the Philippines, and South Africa. In 1996 Dr. Lawrence became founding director of the Center for a Livable Future at the Bloomberg School of Public Health, an interdisciplinary group of faculty and staff that examines the relationships among diet, food production systems, the environment, and human health.

Linda H. Bearinger, PhD, RN, FAAN, is professor in the University of Minnesota's School of Nursing and director of the Center of Adolescent Nursing, with joint appointments in the Schools of Medicine and Public Health. She has worked in adolescent health for more than 30 years, in schools, clinics, and public health settings. In her work with vulnerable youth, she has provided services ranging from home visiting and school health to program development in numerous community settings. Her research focuses on strategies for protecting vulnerable youth from potentially lifelong problems associated with risky behaviors. Dr. Bearinger lectures and consults nationally and internationally on youth development and the translation of research to practice and policy. She has served on adolescent health expert panels for the World Health Organization, UNICEF, the National Institutes of Health, and the federal Maternal and Child Health Bureau of the Health Resources and Services Administration, U.S. Department of Health and Human Services. Based on her leadership in the field of adolescent health, Dr. Bearinger was named 2004 Adele Hoffman Visiting Research Professor in Adolescent Medicine and Health—the first nurse ever to receive this award from the Society for Adolescent Medicine. She has authored more than 40 peer-reviewed publications, all of which focus on youth issues, as well as articles on the training of health professionals for work with adolescents. She received a BSN in nursing from St. Olaf College, an MS in community health nursing from the University of Colorado, and a PhD in educational psychology from the University of Minnesota.

Shay Bilchik, JD, serves as research professor and director of Georgetown University's Center for Juvenile Justice Reform. Housed in the Georgetown Public Policy Institute, the Center is supporting juvenile justice reform through a multisystems approach. The primary activity of the Center is the engagement of public agency leaders in short, intensive periods of study focused on the key elements of a strong reform agenda. Prior to his current position, Mr. Bilchik was president and CEO of the Child Welfare League of America (CWLA). In that position, he was instrumental in formulating CWLA's child welfare financing reform initiative; began a series of program initiatives and collaborations to strengthen supports for Native American children and families; was an outspoken critic of the death penalty for juveniles; and spearheaded CWLA's support for gay, lesbian, bisexual, transgender, and questioning youth, and the adoption of children by gay parents. In 2001, 2004, 2005, and 2006, he was named among *The NonProfit Times* Power and Influence Top 50 for making his mark in the public policy arena and championing child welfare issues. At the request of the governor of Maryland, Mr. Bilchik served for three years as chair of the State Advisory Board to the Department of Juvenile Justice. Cardinal Theodore McCarrick also appointed him to chair the Child Protection Advisory Board of the Archdiocese of Washington, DC. From March 2003 through February 2007, he chaired the National Collaboration for Youth, a coalition of more than 40 national youth-serving organizations. He has also served on the Ad Council's Children's Campaign Advisory Board since April 2003. Prior to his position at CWLA, he served as Office of Juvenile Justice and Delinquency Prevention Administrator from 1994 to 2000; was an Associate Deputy Attorney General within the U.S. Department of Justice; and held varied positions in the Miami, Florida State Attorney's Office from 1977 to 1993. Mr. Bilchik earned his BS and JD degrees from the University of Florida.

Sarah S. Brown, MPH, is co-founder and CEO of the National Campaign to Prevent Teen and Unplanned Pregnancy. Previously she was a senior study director at the Institute of Medicine, where she led numerous studies in the broad field of maternal and child health. Her last major report at the IOM resulted in the landmark volume, *The Best Intentions: Unintended Pregnancy and the Well-being of Children and Families.* She has served on the boards of many influential national organizations including the Guttmacher Institute, the Population Advisory Board of the David and Lucile Packard Foundation, the American College of Obstetricians and Gynecologists, the DC Mayor's Committee on Reducing Teenage Pregnancies and Out-of-Wedlock Births, and *Teen People* magazine. She speaks frequently on issues of teen sex and unplanned pregnancy, and regularly appears in the television, radio, and print media. Ms. Brown has received numerous awards, including the Institute of Medicine's Cecil Award for Excellence in Research; the John MacQueen Award for Excellence in Maternal and Child Health from the Association of Maternal and Child Health Programs; and the Martha May Elliot Award of the American Public Health Association. She holds an undergraduate degree from Stanford University and a Masters in Public Health degree from the University of North Carolina.

Laurie Chassin, PhD, is Regents Professor of Psychology at the Prevention Research Center of Arizona State University. Her research interests include understanding the development of substance abuse/dependence in adolescence and adulthood (cigarette smoking, alcohol use, and illegal drug use).

Dr. Chassin conducts longitudinal studies of children and families at risk for substance abuse/dependence and associated mental health disorders. She received her PhD from Columbia University.

Thomas G. DeWitt, MD *(Board on Children, Youth, and Families liaison),* is Carl Weihl Professor of Pediatrics, director of the Division of General and Community Pediatrics, and associate chair for education in the Department of Pediatrics at the Cincinnati Children's Hospital Medical Center, University of Cincinnati College of Medicine. He is a peer reviewer for many medical journals, including *Pediatrics*, the *New England Journal of Medicine*, and the *American Journal of Public Health*. Having served as president of the Academic Pediatric Association and chair of the Steering Committee of the American Academy of Pediatrics' Pediatric Research in Office Settings (PROS) network and the Committee on Pediatric Education, he recently completed service on the National Academy of Sciences' Board on Children, Youth, and Families' Committee on Adolescent Health and currently is a member of the United States Preventative Services Task Force and the ACGME Pediatric Residency Review Committee. With over 70 published articles and chapters, he is known nationally and internationally for his work in the areas of faculty development and community-based education and research. He has a BA from Amherst College, an MD degree from University of Rochester, and completed a pediatric residency and Robert Wood Johnson fellowship at Yale.

Nancy Dubler, LLB, is Bioethics Consultant at Montefiore Medical Center, Bronx NY and Professor Emerita, the Albert Einstein College of Medicine. Professor Dubler works primarily in Clinical Ethics Consultation and in Bioethics Mediation. She lectures extensively and is the author of numerous articles and books on termination of care, home and long-term care, geriatrics, adolescent rights and interests, prison and jail health care, and AIDS. She founded the Montefiore Medical Center Division of Bioethics the Clinical Ethics Consultation Service. She also founded the Certificate Program in Bioethics and Medical Humanities, Her most recent books are *The Ethics and Regulation of Research with Human Subjects* (Coleman, Menikoff, Goldner and Dubler, Lexis/Nexis, 2005); *Bioethics Mediation: A Guide to Shaping Shared Solution* (co-authored with Carol Lieberman) United Hospital Fund, New York, New York, 2004); and *Ethics for Health Care Organizations: Theory, Case Studies, and Tools* (with Jeffery Bluestein and Linda Farber Post, 2002). She consults frequently with federal agencies, national working groups, and bioethics centers.

Burton L. Edelstein, DDS, MPH, is a board-certified pediatric dentist and professor in the College of Dental Medicine and the Mailman School of

Public Health at Columbia University in New York City. At the dental school, he is chairman of the Section on Social and Behavioral Sciences. He is founding director of the Children's Dental Health Project, a nonprofit policy organization in Washington, DC, that advances children's oral health and access to dental care. Dr. Edelstein practiced pediatric dentistry in Connecticut and taught at Harvard University for 21 years before committing to full-time health policy practice. He has served as a Robert Wood Johnson Health Policy Fellow in the U.S. Senate, worked with the U.S. Department of Health and Human Services on its oral health initiatives, chaired the U.S. Surgeon General's Workshop on Children and Oral Health, and authored the child section of the U.S. Surgeon General's report on oral health in America. Dr. Edelstein is a graduate of the State University of New York, Buffalo, School of Dentistry; Harvard School of Public Health; and the Boston Children's Hospital pediatric dentistry residency program.

Harriette B. Fox, MSS, is CEO of Incenter Strategies, the National Alliance to Advance Adolescent Health, whose mission is to achieve fundamental improvements in the way that adolescent health care is financed and delivered. She formerly was co-director of the Maternal and Child Health Policy Center and president of Fox Health Policy Consultants. Ms. Fox has more than 30 years of experience in child and adolescent health policy research and analysis, strategic planning, and state technical assistance. Her work currently focuses on the development of sustainable models of integrated physical and behavioral health care for adolescents and improvements in training for providers who serve them. A widely published author, Ms. Fox has directed numerous studies of health care access by low-income youth and youth with complex physical and mental health problems, focusing on Medicaid and SCHIP policies, private health insurance coverage, and managed care, and design of public programs serving children and adolescents. Ms. Fox holds a master of social services degree from the Bryn Mawr Graduate School of Social Work and Social Research.

Charles E. Irwin, Jr., MD, is professor and vice chairman of Pediatrics and Director of the Division of Adolescent Medicine at the University of California, San Francisco (UCSF) School of Medicine. He is a faculty member of the Institute for Health Policy Studies at UCSF and directs both the Public Policy Analysis and Education Center for Middle Childhood, Adolescent and Young Adult Health and the National Adolescent Health Information Center. His research has focused on risky behaviors during adolescence and on methods of identifying adolescents who are prone to initiate health-damaging behaviors during the second decade of life. Most recently his work has expanded to include interventions for improving the delivery of clinical preventive services for adolescents and young adults and improving health outcomes. Dr. Irwin is the author of more than 100 publications and the editor of several texts focusing on pediatric and adolescent health. He has been recognized by the American Academy of Pediatrics with the Adele Hofmann Lifetime Achievement Award in Adolescent Health (1998), the Society for Adolescent Medicine's Outstanding Achievement Award (1999) and the Swedish Society of Medicine (1997). Dr. Irwin served as the first chair of the American Board of Pediatrics' Sub-board of Adolescent Medicine (1991–1998) and the president of the Society for Adolescent Medicine (2002–2003). In 2004, he assumed the position of editor-in-chief of the *Journal of Adolescent Health*. Dr. Irwin received a BS degree in biology from Hobart College, a BMS degree from Dartmouth Medical School, and an MD degree from the University of California, San Francisco.

Kelly Kelleher, MD, MPH, is professor of pediatrics, psychiatry, and public health in the Division of Behavioral and Developmental Pediatrics in the Colleges of Medicine and Public Health at The Ohio State University. He is Director of the Center for Innovation in Pediatric Practice at the Nationwide Children's Hospital. He earned his MD from The Ohio State University, completed his pediatric residency at Northwestern University, and obtained an MPH in epidemiology from The Johns Hopkins University. Dr. Kelleher's research interests focus on accessibility, effectiveness, and quality of health care services for children and their families, especially those affected by mental disorders, substance abuse, or violence. He has a long-standing interest in formal outcomes research for mental health and substance abuse services. He is currently a study section member at the National Institute of Drug Abuse and on the Steering Committee of the Mental Health Services Task Force for the American Academy of Pediatrics.

Genevieve Kenney, PhD, is a principal research associate and health economist in the Health Policy Center at The Urban Institute in Washington, DC. She is a nationally renowned expert on The State Children's Health Insurance Program (SCHIP), Medicaid, and the broader coverage and health issues facing low-income children and families. She has published on a range of issues related to these topics, including the impacts of SCHIP and Medicaid on insurance coverage, crowd out, and access to care; take up and barriers to enrollment; managed care impacts; access and use patterns related to socioeconomic status, race, ethnicity, and language; effects of premium increases; and how parents' health and coverage status affects their children. Dr. Kenney is regularly called upon by Medicaid and SCHIP officials from around the country and by congressional staff to provide input on policy issues related to insurance coverage for children. She was a lead researcher on two major evaluations of the SCHIP: a congressionally mandated evaluation for the United States Department of Health and Human

Services and an evaluation supported by a number of private foundations. Dr. Kenney is a graduate of Smith College and received a PhD in economics and an MA in statistics from the University of Michigan.

Julia Graham Lear, PhD, is research professor in the Department of Prevention and Community Health and director of the department's Center for Health and Health Care in Schools at The George Washington University School of Public Health and Health Services. Her research interests center on the organization and delivery of health and prevention services for children, particularly in schools. Dr. Lear has assessed best practice in implementing school-based health centers and approaches to integrating traditional school health programs into schools and communities, and is currently working on web-based surveys, cultural competence, and oral health. She received her PhD in law and diplomacy from Tufts University. Dr. Lear chairs the District of Columbia School Health Advisory Committee and serves on advisory boards for a number of organizations, including the National Education Association Health Information Network and the National Coordinating Council for School Health. Dr. Lear's work in school health has been recognized with the Achievement Award from the National Assembly on School-Based Health Care, the Integrity Award from the U.S. Department of Health and Human Services, and the Martin C. Ushkow Community Service Award from the American Academy of Pediatrics.

Eduardo Ochoa, Jr., MD, is associate professor of pediatrics at the Department of Pediatrics, College of Medicine, and the assistant dean for minority affairs of the College of Public Health, at the University of Arkansas for Medical Sciences. He is a general pediatrician and an expert in reaching out to the Latino community. Dr. Ochoa previously was Chief Resident in Pediatrics at Arkansas Children's Hospital. He is a board member of Just Communities of Central Arkansas, La Casa Health Network and Arkansas Advocates for Children and Families, and is the President of the Arkansas Chapter of the American Academy of Pediatrics. Dr. Ochoa received his bachelor's degree from Princeton University and his MD from Texas Tech University, and completed his pediatric residency at Arkansas Children's Hospital. He has worked on studies involving racial and ethnic health disparities, disease prevention, health promotion, and health education among emerging Hispanic communities in Arkansas. He, along with a colleague, conducted a legislatively enabled, comprehensive descriptive analysis of health disparities in Arkansas.

Frederick P. Rivara, MD, MPH, currently holds The Children's Hospital Guild Association Endowed Chair in Pediatrics and is professor of pediatrics at the University of Washington School of Medicine; Adjunct Professor of Epidemiology in the University of Washington School of Public Health; and vice-chair of the Department of Pediatrics and head of the Division of General Pediatrics at the University of Washington School of Medicine. He is editor of the *Archives of Pediatrics and Adolescent Medicine*. Dr. Rivara's current research interests include preventing intimate partner violence, reducing alcohol-related trauma, determining the long-term outcomes of children with traumatic brain injuries, and studying the effectiveness of trauma systems in the care of pediatric and adult trauma patients. He served as founding director of the Harborview Injury and Research Center in Seattle for 13 years and founding president of the International Society for Child and Adolescent Injury Prevention. His contributions to the field have spanned 30 years. Dr. Rivara has received numerous honors, including the Charles C. Shepard Science Award from CDC, the American Public Health Association's Injury Control and Emergency Health Services Section Distinguished Career Award, and the American Academy of Pediatrics' Section on Injury and Poison Prevention Physician Achievement Award. He is a member of the Institute of Medicine Section 09 for public health, biostatistics, and epidemiology. Dr. Rivara received his MD from the University of Pennsylvania School of Medicine.

Vinod K. Sahney, PhD, is currently senior vice president and chief strategy officer for Corporate Strategy, Planning, and Business Development at Blue Cross Blue Shield of Massachusetts. He was a leader in the founding of the Massachusetts-based Institute for HealthCare Improvement (IHI) and currently serves on its Board of Directors. Dr. Sahney has also served as visiting professor at the Harvard University School of Public Health for the past 31 years. He was previously at Henry Ford Health System in Detroit, where he was Senior Vice President for Planning and Strategic Development. He is an elected member of both the Institute of Medicine and the National Academy of Engineering. Dr. Sahney has published more than 50 articles in peer-reviewed journals and authored two books and ten chapters in books on health care administration. He holds a PhD from the University of Wisconsin, Madison; a master's degree from Purdue; and a bachelor's degree from the Birla Institute of Technology in Ranchi, India.

Mark A. Schuster, MD, PhD, is chief of general pediatrics and vice chair for health policy research in the Department of Medicine at Children's Hospital Boston and Professor of Pediatrics at Harvard Medical School. He previously served in similar positions at UCLA and was Director of Health Promotion and Disease Prevention at RAND, where he held the RAND Distinguished Chair in Health Promotion. He also founded and led the UCLA/RAND Center for Adolescent Health Promotion, a community-based participatory research center funded by the CDC. Dr. Schuster conducts research primarily on child, adolescent, and family issues. Currently, he is leading studies to develop and evaluate a worksite-based parenting program for parents of adolescents to foster healthy sexual development and sexual risk prevention; partner with a school district to prevent obesity; examine the impact of government-mandated paid family leave insurance on families of children with chronic illness; and understand the experiences of children with HIV-infected parents. He leads the Los Angeles site of "Healthy Passages," a longitudinal study of factors that influence substance use, violence, injuries, physical activity, nutrition, sexual behavior, and mental/physical health among ~5,000 youth. He has also conducted research on quality of health care. Dr. Schuster is co-author of *Everything You Never Wanted Your Kids to Know About Sex (But Were Afraid They'd Ask): The Secrets to Surviving Your Child's Sexual Development from Birth to the Teens* (Crown; 2003) and co-editor of *Child Rearing in America: Challenges Facing Parents of Young Children* (Cambridge University Press; 2002). He received his BA from Yale, his MD from Harvard Medical School, his MPP from the Kennedy School of Government at Harvard, and his PhD from RAND Graduate School. He did his pediatrics residency at Children's Hospital Boston and his fellowship with the Robert Wood Johnson Clinical Scholars Program at UCLA.

Lonnie Sherrod, PhD, received his PhD from Yale University in 1978. He is currently executive director of the Society for Research in Child Development (SRCD). He has been professor of psychology in Fordham University's Applied Developmental Psychology Program, executive vice president of the William T. Grant Foundation, a private independent foundation that funds research on child and youth development, and has served on the staff of the Social Science Research Council, which builds areas of new interdisciplinary research. He edits *The Social Policy Reports*. He has been on the Board of the Federation of Cognitive, Behavioral and Psychological Sciences; has been chair and a member of the Committee on Child Development, Public Policy and Public Information of the Society for Research in Child Development; has been on the Executive Council of Division 7 of the American Psychological Association; has served as liaison to the Committee on Children, Youth and Families; and has been on the Program Committee for the Administration on Children, Youth and Families biennial Conference on Head Start Research. He frequently serves as reviewer for the National Science Foundation, the William T. Grant Foundation, and other funders. He is on the editorial boards of the *International Journal of Behavioral Development*, *NHSA Dialogue*, and *Children's Services: Social Policy, Research and Practice*.

Matthew Stagner, PhD, is executive director of Chapin Hall at the University of Chicago, a multidisciplinary policy research center with a staff of more than 100. His areas of research interest include youth risk behaviors and youth development, child welfare services, family formation policy, and the systematic review of evidence for policy making. Until September 2006, Dr. Stagner was director of the Center on Labor, Human Services, and Population at the Urban Institute in Washington, DC. He previously directed the Division of Children and Youth Policy, in the Office of the Assistant Secretary for Planning and Evaluation, U.S. Department of Health and Human Services. He holds a PhD from the Irving B. Harris School of Public Policy Studies at the University of Chicago and an MPP from Harvard University's John F. Kennedy School of Government.

Leslie R. Walker, MD, FAAP, is associate professor and chief of the Adolescent Medicine Section in the Department of Pediatrics at the University of Washington, Seattle, and Seattle Children's Hospital. Until February 2007, she was associate professor and chief of adolescent medicine in the Department of Pediatrics at Georgetown University Medical Center. Dr. Walker is an adolescent medicine specialist with interest in mental health and substance abuse services for teenagers and support services for their parents. She is an expert in adolescent development, adolescent psychosocial issues, mental health, and substance abuse treatment. Dr. Walker's research has been in transitional health care, pregnancy prevention, and substance abuse. She received her BA from Stanford University and her MD from the University of Illinois in 1990. She received her pediatric training at the University of Chicago and completed her adolescent medicine fellowship at the University of California, San Francisco, in 1996. She currently serves on the Board of Directors for the Society for Adolescent Medicine and the Board of Directors for the Youth Suicide Prevention Program.

STAFF

Jennifer Appleton Gootman is a senior program officer at the Board on Children, Youth, and Families, Division of Behavioral and Social Sciences, the National Academies, where she is currently study director for the study on adolescent health care. She recently completed a study on *Contributions from the Behavioral and Social Sciences to the Reduction and Prevention of Motor Vehicle Crashes Involving Teen Drivers*. Prior to that she directed a study for the Food and Nutrition Board—*Food Marketing to Children and Youth: Threat or Opportunity?*—that examines the influence of food and beverage marketing on the diets and health of children and youth. Just before directing this study, she took leave from the National Academies to participate in the Ian Axford Fellowship in Public Policy, working in New

Zealand to examine and publish a report on New Zealand's national youth development strategy and related child and youth policies. Prior to this fellowship, she directed and disseminated two studies—*Community Programs to Promote Youth Development* and *Working Families and Growing Kids*—for the Board on Children, Youth, and Families. She was previously a social science analyst for the Office of Planning and Evaluation in the U.S. Department of Health and Human Services. Her work focused on child and family policy for low-income families, including welfare reform, child care, child health, youth development, and teen pregnancy prevention issues. She has directed a number of community youth programs in Los Angeles and New York City, involving young people in leadership development, job preparedness, and community service. She received her BA in education and fine arts from the University of Southern California and her MA in public policy from the New School for Social Research.

Leslie J. Sim is a program officer for the Board on Children, Youth, and Families, working on studies on adolescent health care and parental depression. Ms. Sim has worked with the Division of Behavioral and Social Sciences and Education and the Institute of Medicine since 2001. During that time, she has progressed through several positions and multiple studies. Her most recent achievements include her role in directing a workshop study and report titled *Influence of Pregnancy Weight on Maternal and Child Health: Workshop Report* (2006), as well as her involvement in the above-mentioned study on adolescent health care. In 2003, Ms. Sim received recognition as a recipient of an Institute of Medicine inspirational staff award. In her earlier work with the Institute of Medicine's Food and Nutrition Board, she provided web support for all Board activities for more than four years and participated in multiple studies on military nutrition and food marketing to children and youth. She previously worked both as a research assistant in the Food Science Department and laboratory assistant for an undergraduate Food Science Laboratory class at North Carolina State University. She received her BS degree in biology with an emphasis on food science from Virginia Tech, and has taken classes in food science and public health from North Carolina State University and A.T. Still University.

Reine Homawoo is senior project assistant for the parental depression study of the Board on Children, Youth, and Families. Ms. Homawoo joined the Board's staff in August 2007 following the completion of several studies within the Institute of Medicine's Board on Military and Veterans' Health. She is currently pursuing a BS in information system management at the University of Maryland University College. Ms. Homawoo has completed courses at Northern Virginia Community College and also received an associate's degree in computer programming (with honors) from the National Center for Computer Studies in Togo, Africa.

April Higgins is a graduate of the University of Memphis, where she studied political science with a minor in philosophy. She joined the staff of the National Academies in July 2006 as senior program assistant for the adolescent health care study. Prior to that time, she worked at the Close-Up Foundation as Capitol Hill Program Coordinator. She has worked with many nonprofit and government organizations, including Girls Inc., YWCA, Habitat for Humanity, and St. Jude Children's Research Hospital.

Rosemary Chalk is director of the Board on Children, Youth, and Families, a collaboration of the National Research Council and the Institute of Medicine. She is a policy analyst who has served as a study director for the National Academies since 1987. She has directed or served as a senior staff member for more than a dozen studies within the National Research Council and the Institute of Medicine, including studies on vaccine finance, the public health infrastructure for immunization, family violence, child abuse and neglect, research ethics and misconduct in science, and education finance. Ms. Chalk has also conducted research projects or policy studies for Child Trends in Washington, DC, and the Congressional Research Service at the Library of Congress. She was program head for the Committee on Scientific Freedom and Responsibility of the American Association for the Advancement of Science from 1976 to 1986. Ms. Chalk holds a BA in foreign affairs from the University of Cincinnati.

Wendy E. Keenan is program associate for the Board on Children, Youth, and Families. She provides administrative and research support for the Board and its various program committees. She also helps organize planning meetings and workshops that cover current issues related to children, youth, and families. Ms. Keenan has been on the National Academies' staff for more than eight years and worked on studies for both the National Research Council and the Institute of Medicine. As senior program assistant, she worked with the National Research Council's Board on Behavioral, Cognitive, and Sensory Sciences. Prior to joining the National Academies, Ms. Keenan taught English as a second language for Washington, DC, public schools. She received a BA in sociology from The Pennsylvania State University and took graduate courses in liberal studies from Georgetown University.

Index

A

Abortion rates, 92
Abortion rights, 180–181
Acceptable health care, 5, 299
Access to care
   access to adolescent medicine specialists, 145
   adolescent perceptions, 38
   challenges for adolescent subpopulations, 97
   cost of care and, 267
   dental care, 161
   fragmentation of current health system as barrier to, 7, 300–301
   health insurance and, 8, 265, 266–269, 274, 285–286, 287, 288, 302
   mental health services, 158
   objectives for adolescent health system, 5, 299
   population patterns and trends and, 6, 17
   primary care, 135
   provider participation in public insurance programs and, 285–286
   racial/ethnic disparities, 137, 177
   recommendations for insurance system, 12–13, 307–308
   right to confidential access, 180–183
   in rural areas, 34–35
   safety-net health services, 6–7, 136, 157, 300
   shortcomings of current health system performance, 6, 299–300
   sources of medical care, 168–172, 299–300
   specialty health services, 136–137, 166, 300
Accidental injury
   adolescent mortality, 53
   health objectives for adolescents, 55
   insurance coverage issues, 8, 302
   mortality, 53, 62–64
   patterns and trends, 6
Adolescence, defined, 2, 23, 25–27
Adolescent health status
   adolescent self-perceptions, 54
   adolescent subpopulations, 96–115
   current state, 1, 17–18, 52, 54, 55–60, 115, 296
   definition, 8–9, 28, 52, 54, 302
   determinants of, 3–4, 18–19, 28, 43–45, 54–55
   mortality and morbidity patterns and trends, 53
   significance of, for adult health, 1, 3–4, 5–6, 17–18, 44, 52, 54, 60–61, 293, 297
   socioeconomic status and, 35
   See also Mental disorders; Mortality

329

Adolescent perceptions and understanding
    access to care, 38
    data collection, 22, 38
    demographic differences in, 38–39
    mental health services, 39
    of parental involvement in health care, 38
    privacy and consent for care issues, 38, 42–43
    self-perceived health, 54
    substance use treatment, 39
Alcohol use
    addiction risk, 90
    age at onset, 89–90
    associated risks, 88, 89
    mortality, 89
    motor vehicle accidents and, 84–85
    outcomes of adolescent health-compromising behavior, 54
    patterns and trends, 6, 87–88, 89, 90
    preventive interventions, 30, 212
    risks among homeless adolescents, 102
    significance of, in adolescent health, 53, 91
    treatment needs, 163–164
American Academy of Pediatrics, 198, 222
American Medical Association, 198
Anxiety and anxiety disorders, 53, 72, 73, 77
Appropriate health care, 5, 299
Assessment of adolescent health
    barriers for vulnerable subpopulations, 202
    goals for improving adolescent health services system, 195–196, 231
    Guidelines for Adolescent Preventive Services, 145, 198–199, 248
    in primary care, 144, 199–201
    privacy and confidentiality in, 202
    public insurance coverage of screening services, 278
    recommendations for adolescent care provider training, 12, 307
    recommendations for monitoring health care system performance, 14–15, 309–310
    recommendations for research, 14, 309
    reimbursement, 201
    screening tools, 172, 174–175, 197–199
    shortcomings of current health system, 8–9, 172–175, 303–304
    standardized screening practices, 198
    strategies for improving adolescent health service system, 197–202, 203
    substance use, 201–202
Asthma
    limitations in normal daily activities due to, 66
    prevalence, 53, 66, 67, 71
    risk factors, 66–67
Attention-deficit hyperactivity disorder, 72, 73, 74, 202

B

Behavioral health in adolescence
    advantages of safety-net health services, 7, 136, 157, 300
    current adolescent health status, 53–54
    developmental significance, 3–4, 17–18, 44, 52, 54, 60–61, 197, 211, 297
    goals for improving adolescent health services system, 196
    health management strategies in primary care, 202–204
    monitoring, 204
    morbidity, 84
    patterns and trends, 6
    primary care assessment, 144
    primary care reimbursement, 143–144
    protective factors, 212
    rationale for early assessment and intervention, 197
    recommendations for adolescent care provider training, 12, 307
    recommendations for improving primary health care, 9–10, 305
    recommendations for monitoring health care system performance, 14–15, 309–310
    risks, 24–25
    shortcomings of current health system performance, 5–6, 7, 301
    significance of, in adolescent health system, 3, 43–44, 211, 297
    See also Risky behavior
Bisexual adolescents. See Lesbian, gay, bisexual, or transgender adolescents
Board certification in adolescent medicine, 254
Body piercing, 84

Brain development, 25
Bullying behaviors, 87

C

Cancer
  mortality, 64
  prevalence, 67–70
  survival rate trends, 70
  type distribution, 70
Case management
  in community-based health centers, 150–151
  recommendations for health insurance coverage, 13, 308
  referral management, 208
Centers for Disease Control and Prevention, 253
Chronic illness
  associated conditions, 65
  causes in adolescence, 53
  comorbidity, 65
  epidemiology, 65–66
  implications for health care system, 66
  mortality, 64
  risks in foster care, 54, 98
  See also Asthma; Cancer; Diabetes
Community-based health centers
  goals for improving adolescent health services system, 195–196
  innovative programs, 150, 226–228
  limitations, 151
  scope of services, 150
  significance of, in adolescent health care system, 150–151
Community-level public health interventions
  disease prevention interventions in, 212
  recommendations for improving, 10–11, 305–306
  significance of, in adolescent health, 4, 44, 195, 298
  youth development promotion, 218
Comorbidity
  mental disorders, 72
  patterns and trends, 6
  special health care needs, 65
Competency domains, 249–251
Conduct disorder, 72, 73, 74–75
Confidentiality and privacy. *See* Privacy and confidentiality

Congenital anomalies, 64
Consent for care
  adolescent concerns, 42–43
  adolescent utilization of health services and, 178–179
  current legal framework, 180–181
  parental concerns, 42, 211
  policy formulation challenges, 42, 43
  recommendations for, 11, 306
Consultation, specialty, 208
Contextual factors
  determinants of adolescent health status, 3, 4, 18–19, 43–45, 54–55, 138, 297, 298
  recommendations for research, 14, 309
Continuing education for health providers, 255
Contraception
  adolescent patterns, 159
  counseling, 159
  insurance coverage, 279, 280
  parental notification, 211
  right to access, 180
Coordination of care
  adolescent primary care, 145, 146
  care management of specialty services, 206–207
  goals for improving adolescent health services system, 194, 196
  recommendations for improving, 9, 10–11, 304, 305–306
  regional approach to resource management, 209
  shortcomings of current system, 7, 300–301
  strategies for improving adolescent health service system, 206–207
  strengthening primary care–specialty care linkages, 207–210
Correctional facilities, 35
Cost of care
  access to care and, 267
  chronic health conditions, 66
  dental care expenditures, 266
  insurance cost sharing arrangements, 285–286
  Medicaid cost-sharing requirements, 277
  mental health services, 282
  recommendations for health insurance system, 13, 308

D

Data collection
  among homeless population, 99
  current health care system, 21–22
  recommendations for monitoring health care system performance, 14–15, 309–310
  shortcomings of current health system, 8–9, 23, 294–295, 303–304
Definition of adolescence, 2, 23, 25–27
Definition of adolescent health status, 8–9, 28, 296, 303
Dental care
  adolescent perceptions of access and quality, 38
  barriers to, 161
  current adolescent health status, 53, 79–82, 84
  fragmentation of current health system as obstacle to, 7, 301
  insurance coverage and, 8, 265, 266, 267–269, 271–272, 284–285, 302
  in juvenile justice system, 114
  juvenile periodontitis, 83–84
  linkage with primary care, 208–209
  opportunities for health promotion in dental practice, 161
  oral disease risk factors, 79
  parental educational attainment and, 162
  preventive interventions, 161, 214
  public insurance coverage, 277
  recommendations for health insurance coverage, 13, 308
  recommendations for improving public health system for adolescent care, 10–11, 305–306
  trauma risk, 84
  trends, 82–83
  unmet needs, 162
  utilization, 161, 265, 269, 271–272
Depression
  among homeless adolescents, 103, 104
  associated behaviors, 73, 74
  current screening and counseling practice, 173
  pharmacotherapy, 202
  prevalence, 72, 73–74
  screening, 198
  See also Mental disorders
Development
  changes in adolescence, 24–25
  developmental delays in foster care children, 98–99
  significance of adolescent experience for later development, 1, 3–4, 5–6, 17–18, 44, 52, 54, 60–61, 197, 211, 293, 296, 297
  violent behavior risk, 85–86
  youth development promotion strategies, 214–219
Diabetes
  health outcomes in adulthood, 67
  prevalence, 53, 67, 71
Diet and nutrition
  adolescent consumption choices, 24–25
  current adolescent intake, 94, 172
  current screening and counseling practice, 173
  food and beverage marketing, 31
  outcomes of adolescent health-compromising behavior, 54
  risky eating behaviors, 94, 95
  See also Obesity
Disease prevention
  communication of behavioral health information, 211–213
  fragmentation of current health system as obstacle to, 7, 300–301
  goals for improving adolescent health services system, 196, 231
  insurance policies and practices and, 265
  in primary care settings, 145–146
  rationale, 172
  recommendations for primary care, 10, 305
  in safety-net health services, 157
  shortcomings of current health system performance, 7, 172–175, 301
  strategies for improving, 211–214
  strengthening protective factors, 212
  See also Health promotion; Preventive interventions; Sexually transmitted disease

E

Early adolescence
  definition, 55
  mortality patterns, 62

Eating disorders, 75, 79, 110
Education and training for health care professionals. *See* Provider education and training
Effective health services
  family and adolescent participation and, 4, 298
  mental health services, 158
  objectives for adolescent health system, 5, 299
  sexual and reproductive health clinics, 160
  substance use treatment, 165
Electronic communication, 211–212, 224
Electronic health records
  confidentiality, 223
  recommendations for, 10–11, 305–306
Emergency care
  adolescent utilization, 6–7, 171, 300
  hospital-affiliated primary care and, 152
  shortcomings of current health system performance, 6–7, 300
Equitable health care delivery, 5, 299

F

Family
  influence on adolescent health behavior, 38
  one- and no-parent homes, 34
  parental involvement in adolescent care, confidentiality and, 221–222
  parental notification effects on adolescent health care utilization, 178–179
  recommendations for adolescent confidentiality and consent for care, 11, 306
  role in preventive intervention, 212
  significance of, in adolescent health, 4, 44, 298
Family medicine as model for adolescent care, 19
Family planning services, 160, 279–280
Federal government
  confidentiality laws, 181–182
  recommendations for confidentiality and consent policies in adolescent health care, 11, 306
  recommendations for health insurance system, 12–13, 307–308
  recommendations for improving primary care, 9, 304
  recommendations for research, 13–14, 309
  training grants, 251
Federal Interagency Forum on Child and Family Statistics, 14–15, 309–310
Fighting, 87
Financial factors
  compensation for adolescent health care specialists, 259
  funding for adolescent care provider training programs, 12, 251, 253, 307
  funding for school-based health centers, 153–156
  recommendations for health insurance system, 13, 308
  recommendations for improving primary health care, 10, 305
  scope of, in adolescent health care, 4, 44–45, 298
  strategies for improving immunization programs, 213
  See also Cost of care
Focus of adolescent health services, 7, 301
Foster care system, adolescents in, 2–3, 35
  abuse and neglect patterns, 97–98
  health risks, 53, 54, 98–99
  insurance coverage after departure, 272
  mental health services, 73
  recommendations for health insurance coverage, 12–13, 307–308
  recommendations for improving primary health care, 9–10, 305
  substance abuse risk, 163
  See also Subpopulations of adolescents
Free time, 35–36

G

Gay adolescents. *See* Lesbian, gay, bisexual, or transgender adolescents
Gender differences
  adolescent health behaviors and attitudes, 38–39
  board certifications in adolescent medicine, 254
  demographic and population patterns, 32, 35
  diabetes prevalence, 67
  health care utilization, 171

mental disorder risk, 72–73, 74, 75
mortality patterns, 62
physical activity, 96
seat belt use, 85
sexual and reproductive health service utilization, 158–160
sexually transmitted disease patterns, 77–78
substance use, 76
suicidal behavior or ideation, 77
Group homes, 35
Guidelines for Adolescent Preventive Services, 145, 198–199, 248

H

Health Insurance Portability and Accountability Act, 181–182
Health promotion
  conceptual evolution in adolescent medicine, 37
  in dental and oral health care, 161
  fragmentation of current health system as obstacle to, 7, 300–301
  goals for improving adolescent health services system, 196, 231
  participants, 210
  in primary care settings, 145–146, 147
  print and electronic resources for, 210–211
  rationale, 172, 195
  recommendations for monitoring health care system performance, 14–15, 309–310
  recommendations for primary care, 10, 305
  in safety-net health services, 157
  shortcomings of current health system performance, 7, 137, 172–175, 301
  significance of intervention in adolescence, 3–4, 17–18, 54, 297–298
  strategies for improving adolescent health service system, 210–212
Health system, adolescent care in
  behavioral and contextual framework, 3–4, 43–45, 137–138, 297–298
  community factors, 4, 298
  conceptual and technical evolution, 36–37
  current models of care, 6–7, 19, 300
  data sources on current state, 21–23
  determinants of adolescent health status, 18–19, 28
  family factors, 4, 298
  financial factors, 4, 298
  focus, 7, 301
  objectives, 4–5, 138–140, 298–299
  perceptions and attitudes, 37–41
  policy factors, 4, 298
  rationale for improving, 15, 310
  recommendations for improving, 10–11, 305–306
  recommendations for research, 13–14, 309
  research needs, 19–20, 294–295
  safety-net services, 136
  salient issues, 2, 20–21, 293–294
  scope of settings and services, 3, 28–29, 37, 299
  sectors, 140–142
  shortcomings of current system, 1, 6–9, 15, 18–19, 142, 293, 299–304, 310
  specialty care services, 136–137
  See also Improving adolescent health services system; Provider education and training
Healthy People 2010 objectives, 6, 55, 145, 196, 296
Heart disease, 64
HIV/AIDS, 78, 101, 111
Homeless population, 2–3, 35
  alcohol and substance use, 102
  associated health risks, 99–100
  data collection challenges, 99
  mental health, 103–104
  patterns and trends, 99
  physical and sexual abuse risk, 100
  recommendations for improving primary health care, 9–10, 305
  risks for lesbian, gay, bisexual, or transgender adolescents in, 104–105
  sexual activity and health, 100–102
  See also Subpopulations of adolescents
Homicide
  access to weapons and, 86
  mortality, 53, 62, 64, 65
  victimization patterns, 87
Hospital-affiliated primary care, 151–152
  innovative programs for adolescent care, 228–229

I

Immigrants, 2–3, 35, 105–107
   access to care, 18
   insurance coverage disparities, 269–271, 272
   insurance coverage patterns, 8, 302
   population patterns, 33
   public insurance eligibility, 274
   recommendations for improving primary health care, 9–10, 305
   See also Subpopulations of adolescents
Immunization. *See* Vaccination and immunization
Improving adolescent health services system
   care management of specialty services, 206–207
   community role, 4, 195, 298
   consideration of special needs and vulnerable populations, 9–10, 194, 305
   coordination of care, 194, 206–207, 231
   family role, 4, 195, 298
   goals, 194, 195–196, 231
   health information technology, 223–225
   health management strategies in primary care, 202–204
   immunization programs and policies, 213–214
   implementation of strategies for, 231–232
   innovative programs, 225–231
   linkages between primary and specialty care, 207–210
   participation and engagement for, 4, 195, 298
   personalized health services, 225
   prevention and health promotion, 194, 195, 210–212, 231
   privacy and confidentiality issues, 194
   provider training, 255–258
   rationale, 1, 15, 18, 194–195, 293, 310
   recommendations for, 9–15, 304–310
   referral practice, 204–206, 207–208
   research needs, 232
   screening and assessment, 197–202, 203, 231
   youth development promotion, 214–219
Inpatient hospital care
   adolescent utilization, 167–168
   mental health and substance abuse treatment insurance coverage, 281–283
   specialized units for adolescents, 167
   treatment teams, 167
Institutionalized adolescents
   population characteristics, 35
   settings, 35
   substance abuse risk, 163
Insurance
   age distribution of coverage patterns among adolescents and young adults, 273, 288
   barriers to health care access, 8, 265, 266–269, 274, 285–286, 287, 288, 302
   confidentiality protection, 223, 287
   cost sharing, 285–286, 287
   coverage patterns and trends, 8, 265, 269–272, 276–285, 288, 302
   current sources and benefit plans, 276–278
   definition of adolescence for, 26–27
   dental services coverage, 284–285
   eligibility, 272–273
   employment characteristics and, 269–271, 272–273
   failure of eligible adolescents to enroll in public programs, 8, 265, 273–276, 302
   health risks related to lack of, 8, 265, 266, 302
   inpatient pregnancy expenses, 168
   mental health and substance abuse treatment coverage, 158–159, 280–284
   preventive services coverage, 278–279, 286–287
   recent reform proposals, 42
   recommendations for improving health care system, 12–13, 307–308
   sexual and reproductive health services coverage, 279–280
   shortcomings of current health system, 7, 18, 265, 276, 278, 287, 288, 300
   source of medical care and, 169–170
   strategies for increasing coverage, 275–276
Internet
   harassment via, 87
   online health services, 224–225
   resources for medical education, 256–257

J

Juvenile justice system, adolescents in, 2–3, 35
  health risks, 53–54, 113, 114
  mental disorder risk among, 113–114
  mental health services, 73
  population patterns, 113–114
  recommendations for health insurance coverage, 12–13, 307–308
  recommendations for improving primary health care, 9–10, 305
  substance abuse risk, 163
  victimization risk, 114
  See also Subpopulations of adolescents

L

Leadership Education in Adolescent Health, 12, 307
Lesbian, gay, bisexual, or transgender adolescents, 2–3, 173
  eating disorders among, 110
  health-related data, 109
  in homeless population, 104–105
  population patterns, 108–109
  psychosocial stressors, 111
  recommendations for improving primary health care, 9–10, 305
  research challenges, 108
  sexual health risks, 111
  social stigma, 107–108
  special issues for transgender teens, 112
  substance abuse, 110
  suicidal behavior or ideation, 109–110
  violence victimization risk, 111
  See also Subpopulations of adolescents
Licensing, certification and accreditation
  adolescent medicine board certification, 254
  continuing education requirements, 255
  inconsistency in national system of, 260
  recommendations for, 11–12, 306–307
  shortcomings of current system, 240, 252, 260
  strategies for improving adolescent health care system, 255–256

M

Managed care
  adolescent utilization, 169
  carve outs, 205–206
  confidentiality concerns, 287
  recommendations for improving public health system for adolescent care, 10–11, 305–306
Maternal and Child Health Block Grant, 181
Maternal and Child Health Bureau, 252, 258
Medicaid
  confidentiality of adolescent health care, 181, 287
  coordination of care, 174
  cost-sharing requirements, 277, 285
  covered services, 276–277, 278–280, 281, 284
  current shortcomings in adolescent health care, 42
  eligibility, 272, 274
  failure of eligible adolescents to enroll in, 273–276
  physician reimbursement, 285–286
  pregnancy care, 168, 272
  preventive care reimbursement, 287
  provider participation, 285–286
  recommendations, 12–13, 307–308
  settings for adolescent medical care and, 169
Mental disorders
  age of onset, 72, 77
  among adolescents in juvenile justice system, 113–114
  comorbidity, 72
  definition and clinical conceptualization, 71
  prevalence, 71–72, 73, 74, 75, 77, 157
  risk factors, 72–73
  risk in adolescence, 53, 54
  risks among homeless adolescents, 103–104
  risks in foster care, 98, 99
  See also Mental health services; *specific disorders*
Mental health services
  adolescent perceptions, 39
  confidentiality concerns of adolescents, 179

effectiveness, 158
evolution of costs and reimbursement, 282
fragmentation of current health system, 7, 301
inpatient hospitalization, 168
insurance and reimbursement, 8, 157–158, 280–284, 286, 302
online, 224–225
primary care reimbursement, 143–144
public insurance coverage, 277, 286
racial differences in service delivery settings, 73
recommendations for health insurance coverage, 13, 308
recommendations for improving public health system for adolescent care, 10–11, 305–306
in schools, 206
screening, 172–173
shortcomings of current health system, 7, 158, 172–173, 301
specialty consultation approach, 208
substance abuse risk, 163
unmet needs, 158
workforce, 157
See also Mental disorders; Specialty care services

Models of care, 6–7, 19–20, 36–37, 300
criteria for evaluating, 195

Mortality
adolescent risk, 53
in adulthood, adolescent health-related behaviors and, 54
causes, 53, 62–64, 65, 172
patterns and trends, 6, 62–65

Motivational interviewing, 203

Motor vehicle accidents
adolescent mortality, 53
alcohol use and, 84–85
causes of risky driving, 84
injury outcomes, 53
mortality, 62, 65, 84
objectives for adolescent health, 55
patterns and trends, 6
prevention strategies, 31
seat belt use and, 85
sleepiness as cause of, 85

N

National Adolescent Health Information Center, 257
National Initiative to Improve Adolescent Health, 29–30
Nurses, 247–248

O

Obesity
in adulthood, 94
associated health risks, 93, 94
associated psychosocial risks, 93
current screening and counseling practice, 173
electronic entertainment and, 35–36
health management strategies in primary care, 203
insurance coverage issues, 8, 302
objectives for adolescent health, 55
patterns and trends, 6, 53, 93–94, 95
prevention, 30–31
Objectives for adolescent health system, 4–5, 6, 135, 298–299
application, 139
components, 138–140
framework for evaluation of adolescent health service models, 195
recommendations for health insurance coverage, 13, 308
recommendations for research agenda, 13–14, 309
shortcomings of current health system performance, 55
shortcomings of current service delivery models, 6–7, 296, 299–300
Office of Technology Assessment, 29
Oral health. *See* Dental care

P

Parental educational attainment, dental health and, 162
Pediatric care, 19
Perceptions and attitudes about adolescent health
adolescents', 22, 38–39, 136
adolescents' self-perceived health status, 54

data sources, 22
health care providers, 40–41
historical evolution, 23–24
parents' perspectives, 39–40
perceptions of drug use, 90
significance of, 37–38
Personalized health services, 225
Pharmacists, 41
Pharmacotherapy
  cost of medications as barrier to, 267
  medication management, 202–203
Physical activity
  electronic entertainment and, 35–36
  health and, 95
  objectives for adolescent health, 55
  outcomes of adolescent health-compromising behavior, 54
  patterns and trends, 6, 95–96
PIPPAH, 258
Policy making
  privacy and confidentiality issues, 42, 43, 302
  recommendations for improving adolescent health care, 10–11, 305–306
  shortcomings of current policy environment, 41–42
  significance of, in adolescent health care, 4, 45, 298
  taxes to discourage alcohol and tobacco consumption, 212
  See also Federal government; State government
Poor families, 2–3
  access to care, 6, 17, 18, 33–34, 97
  chronic health condition risk, 65–67
  insurance coverage, 8, 265, 275–276, 302
  Medicaid cost-sharing requirements, 277
  population patterns, 34
  racial/ethnic patterns, 6, 34, 296
  recommendations for health insurance coverage, 13, 308
  recommendations for improving primary health care, 9–10, 305
  See also Socioeconomic status
Population-based health care delivery, 210
Population patterns and trends, 6, 17, 32–33, 34–35, 97, 296
Pregnancy, dental care in, 272
Pregnancy in adolescence
  abortion rates, 92
  associated risks, 91
  consent for care and confidentiality laws, 180
  fetal loss rates, 92–93
  health objectives for adolescents, 55
  incidence, 91
  inpatient hospital utilization, 167–168
  insurance reimbursement, 168
  oral disease risk and, 79
  patterns and trends, 6, 53, 91–92
  risks among homeless, 101, 102
Preventive interventions
  current insurance coverage and reimbursement, 278–279, 286–287
  disincentives for insurance providers, 286–287
  health management strategies in primary care, 203
  interaction and coordination among social service sectors, 174
  rationale, 195
  recommendations for health insurance coverage, 13, 308
  screening and assessment, 197–202
  seat belt use, 85
  shortcomings of current health system performance, 137
  See also Disease prevention; Health promotion
Primary care
  adolescent medicine specialists, 144–145
  behavioral health assessment and monitoring, 144, 204
  in community-based health centers, 150–151
  goals for improving adolescent health services system, 195–196, 231
  health management strategies, 202–204
  hospital-affiliated, 151–152
  medication management, 202–203
  private office-based, 143–147
  provider–patient relationship in, 203–204
  recommendations for improving, 9–10, 305
  recommendations for research, 14, 309
  referrals to specialty care, 204–206, 207–208
  reimbursement, 143–144, 145, 146, 201
  safety-net programs, 143–147
  school-based, 152–156
  scope of services, 142, 143

INDEX

settings for, 143
shortcomings of current health system performance, 6, 18, 135, 145–147
specialty care linkages, 142, 157, 207–210
strategies for improving adolescent health services system, 199–201, 231

Privacy and confidentiality
adolescent candor and, 178
adolescent concerns, 38, 42–43
adolescent utilization of health services and, 177–179, 219, 220, 300–301
adult protections, 219
conceptual approaches to adolescent care, 219–220
consent for care law and, 180–181
electronic health records and, 223
insurance issues, 223, 287
legal framework, 181–183, 219
parental concerns, 42
parental involvement in adolescent care, 221–222
policies of health care professional organizations, 222
policy issues, 42, 43, 302
provider attitudes and beliefs, 43, 219, 301
provider communication with adolescent, 220
recommendations for, 11, 306
sexual and reproductive health service utilization and, 160
significance of, in adolescent health care, 137, 183, 219, 301–302

Protective factors, 212

Provider education and training
adolescent medicine specialists, 144–145, 252–255
certification standards, 255–256
challenges, 258–261
competency domains, 249–251
conceptual evolution, 243–244
continuing education, 255
current models, 252–256
doctoral programs, 255
economic disincentives, 259
funding for training programs, 12, 251, 253, 307
future demand and supply, 244–245
goals, 241, 261

importance of, for adolescent health care system, 4, 44, 240–241, 261, 298
innovative programs, 240, 256–258
interdisciplinary programs, 12, 252–253, 307
leadership programs, 252–253
levels of expertise in adolescent medicine, 245–246
master degree programs, 255
patient simulations, 256
postresidency fellowships, 253–254
primary care physicians, 144–145
provider attitudes and beliefs, 41, 246–248
recommendations for, 11–12, 306–307
recommendations for research, 14, 309
for screening and counseling, 174
shortcomings of current health system, 8, 240, 241, 244, 246–248, 249, 258, 302–303
for specialty care services, 167
substance abuse treatment, 164–165
train-the-trainer programs, 256–257
See also Licensing, certification and accreditation

Provider–patient relationship
adolescent primary care, 145
adolescents' confidentiality beliefs and, 177–178
clinical significance, 203–204
confidentiality discussions, 220
participation and engagement, 4, 195, 298
provider perception, 41
recommendations for adolescent care provider training, 12, 307

Provider performance measurement
primary care services, 10, 305
recommendations for monitoring health care system performance, 14–15, 309–310
recommendations for research, 13–14, 309
standards and guidelines, 248
See also Licensing, certification and accreditation

Psychosocial functioning
changes in adolescence, 24, 25
dating violence, 86–87
individual differences in adolescents, 41

risks for lesbian, gay, bisexual, or transgender adolescents, 107–108, 111
See also Mental disorders; Mental health services

Q

Quality of care
adolescent primary care, obstacles to, 145
impediments to, in current adolescent health system, 18–19
insurance and, 8, 265, 302
racial/ethnic disparities, 137
in safety-net settings, 7, 300
U.S. health system, 31

R

Race/ethnicity
access to care and, 6, 17, 18, 33, 97, 137, 296
adolescent health status patterns and trends, 53
adolescent pregnancy, 53, 91, 92–93
alcohol and substance use and, 76, 85, 90
asthma prevalence, 66
cancer incidence and survival, 70
diabetes prevalence, 67
disparities in health care delivery, 177–178
insurance coverage patterns and disparities, 8, 265, 269–271, 272, 302
mental disorder risk, 73
mental health service delivery settings, 73
mortality patterns, 62, 64
obese and overweight patterns in adolescence, 93
oral health care needs, 79–82, 83, 162
parental attitudes toward sexual behavior and sexual health, 40
physical activity patterns, 96
population patterns and trends, 6, 17, 32–33, 97, 296
poverty and, 6, 34, 296
provider workforce diversity, 242–243
quality of care and, 137
recommendations for improving primary health care, 9–10, 305
sexual and reproductive health service utilization, 159
sexually transmitted disease patterns, 77–78, 79
suicidal behavior or ideation, 77
tobacco use, 89
violent crime victimization, 87
See also Subpopulations of adolescents
Referrals
goals for improving adolescent health services system, 195–196
strategies for improving, 204–206, 207–208
substance abuse, from schools, 162–163
Regional resource management, 209
Reimbursement
care management, 206
immunization policies, 213
mental health services, 157–158
preventive care, 287
private office-based primary care, 143–144, 145, 146
provider participation in public insurance programs and, 285–286
recommendations for health insurance system, 13, 308
for screening and counseling, 174, 201
Research
current shortcomings, 19–20, 294–295
for improving adolescent health services system, 232
notable past work, 29–31
recommendations for, 13–14, 309
recommendations for monitoring health care system performance, 14–15, 309–310
See also Data collection
Risky behavior
adolescent morbidity, 53
assessment, 201–202
comorbidity risk, 6
current screening and counseling practice, 173
health management strategies in primary care, 202–204
morbidity, 84
normal adolescent development and, 24, 25

INDEX 341

oral disease risk, 79
primary care intervention, 147
rationale for early identification and
    intervention, 197
scope of, 53, 115
screening strategies, 197–201
significance of, in adolescent health, 3–4,
    5–6, 17–18, 52, 54, 91, 115, 172,
    197, 211, 296, 297
unsupervised nonschool hours and, 35
See also Alcohol use; Behavioral health
    in adolescence; Sexually transmitted
    disease; Substance abuse
Rural areas
    access to care, 34, 97
    agricultural workers, 106–107
    obese and overweight patterns in
        adolescence, 93–94
    physical activity patterns in, 96
    population patterns and trends, 31–35,
        97

S

Safety-net providers
    advantages of, in adolescent care, 7,
        136, 156–157, 300
    community-based health centers,
        150–151
    current research base, 147
    definition and characteristics, 147
    quality of care, 7, 156, 300
    recommendations for improving, 9, 304
    scope of care settings, 147
    shortcomings of current health system
        performance, 6–7, 299–300
    significance of, in adolescent health care
        system, 7, 156, 300
School-based health centers
    characteristics, 153
    clients, 152
    funding, 153–156
    in innovative integrated health
        programs, 226–227
    mental health services, 206
    number of, 152
    quality of care, 7, 300
    rationale, 152, 153
    services, 153

significance of, in adolescent health care
    syste, 152
sponsors, 153
strengths and weaknesses, 6–7, 299–300
substance abuse referrals from, 162–163
School-based insurance coverage, 276
Sex education, 40, 158
Sexual abuse risk for homeless adolescents,
    100
Sexual and reproductive health
    adolescent utilization of health services,
        158–160
    among lesbian, gay, bisexual, or
        transgender adolescents, 111
    current insurance coverage, 279–280
    current screening and counseling
        practice, 173
    dating violence, 86–87
    effectiveness of clinic services, 160
    family influences on adolescent health
        behavior, 38
    fragmentation of current health system,
        7, 301
    guidance and counseling, 158
    information technology, 224
    objectives for adolescent health, 55
    outcomes of adolescent health-
        compromising behavior, 54
    parental attitudes and perceptions, 40
    primary care reimbursement, 143–144
    privacy concerns of adolescents, 160,
        178–179
    public insurance coverage, 277
    recommendations for health insurance
        coverage, 13, 308
    recommendations for improving public
        health system for adolescent care,
        10–11, 305–306
    right to access to health care, 180–181
    risks among homeless adolescents,
        100–102
    risks for lesbian, gay, bisexual, or
        transgender adolescents, 105
    risky behaviors, 77
    sexual activity of adolescents, 40, 77
    shortcomings of current health system
        performance, 7, 301
Sexually transmitted disease
    consent for care and confidentiality laws,
        180

current insurance coverage for screening, 279, 280
    patterns and trends among adolescents, 53, 77–79
    risk, 77
    risk for adolescents in juvenile justice system, 114
    risks among homeless adolescents, 100, 101–102
    risks for lesbian, gay, bisexual, or transgender adolescents, 111
    screening for, 198
Single-parent families, 34, 38
Sleep patterns, 85
Society for Adolescent Medicine, 210–211, 213, 222
Sociocultural context
    perception and status of adolescents, 23–24
    significance of, in health care delivery, 28
Socioeconomic status
    adolescent health status and, 35
    emergency department admissions and, 168
    insurance coverage patterns and disparities, 8, 269–271, 272, 302
    insurance eligibility, 272–273, 274–275
    mental disorder risk, 72
    mortality patterns, 64
    significance of, as adolescent health factor, 4, 298
    See also Poor families
Solution-focused interviewing, 203
Special health care needs, 65. *See also* Chronic illness
Specialists, adolescent medicine, 144–145
Specialty care services
    access, 136–137, 166, 300
    adolescent medicine board certification, 254
    adolescent perceptions, 136
    care management, 206–207
    competency domains, 250–251
    consultation, 208
    directories, 205
    economic disincentives for adolescent health care specialists, 259
    goals for improving adolescent health services system, 196
    primary care and, 142, 157, 207–210

provider preparation for, 167
    purpose, 142
    recommendations for improving, 9, 304
    regional resource management, 209
    scope of, for adolescent care, 242
    service agreements, 209
    shortcomings of current system, 166–167
    strategies for improving referral practice, 204–206, 207–208
    See also Dental care; Mental health services; Sexual and reproductive health; Substance abuse treatment
Standards of care
    competency domains, 249–251
    provider implementation and adherence, 248–249
    recommendations for, 13–14, 309
    screening practices, 198
State Children's Health Insurance Program
    confidentiality of adolescent health care, 181, 287
    covered services, 277, 279, 280, 281–283, 284–285
    current shortcomings in adolescent health care, 42
    dental care coverage, 267
    eligibility, 272, 274
    failure of eligible adolescents to enroll in, 273–276
    provider participation, 285–286
    recommendations for, 12–13, 307–308
    reimbursement rates, 169
State government
    confidentiality laws, 182–183
    interaction and coordination among social service sectors, 174
    recommendations for health insurance system, 12–13, 307–308
    recommendations for improving primary care, 9, 304
Subpopulations of adolescents
    advantages of school-based health care delivery, 153
    barriers to assessment, 202
    comorbidity risk, 6, 296
    goals for improving adolescent health services system, 196
    insurance coverage disparities, 269–271
    population patterns, 35
    primary care services, 146

INDEX

public perceptions and attitudes, 37
recommendations for adolescent care provider training, 12, 307
recommendations for health insurance system, 12–13, 307–308
recommendations for improving primary health care, 9–10, 305
recommendations for monitoring health care system performance, 14–15, 309–310
safety-net health care, 150
scope, 2–3, 27
special needs and vulnerabilities, 4, 6, 18, 27, 52, 96–97, 296, 298
unmet oral health needs, 162
See also Foster care system, adolescents in; Homeless population; Immigrants; Juvenile justice system, adolescents in; Lesbian, gay, bisexual, or transgender adolescents; Poor families

Substance abuse
among adolescents in juvenile justice system, 113–114
among lesbian, gay, bisexual, or transgender adolescents, 110
associated risks, 88
clinical disorders, 75–76
current screening practice, 173
depression and, 74
health management strategies in primary care, 203
mental disorder risk, 72
outcomes of adolescent health-compromising behavior, 54
patterns and trends, 76, 87, 90–91
racial/ethnic differences in emergency room screening, 176
risk in institutional settings, 163
risks among homeless adolescents, 102, 103
risks in foster care, 98
screening and assessment, 198, 201–202
significance of, as adolescent health risk, 53, 91
See also Substance abuse treatment

Substance abuse treatment
adolescent attitudes and perceptions, 39
adolescent-specific provider certification, 164–165

confidentiality concerns of adolescents, 179
consent for care and confidentiality laws, 180
current insurance coverage, 280–284
effectiveness, 165–166
fragmentation of current health system as obstacle to, 7, 301
insurance coverage issues, 8, 302
need, 163–164
outcome indicators, 164
public insurance coverage, 277
recommendations for health insurance coverage, 13, 308
recommendations for improving public health system for adolescent care, 10–11, 305–306
relapse risk, 165–166
schools as referral sources, 162–163
shortcomings of current system, 164–165
See also Specialty care services; Substance abuse

Suicidal behavior or ideation
access to weapons and, 86
alcohol use and, 89
among lesbian, gay, bisexual, or transgender adolescents, 109–110
depression and, 73
mortality, 53, 62, 65, 77
prevalence, 77
risks among homeless adolescents, 104
screening for, 198

T

Technology, health information, 10–11, 223–225, 305–306
Text messaging, 211–212, 224
Time use patterns, adolescent, 35–36
Title X, 181
Tobacco use
dependency, 76
health consequences, 89
mortality, 54, 88
oral disease risk, 79
patterns and trends, 6, 88, 89, 172
secondhand smoke exposure, 88–89
significance of, in adolescent health, 53, 91
strategies for discouraging, 212

Training and education for health care professional. *See* Provider education and training
Transgender adolescents. *See* Lesbian, gay, bisexual, or transgender adolescents

U

U.S. Preventive Services Task Force, 199
Utilization of health care resources
    confidentiality concerns of adolescents and, 177–179, 219, 220, 300–301
    emergency care, 6–7, 171, 300
    insurance coverage and, 8, 265, 266, 267–269, 272, 285, 302
    sources of care, 168–172, 299–300

V

Vaccination and immunization, 143, 213–214, 278–279

Violent behavior
    adolescent victims, 86–87, 105
    dating violence, 86–87
    developmental patterns, 85–86
    victimization risk for lesbian, gay, bisexual, or transgender adolescents, 111
    See also Homicide

W

Weapons access and use, 53, 86
Workforce, health care
    current structure and capacity, 242–246
    diversity rationale, 242–243
    need for multidisciplinary approach to adolescent care, 242, 249
    shortcomings of current system, 240
    supply concerns, 244–245
    See also Provider education and training